# THE FAMILY THERAPY OF DRUG ABUSE
# AND ADDICTION

THE GUILFORD FAMILY THERAPY SERIES
Alan S. Gurman, *Editor*

ETHNICITY AND FAMILY THERAPY
Monica McGoldrick, John K. Pearce, and Joseph Giordano, *Editors*

PATTERNS OF BRIEF FAMILY THERAPY: AN ECOSYSTEMIC APPROACH
Steve de Shazer

THE FAMILY THERAPY OF DRUG ABUSE AND ADDICTION
M. Duncan Stanton, Thomas C. Todd, and Associates

FROM PSYCHE TO SYSTEM: THE EVOLVING THERAPY OF
CARL WHITAKER
John R. Neill and David P. Kniskern, *Editors*

NORMAL FAMILY PROCESSES
Froma Walsh, *Editor*

HELPING COUPLES CHANGE: A SOCIAL LEARNING APPROACH TO
MARITAL THERAPY
Richard B. Stuart

*In Preparation*

THE PROCESS OF CHANGE
Peggy Papp

THE PRACTICE OF THEORY IN FAMILY THERAPY
Larry Constantine

CONTEMPORARY MARRIAGE
Henry Friedman, Carol Nadelson, and Derek Polonsky, *Editors*

PARENT–ADOLESCENT CONFLICT
Arthur Robin and Sharon Foster

DEPRESSED FAMILIES
David Rubinstein

# THE FAMILY THERAPY OF DRUG ABUSE AND ADDICTION

M. DUNCAN STANTON, THOMAS C. TODD,
AND ASSOCIATES

*Philadelphia Child Guidance Clinic,*
*Philadelphia Veterans Administration Hospital,*
*and the University of Pennsylvania*

*Foreword by Salvador Minuchin*

THE GUILFORD PRESS
*New York, London*

© 1982 The Guilford Press, New York

A Division of Guilford Publications, Inc.

200 Park Avenue South, New York, N.Y. 10003

Printed in the United States of America

Fourth printing, December 1986

LIBRARY OF CONGRESS CATALOGING IN PUBLICATION DATA

Stanton, M. Duncan.

    The family therapy of drug abuse and addiction.

    (The Guilford family therapy series)

    Bibliography: p.

    Includes index.

    1. Drug abuse—Therapy.   2. Narcotic habit—Therapy.   3. Family psychotherapy.  I. Todd, Thomas C.  II. Title.   III. Series: Guilford family therapy series. [DNLM: 1. Family therapy. 2. Substance dependence—Therapy. WM 270 S792f]

RC564.S73       616.86'3'06     81-6602

ISBN 0-89862-037-6       AACR2

To Louise Richards, PhD, Daniel J. Lettieri, PhD, Joan D. Rittenhouse, PhD,
and Jack Blaine, MD, of the National Institute on Drug Abuse.
Each of them served as our Project Officer at some time during the life
of the Addicts and Families Program. Their foresight, commitment, and support
through the years allowed us to prevail with what, at times,
seemed like an impossible task.

# CONTRIBUTORS

HENRY BERGER, MD, Clinical Supervisor, Addicts and Families Program, Philadelphia Child Guidance Clinic, Philadelphia, Pennsylvania; private practice, Philadelphia, Pennsylvania

ESTHER K. CARR, (formerly) Research Associate, Addicts and Families Program, Philadelphia Child Guidance Clinic, Philadelphia, Pennsylvania

LINDA COOK, Research Associate, Addicts and Families Program, Philadelphia Child Guidance Clinic, Philadelphia, Pennsylvania

H. CHARLES FISHMAN, MD, Director of Training, Family Therapy Training Center, Philadelphia Child Guidance Clinic, Philadelphia, Pennsylvania

JAY HALEY, MA, Director, Family Therapy Institute of Washington, D.C.; Consultant, Addicts and Families Program, Philadelphia Child Guidance Clinic, Philadelphia, Pennsylvania

H. ELTON HARGROVE, MSW, Senior Drug Counselor, Drug Dependence Treatment Center, Philadelphia Veterans Administration Medical Center, Philadelphia, Pennsylvania

DAVID B. HEARD, PhD, Private practice, Albuquerque, New Mexico; (formerly) Family Therapist, Addicts and Families Program, Philadelphia Child Guidance Clinic, Philadelphia, Pennsylvania

SAM KIRSCHNER, PhD, Director, Institute for Comprehensive Family Therapy, Lansdale, Pennsylvania; (formerly) Family Therapist, Addicts and Families Program, Philadelphia Child Guidance Clinic, Philadelphia, Pennsylvania

JERRY I. KLEIMAN, PhD, Private practice, Manhasset, Long Island, New York; (formerly) Family Therapist, Addicts and Families Program, Philadelphia Child Guidance Clinic, Philadelphia, Pennsylvania

GARY LANDE, MD, Private practice, Philadelphia, Pennsylvania; (formerly) Clinical Supervisor, Addicts and Families Program, Philadelphia Child Guidance Clinic, Philadelphia, Pennsylvania

DAVID T. MOWATT, EdD, Family Therapist, Addicts and Families Program, Philadelphia Child Guidance Clinic, Philadelphia, Pennsylvania; private practice, Philadelphia, Pennsylvania

CHARLES P. O'BRIEN, MD, PhD, Chief of Psychiatry, Philadelphia Veterañs Administration Medical Center; Professor of Psychiatry, University of Pennsylvania School of Medicine; (formerly) Director, Drug Dependence Treatment Center, Philadelphia Veterans Administration Medical Center, Philadelphia, Pennsylvania

PAUL RILEY, Family Counselor, Outpatient Department and Addicts and Families Program, Philadelphia Child Guidance Clinic, Philadelphia, Pennsylvania

BERNICE L. ROSMAN, PhD, Director of Research, Philadelphia Child Guidance Clinic, Philadelphia, Pennsylvania

SAMUEL M. SCOTT, Director of Training and Service to the Retarded, and Family Therapist–Supervisor, Addicts and Families Program, Philadelphia Child Guidance Clinic, Philadelphia, Pennsylvania

M. DUNCAN STANTON, PhD, Director, Addicts and Families Program, Philadelphia Child Guidance Clinic, Philadelphia, Pennsylvania; Associate Professor of Psychology in Psychiatry, University of Pennsylvania School of Medicine, Philadelphia, Pennsylvania

FREDERICK STEIER, MS, Research Coordinator, Addicts and Families Program, Philadelphia Child Guidance Clinic, Philadelphia, Pennsylvania; Lecturer, Annenberg School of Communications, University of Pennsylvania, Philadelphia, Pennsylvania

THOMAS C. TODD, PhD, Chief Psychologist, Harlem Valley Psychiatric Center, Wingdale, New York; Research Psychologist, Addicts and Families Program, Philadelphia Child Guidance Clinic, Philadelphia, Pennsylvania

PETER URQUHART, Family Counselor, Outpatient Department, Philadelphia Child Guidance Clinic, and (formerly) Family Counselor, Addicts and Families Program, Philadelphia Child Guidance Clinic, Philadelphia, Pennsylvania

JOHN M. VAN DEUSEN, MAC, Co-Director, CONTEXTS, Ardmore, Pennsylvania; (formerly) Research Coordinator and Research Associate, Addicts and Families Program, Philadelphia Child Guidance Clinic, Philadelphia Pennsylvania

GEORGE E. WOODY, MD, Director (and former Medical Director), Drug Dependence Treatment Center, Philadelphia Veterans Administration Medical Center, Philadelphia, Pennsylvania

# FOREWORD

This book challenges the theory and practice of many programs for drug abusers. In a field where most programs focus on self-responsibility, proximity, group cohesion, and symmetry, the authors emphasize the mutual responsibility of family members in family functioning and develop a therapeutic method that focuses on hierarchical restructuring and distancing.

I was touched by the similarity between their work and my work at Wiltwyck with disorganized families who have delinquent children.[103] In both projects a group of concerned therapists commit themselves to help people who have given up hope; in both, the social context responsible for creating the conditions for deviancy denies responsibility and blames the patient; in both, the emotional draining of the therapist can be overcome only through esprit de corps and a commitment to social action.

A stubborn refusal to accept defeat, a freedom to use one's own authority and leadership, a flexibility to bend in crisis, a capacity for anger and compassion are essential prerequisites to work with drug abusers. Without these personal ingredients, therapy with the socially deviant is destined to fail.

But the therapist's repertoire needs a map that is clearly formulated to prevent him from getting lost in the labyrinth of partial truth that is the reality of deviancy.

This book offers the woof and warp of therapy. The result is a well-balanced mixture of erudition and practicality ranging from a thorough review of the literature to a focus on the minutiae of the therapeutic session. A precise conceptual model is presented that is offset and often challenged by the details and refinements in the clinical chapters—theory and praxis growing, challenging, and expanding each other. The reader is drawn to the description of the therapeutic dance: the matching of wits between two experts, the addict and the therapist, in the manipulation of reality. Concrete maneuvers are utilized, first to engage the addict and get him to bring his family, and then to accommodate and challenge, as the initial process of joining shifts to the development and management of therapeutic crises. Lastly, as a measure of the authors' commitment to family healing, there is a description of their more recent work focusing on home detoxification.

The complexity of therapy with the drug abuser and his family is reflected in the balance between the authoritative way the rules of therapy are presented and the sensitivity of the therapist to the family idiosyncracies that transcend these rules; that is, "After ascertaining the composition of the family, *but prior to suggesting that they be brought in*, the therapist must inquire how much they know about the drug problem." Or, as in Principle 12, "The rationale for family treatment should be presented in such a way that, in order to oppose it, family members would have to state openly that they want the index patient to remain symptomatic." Expanding these rules in the clinical chapters are the discrete interventions by which the therapist supports the competence and autonomy of the index patient. This balance emphasizes a "how-to" therapy that facilitates the therapist's creative freedom.

Therapists are notorious story tellers and the aesthetic of therapy or of its telling doesn't guarantee efficient treatment procedures. What makes this work significant is not only the authors' commitment to cure, but also to assess their results. It is the combination of this three-pronged approach—a theoretical formulation, a procedure for treatment, and a methodology for measuring the effectiveness of their intervention—that makes this book a model in the field.

Salvador Minuchin

# PREFACE

The work described herein has its roots in several different sources. Interest in drug abuse initially arose for the first author (Stanton) when he served as an Army psychologist in Vietnam in 1969. He was assigned to a psychiatric team that, 1 month before his arrival, had established the first systematic program in that country for treating drug problems among servicemen. In addition to clinical duties, Stanton also undertook research to assess the extent of drug use in Vietnam—both among soldiers within the country and among those entering from the United States.[144] (Even though the use of drugs had become widespread among servicemen in that theatre, there was general ignorance about it at higher levels, and, among those who did have some knowledge, a certain amount of energy often was devoted to suppressing relevant findings and testimony when these emerged.[145, 156]) Upon returning home, Stanton was called upon to advise on policy and to assist in the establishment of numerous drug-abuse programs within the Army medical system. In responding to the demands of these various contexts, he eventually developed a kind of inadvertent expertise that had been neither foreseen nor originally intended.

Prior to overseas duty Stanton had been flirting with family therapy for several years, partly because he was placed in charge of a child guidance service on an Army post and was discovering the futility of individual child treatment. This interest was rekindled after Vietnam and he started seeing families and couples almost exclusively—many of whom had drug or alcohol problems—while at Fort Meade, Maryland, and Walter Reed General Hospital. He thus began to develop a much keener appreciation of family patterns surrounding substance abuse. He was also directly influenced during this period by several training experiences he had with Virginia Satir, MSW, and D. Ray Bardill, DSW, and indirectly by the writings of Jay Haley, MA.

In 1972 Stanton took the position of Associate Clinical Director of the University of Pennsylvania psychiatry service at Philadelphia General Hospital. He continued to see families, including those of drug addicts. Also important were weekly meetings and live case presentations with Ivan Boszormenyi-Nagy, MD, a consultant to the program, and Nobu Miyoshi, MSW. As noted in Chapters 1 and 6, certain facets of this experience had a lasting impact on the work that emerged later.

Thomas Todd migrated to Philadelphia from New York (New York University and the Staten Island Mental Health Center) for a postdoctoral fellowship sponsored jointly by the Philadelphia Child Guidance Clinic (PCGC) and the University of Pennsylvania ("Penn") Department of Psychiatry. The Penn component of this position involved work with Lester Luborsky, PhD, on psychotherapy research; Todd had a combined clinical and research–statistics background and was particularly interested in outcome research. After a year, he switched his activities almost entirely to PCGC, where he performed family therapy and became part of the original team, under Salvador Minuchin, MD, studying and treating psychosomatic families.

In addition to considerable input from Minuchin, Todd's development as a therapist was directly influenced both by Haley and by Harry Aponte, MSW. As noted further on, Haley's particular approach later became especially relevant to the work presented in these pages.

The bulk of the material in this book is derived from what came to be known as the Addicts and Families Program (AFP). The initial collaboration leading to the AFP occurred in the fall of 1972. Stanton had come to Philadelphia with this work in mind, had worked out a basic research design, and was planning to apply for a National Institute on Drug Abuse (NIDA) grant. Because of PCGC's work with lower-income and minority families, its sizable staff of family therapists, its inclination toward research, and its affiliation with Penn, it was a logical institution with which to couple. A mutual colleague, Byron Fiman, PhD, put Stanton and Todd in touch and they began to refine the design, with additional input from Luborsky, Jim Mintz, PhD, and Karl Rickels, MD. In December, they also undertook a survey (described in Appendix A) among addicts at the Philadelphia Veterans Administration (VA) Hospital Drug Dependence Treatment Center on the frequency of contact with their families of origin.

Early on, a decision had to be made as to which of several drug-abuse programs affiliated with Penn would be most appropriate for carrying out the studies. Albert Stunkard, MD, who was chairman of the Department of Psychiatry at that time, recommended the program at the Philadelphia VA Hospital. This made sense for a number of reasons: (1) VA staff were interested—the director of the program, Charles P. O'Brien, MD, PhD, had taken part of his psychiatric residency at PCGC and also saw families privately; (2) several staff members, most notably Karen Barton, MSW, and H. Elton Hargrove, MSW, were treating a few addicts' families on an ongoing basis; (3) the program was in close proximity to Penn, PCGC, and Philadelphia General Hospital; (4) the program was fast developing an excellent reputation for its research accomplishments. Thus the final grant proposal included contributions from O'Brien, Barton, and the drug program's medical director, George Woody, MD. It was submitted for funding in early 1973, was deferred once—following a site visit—and eventually funded in 1974.*

The original plan was to house the AFP at Philadelphia General Hospital and to have PCGC therapists assigned to it part-time. At the suggestion of Minuchin, however, it was decided to move the complete project to PCGC's new building adjoining both Penn and the Children's Hospital of Philadelphia. Thus Stanton joined PCGC full-time in July of 1974, dividing his efforts between the AFP and the outpatient department. Concomitantly, Todd split his time between the AFP, the inpatient service, and his duties in directing PCGC's clinical psychology internship.

A number of considerations went into the development of a clinical team to carry out this work. Todd initially served as a clinical supervisor; when he departed PCGC for the Harlem Valley (New York) Psychiatric Center in 1975, Henry Berger, MD, a senior supervisor within the Clinic, assumed his supervisory duties. Haley had earlier been a supervisor in the treatment of addicts' families through a joint clinical–research project with Eagleville Hospital and Rehabilitation Center. He then served as a supervisor–consultant on the AFP for a year, later continuing to consult, through 1977, from the Family Therapy Institute, which he and his wife Cloé Madanes had established in Washington, D.C. He was succeeded as a therapy supervisor by Gary Lande, MD, who had worked both on the Eagleville project and in Haley's Schizophrenia Project, and was also on

*The grant was awarded by the National Institute on Drug Abuse (Grant No. DA 01119) and entitled "Family Characteristics and Therapy of Heroin Addicts."

the staff of PCGC's Family Therapy Training Center. The nine
therapists involved in the AFP were Gerald Hawthorne, David B.
Heard, PhD, Sam Kirschner, PhD, Jerry I. Kleiman, PhD, David T.
Mowatt, EdD, Paul Riley, Alexander Scott, MSW, Samuel M. Scott,
and Peter Urquhart. In addition to interest in this work, and a
minimum of 1 year's family therapy experience, each was recruited
for one or more of the following reasons: (1) prior experience with
drug abusers and/or their families; (2) prior experience on the
Schizophrenia Project; (3) a certain "streetwise" facility; (4) the
ability not to become rigid when working with "manipulative" clients;
(5) clearly demonstrated skill or potential as a family therapist. This
group, then, was composed of an interesting mixture of savvy paraprofessionals and young professionals, providing a diversity that has
carried over to the present volume.

The people most actively involved in the work as it interfaced
with the VA Hospital Drug Dependence Treatment Center (DDTC)
were Woody and Hargrove, with continuing input also from O'Brien
and Mintz. All of them collaborated in the treatment and research
throughout the life of the program.

In all, over 70 people have worked part-time, full-time, or served
as consultants within the AFP. While many were clinicians, the
majority functioned in research or administrative–clerical capacities.
Most of the research facets—such as family interactions and family
perceptions studies—will not be dealt with herein. However, several
research staff were key to the clinical work, particularly John M. Van
Deusen, MAC, and Esther K. Carr, who joined the AFP at its inception in the role of Research Associates. Van Deusen maintained a
theoretical and operational interest throughout most of the study and
eventually became Research Coordinator. He was succeeded by Frederick Steier, MS, in 1977, who was later assisted by Linda Cook. All of
these people have coauthored chapters in this book.*

The clinical or treatment part of the AFP extended over nearly
3 years, from the fall of 1974 to the summer of 1977. Posttreatment
follow-up research on the cases continued through July 1981, al-

*Special appreciation is accorded Mary Roken, Eleanor Mullen, and Kathy
Brennan for their unstinting efforts in carrying out the extensive secretarial and
administrative duties required to bring this book to fruition. In addition, we wish to
thank Salvador Minuchin, MD, and Alan Gurman, PhD, for careful reading of an
early version of the manuscript and providing invaluable suggestions for improving it.

though data analyses from the latter 2 years of follow-ups have not been completed as of this writing.*

The material presented on families of adolescent drug abusers (e.g., Chapter 13) is derived primarily from the clinical experience of H. Charles Fishman, MD, and M. Duncan Stanton, PhD. A sizable proportion of the adolescent cases seen by Fishman were, in fact, treated in conjunction with a PCGC (nontherapy) research project on such patients directed by Bernice L. Rosman, PhD. The project ran from 1977 to 1980.†

The family therapy model applied in this work had two major influences. First, many of the treatment concepts are derived from the work of Minuchin and colleagues at PCGC, particularly as represented in the aforementioned Psychosomatic Research Project.‡ This project combined a systematic therapy approach, videotaped family interaction evaluation, and treatment outcome within a single research program. In addition to the therapeutic principles that emerged from (or were enhanced by) it, the project served as a model for the AFP and adolescent drug abusers' project in both its operational–administrative facets and as a source for comparisons between psychosomatic and addicts'–abusers' families.

Haley was the second major source of our ideas. He introduced to the AFP concepts and methods that he had worked out with families of schizophrenics, first in Palo Alto and later in the Schizophrenia Project at PCGC.§ In addition to having helped develop structural family therapy, Haley contributed many ideas that are

*Funding for these follow-up studies was granted during 1976 through 1978 by the Governor of Pennsylvania's Public Health Trust Fund (Grant No. 56772), and during 1978 through 1981 by the National Institute on Drug Abuse (Grant No. DA 02117).

†Therapists serving on this project, which was entitled "Adolescent Substance Abuse in Three Family Contexts" (NIDA Grant No. 5 R01 DA 01629), were Janet Berson, PhD, Susan Bogas, PhD, Barbara Bryant, Jorge Colapinto, Lic., Kenneth Covelman, PhD, Jody Cox, MSW, H. Charles Fishman, MD (who also served as the clinical supervisor), Hector Goa, MD, Jay Lappin, MSW, Barbara Penn, David Treadway, MEd, and Peter Urquhart.

‡Psychosomatic Research Project staff, in addition to Minuchin and Todd, included Lester Baker, MD, Ronald Liebman, MD, Leroy Milman, MD, and Bernice L. Rosman, PhD. The cases were treated clinically by 16 different therapists.

§Members of the PCGC Schizophrenia Project were Charles Billings, MD, Harold Cohn, MD, H. Charles Fishman, MD, Paul Gross, MD, David B. Heard, PhD, David Hunt, MD, Gary Lande, MD, Lawrence Miller, MD, David T. Mowatt, EdD, Lee Petty, MD, Alberto Rish, MD, Meyer Rothbart, MD, and Frances Ziegler, MSW.

uniquely his own.[64,65,66] A summary of his therapy appears in Chapter 6, and a case example in Chapter 7.

Throughout the life of the AFP, of course, many new ideas, therapeutic procedures, and findings emerged, traceable directly to our unfolding experience. From the start we were concerned with what "worked" rather than what was theoretically interesting. This statement may seem obvious, but too often we have seen others become so enamored of family dynamics that the means for effecting change escape them. Furthermore, it has unfortunately not been characteristic of most programs to evaluate their degree of success in any objective fashion. We feel one of the strengths of the AFP was its continuous attempt to monitor its own effectiveness in order to further develop the techniques.

M. Duncan Stanton<br>Thomas C. Todd

# CONTENTS

# SECTION III. OTHER DIMENSIONS OF THERAPY

# THE FAMILY THERAPY OF DRUG ABUSE
# AND ADDICTION

# INTRODUCTION

M. DUNCAN STANTON
THOMAS C. TODD


PROBLEMS OF SUBSTANCE abuse and drug addiction have become increasingly prevalent in North America and throughout the world since at least the mid-1960s. In some parts of the United States, and in certain other contexts such as among soldiers in Vietnam, they have at times reached epidemic proportions. Certainly they have impacted on the mental health system, and Nicholas Cummings,[35] in his presidential address to the American Psychological Association, has noted that (1) 1 of every 11 Americans, and 1 of every 6 teenagers, suffers from a severe addictive problem, and (2) 23% of psychotherapy patients suffer either from addictive problems or from emotional problems substantially exacerbated by alcohol or drug abuse (although only 3.5% were so identified by their own therapists).

The trend in substance abuse has been met by at least two major, and related, responses in the United States: the establishment of a number of local, state, and federal drug-abuse agencies (e.g., the National Institute on Drug Abuse, the National Institute on Alcohol Abuse and Alcoholism), and the development of a number of treatment modalities specifically geared to addiction. The latter includes the birth of many therapeutic communities for treating addiction, the monitoring and screening of drug use through urinalysis, and the implementation of procedures that provide pharmacological substitutes, such as methadone maintenance. These modalities have met with varying degrees of success, depending on a multitude of factors. However, nearly all of them address addiction as primarily a problem in the individual, that is, one that is located either in the "body" or the "personality." Little attention has been given to the interpersonal aspects of addiction, except as it is influenced by the peer group, or as it is dealt with in certain family-oriented self-help groups such as Al-Anon and Families Anonymous. Even though literature on families of drug addicts emerged as early as the 1950s,[52, 98, 199] until recent years[147] very little attention has been directed toward family factors within the overall field. Consequently, the purpose of this book is, in part, to identify some of the patterns that occur in families of drug abusers, and more importantly, to present rationales, strategies, and techniques for changing such patterns and the drug-related cycle embedded within them.

It may be obvious that we have intended this as an *integrated* text, with continuity across its pages, rather than a compendium of separate chapters. Of course there are variations in style and, to some extent, emphasis, since the various chapters were penned by different combinations of authors. Nonetheless, there has been much cross-fertilization among those Philadelphia Child Guidance Clinic staff working with drug problems, and the content of their writings derives from a shared body of data.

The book is divided into three sections. The lead-off chapter in Section I is the fruit of seven "marathon" sessions—most of which extended far into the night—held in the summer and fall of 1977. The task that the nine authors set for themselves was to bring some sort of conceptual synthesis to their experience, to define a theoretical platform upon which the remainder of the clinical material could rest. The resulting document became known as the "cornerstone" paper[170] and Chapter 1 is a revised and updated version of the original publication.

Section I also includes a description of the context of the work and several chapters dealing with the means for getting these (usually resistant) families into therapy.

The bulk of the book's clinical material is presented in Section II. This includes an overview and a comment on the therapy model, four case studies, a model for home detoxification, techniques for treating families with an adolescent drug abuser, a look at crisis resolution across many cases, and a discussion among therapy supervisors of the treatment process.

Section III covers the impact of the treatment program and administrative procedures on therapy, followed by a chapter each on therapy outcome results and directions for the future.

This book is primarily for clinicians.* While most therapists do not specialize in treating families of drug abusers, the majority of them are encountering such problems more and more frequently in their

---

*Readers who are research-minded will find technical material treated more comprehensively, and in greater detail, in the various appendices.

general practice. The principles, techniques, and therapy model set forth are designed to help them in such situations. In addition, much of the book's substance is relevant to the treatment of cases that do *not* manifest a substance-abuse problem. The material on engaging resistant families (Chapter 5), ascribing noble intentions or "noble ascriptions" (Chapter 6), inducing crises (Chapters 6 and 9), developing family tasks (Chapter 12), and effecting a working alliance (Chapter 13), in particular, is generic enough to apply to a spectrum of clinical problems extending well beyond the area of substance abuse.

Regarding drug problems, it should be noted that, to date, not a great deal has been written on the actual treatment of drug abuse from a family viewpoint. There is an especial shortage of "how-to" information pertaining to the operations of therapy. Thus the family-oriented therapist has been left to his own resources if he wanted to progress from an "understanding" of drug abusers' families to the adventure of bringing about change.* Consequently, we have attempted in these pages to present some strategies and techniques that we hope will not lessen the adventurous nature of the trip, but will help the therapist keep from getting lost or discouraged as he sails these newly chartered waters.

*The masculine pronoun is used here and later in the text primarily for purposes of convenience. To paraphrase Haley,[66] therapists and clients come in both sexes, and the authors acknowledge the inequity of the traditional use of the masculine pronoun.

The terms "abusers' families" and "addicts' families" are used throughout the book also for convenience. However, as our colleague Marianne Walters, MSW, emphasizes (personal communication, March 1981), the more proper term would be "families with an addicted member," making it clear that not everyone in the family is addicted.

SECTION I

# PRETHERAPY ASPECTS

# 1

# A CONCEPTUAL MODEL

M. DUNCAN STANTON/THOMAS C. TODD/
DAVID B. HEARD/SAM KIRSCHNER/JERRY I. KLEIMAN/
DAVID T. MOWATT/PAUL RILEY/SAMUEL M. SCOTT/
JOHN M. VAN DEUSEN

THE DRAMA of drug addiction is obvious. It fills the stage with violence, stealing, arrests, intense emotional highs, periods of desperate craving, and possible death from overdose. Less obvious, however, is the stability that actually underlies these fluctuations—a stability that includes both the addict and his family. These phenomena are stable in their predictability, their repetitiveness, and in the function they serve for the people involved. This chapter is an attempt to identify some of the elements within the process and integrate them into a conceptual model.

Our plan is to lead the reader through the evolution of some ideas that have emerged from our observations and research, and to integrate these, whenever possible, with the work of other investigators. The focus will be on a class of factors that have not always been considered in the drug-abuse field and appear to be quite potent, especially as they relate to the maintenance of addiction. We wish to emphasize that, although we are applying a particular framework to compulsive drug use, we are not denying the importance of physiological variables in addiction; we recognize that a drug can be extremely powerful in its own right. It is also accepted that—in addition to the family—economic, environmental, and conditioning determinants are also crucial.

This chapter is a revision of a paper by the authors entitled "Heroin Addiction as a Family Phenomenon: A New Conceptual Model" and is reprinted with permission from the *American Journal of Drug and Alcohol Abuse*, 1978, 5, 125–150. © Marcel Dekker, Inc.

Appreciation is extended to Jim Mintz, PhD, Salvador Minuchin, MD, Braulio Montalvo, MA, and Bernice L. Rosman, PhD, for their helpful comments on an earlier version of this chapter.

## RESEARCH ON ADDICTS' FAMILIES

Drug abuse generally has its origins in adolescence. It is tied to the normal, albeit troublesome, process of growing up, experimenting with new behaviors, becoming self-assertive, developing close (usually heterosexual) relationships with people outside the family, and leaving home. Kandel et al.,[76] extrapolating from their data, propose that there are three stages in adolescent drug use and each has different concomitants. The first is the use of legal drugs, such as alcohol, and is mainly a social phenomenon. The second involves use of marijuana and is also primarily peer-influenced. The third stage, frequent use of other illegal drugs, appears contingent more on the quality of parent–adolescent relationships than on other factors. Thus, it is concluded that more serious drug abuse is predominantly a family phenomenon, which corresponds to the conclusion by Blum et al.[17] that the peer group has little or no influence as long as the family remains strong.

At least five literature reviews have been published that deal with family factors in drug addiction.[67, 80, 127, 134, 150] These reviews describe a prototypic pattern for male addicts' families in which the mother is involved in an indulgent, enmeshed, overprotective, overly permissive relationship with the addict, who is put in the position of a favored child. Often he is "spoiled."[198] He is reported by the mother to have been the "easiest to raise" of the children and was generally "good" as a child.[51, 179] Fathers of male addicts are reported to be detached, uninvolved, weak, or absent.* Compared with normals, the father–son relationships in addicts' families are described by the addict as being quite negative, with harsh and inconsistent discipline, especially for those who inject heroin versus those who inhale it.[41,84,93] A disproportionate number of fathers are reported to have a drinking problem.[22, 43, 58, 105, 122, 164, 179, 198]† Schwartzman[130] describes two types of addict fathers, a "straw man" type who is authoritarian, violent, but easily controlled by mother, and a distant type who is clearly secondary to mother in terms of power within the family. Interestingly,

*As noted in Chapter 6, caution should be exercised regarding these conclusions, as Kaufman and Kaufmann[78] noted enmeshed father–child relationships in 40% of their cases—particularly within certain ethnic groups. Further, Alexander and Dibb[2] feel the father (rather than the mother) assumes the overinvolved role in some middle-class families, a pattern we also found in approximately 5% of the Addicts and Families Program (AFP) families.

†Of course the statistical distributions in these and other studies cited in this section are overlapping (e.g., some "normal" families will also show such patterns).

Rosenberg[123] reports that siblings of male addicts are more likely to have a positive relationship with the father. In contrast to males, female addicts seem to be in overt competition with their mothers (whom they see as overprotective and authoritarian), while their fathers have been reported to be inept, indulgent of them, sexually aggressive, and often alcoholic; the probability of incest is much greater than normal,[36, 43, 190] with estimates running as high as 90%.[78] A high incidence of parental deprivation is reported for families of both sexes, many of whom have experienced separation or death of a parent—most commonly father—before age 16.[39,43,67,80,111,123,182] However, this incidence appears to be changing in recent years, so that rates in addicts' families are now more comparable to the overall population.[151] In general, research in this area has progressed from reports by the user about his family, to dyadic (e.g., mother–child) assessments, to triadic (parents and child) concepts, and, with the more sophisticated studies, to assessments of the interactional behavior of the whole family.

*ADDICT-FAMILY CONTACT*

One area that has tended to be overlooked or unrecognized in the drug-abuse field is the extent to which "hard" drug users are involved and in contact with the people who raised them. For adolescents such involvement is natural and developmentally appropriate, since they are still minors and are generally not expected to have left home. On the other hand, it is not necessarily obvious that addicts in their late 20s and early 30s would still be involved with their families of origin. Their age, submersion in the drug subculture, frequent changes in residence, possible military service, and so forth, would seem to imply that they are cut off, or at least distanced, from one or both parents.

On the other hand, there is a preponderance of evidence (presented in Appendix A) that, despite their protestations of independence, the majority of addicts maintain close family ties. Even if they do not reside with their parents, they may live nearby, and their frequency of contact is much higher than that occurring among comparable "normals," other psychiatric patient groups, or even polydrug abusers. Fifteen of 17 reports on living arrangements, and 7 of 7 reports on frequency of family contact attest to this pattern (these studies are reviewed in Appendix A). For example, Perzel and Lamon[113] found that 64% of heroin addicts were in daily telephone contact with at least one parent, compared to 51% of polydrug abusers and 9% of normals. Further, this appears to be an international phenomenon, as similar rates of addicts living with parents have been found in Puerto Rico, Italy, England, and Thailand, in addition to North America. In sum, it would appear that at least two-thirds of male hard drug users under age 35 live with the people that raised them and 80–85% are in at least weekly contact with these same parental figures. In fact, we have observed these intense entanglements so often in our clinical work that we are by now skeptical when *any* addict tells us that he does not see his parents regularly. We tend to regard such responses as moves to protect the family rather than as valid in their own right (see Chapters 4 and 5).

Of course, either living with parents or seeing them regularly is not necessarily an indication of dysfunction. Depending on the cultural and ethnic milieu, such arrangements can be quite natural, and maintaining regular family involvement certainly does not mean one will become a drug addict. What may be more important is the quality and the operational–functional structure within families who develop drug-abusing offspring, with consideration also given to their stage in the family life cycle. Overinvolvement, then, can only be considered an indirect measure of family dysfunction. However, there is some evidence that it can have meaning and value in terms of determining both the prognosis for existent treatment paradigms and the direction for new therapeutic modes. For example, Vaillant[182] found that addicts who became abstinent did not live with their parents, and Zahn and Ball's[196] data indicate that cure was associated with not living with parents or relatives. Both reports noted a correlation between living in the home of relatives and continued addiction. Further, in a comparison of posttreatment outcomes by Stanton *et al.*,[171] significant correlations were found between regularity of contact with a parent and the extent of use of illegal drugs (.20), as well as use of marijuana (.23); the correlations were similar when measured against whether the addict lived with his parents (all illegal drugs, .21; marijuana, .22). These results imply that being closely involved with one's family of origin is not necessarily healthy, especially among young men aged 20 to 35.

## FAMILY OF PROCREATION

Concerning marriage and the family of procreation, it has generally been concluded that the (usually heterosexual) dyadic relationships that addicts become involved in are a repetition of the nuclear family of origin, with roles and interaction patterns similar to those seen with the opposite-sex parent.[67, 134, 177, 190, 194] In a certain number of these marriages both spouses are addicted, although it is more common for either one or both to be drug-free at the beginning of the relationship.[48, 190] If the marital union is formed during addiction, it is more likely to dissolve after methadone treatment than if initiated at some other time.[1] Also, nonaddicted wives tend to find their husbands' methadone program to be more satisfactory than do addicted wives.[27] Equally important, the rate of marriage for male addicts is half that which would be expected, while the rate for multiple marriages is above average for both sexes.[109] In line with the observations of Chein et al.[25] and Scher,[129] we have noted (e.g., in references 154, 158, and 170) how parental permission is often quite tentative for the addict to have a viable marital relationship. Although he attempts flight into marriage, there is often a considerable pull or encouragement for him to go back. Consequently, he usually returns home, defeated, to his parents.

## BACKGROUND

While much of the aforementioned research on drug abusers' families was helpful to us when we set out to examine such families ourselves, we also found these studies to be limited in the kinds of data they provided, at least in terms of a systemic paradigm. This section briefly notes the experiential and observational sources that became the bases of our conceptualizations.

The formulations to be presented are based upon actual behavioral observations of drug abusers' families "in action"—either in family treatment of while performing prescribed tasks together. The data bank includes over 450 videotapes of such interactional sessions. These were scrutinized by groups of from 2 to 12 of us, either directly at the time of recording or jointly afterward. Particular attention was paid to repetitive behavioral sequences, formation of coalitions, and other observable patterns. They were also viewed within the context of events occurring simultaneously outside the research site, whether in the home, the methadone clinic, or elsewhere. Certain of the videotapes have been condensed and edited for training or scientific purposes, and have been reviewed dozens of times.

The patterns we have observed with these families may differ more in degree than in kind, when compared with other addicts' families. We state this based on (1) reports published by other investigators (cited herein) showing similar patterns with addict groups different from our own, and (2) the experience that four of us have had over the past 9 to 13 years with a broad cross-section of families of drug abusers. The latter has involved clinical work within a total of eight different drug-treatment settings in several metropolitan areas, including two multimodal (methadone) clinics, a detoxification program, a day treatment program, an inpatient program, a therapeutic community, and two adolescent-oriented outpatient clinics. Our conceptualizations draw upon this broad experience and are not limited only to the kind of families treated within the AFP. While exceptions certainly exist, we have tried to develop a model that applies to the majority of drug addicts—particularly males under age 35—at least as far as basic elements and behavioral patterns are concerned.

## ELEMENTS TOWARD THE CONSTRUCTION OF A MODEL

Before presenting our model, certain aspects of it require clarification. In this section discussion is devoted to the ways in which our observations led us along a path toward the formulations from which the model has been constructed.

### FEAR OF SEPARATION

It is commonly recognized that drug addicts usually present as dependent and inadequate individuals who frequently "screw up." They seem not to function because they are too dependent and not ready to assume responsibility—as if they want to be taken care of. They fear being separate or separated. At the outset of our work we observed this characteristic and it was not obvious to us how or whether it fit into the total family system. On looking further, however, we started to notice that when the addict began to succeed—whether on the job, in a treatment program, or elsewhere—he was in a sense heading toward leaving the family, either directly or by developing more autonomy in general. What was interesting was that at this point some sort of crisis would almost inevitably occur in the family, such as parents having a fight or a separation, one parent developing symptoms, or a sibling becoming a problem. On the heels of this the addict would revert back to some kind of failure behavior and the other family problem would dissipate. We observed this pattern so frequently that it became clear to us that not only did the addict fear separation from the family, but the family felt likewise toward him. Their behavior told us this was an *interdependent process* in which his failure served a protective function of maintaining family closeness. The family's "need" for him was equal to or greater than his "need" for them. The members seemed to cling to each other for confirmation or perhaps a sense of "completeness" or "worth."

Concerning the relation between fear of separation and the onset of difficulties in adjustment, the addict does not generally become problematic until adolescence.[51, 83, 134, 179, 195, 200] It is at this point that he should be expected to actively engage in heterosexual and other intense outside relationships. If he does, however, he becomes less available and less attached to his family. Since he seems to be badly needed by the family, his threatened departure can cause panic. Consequently, the pressure on him not to leave is so powerful that the family will endure (and even encourage) terrible indignities, such as his lying, stealing, and the public shame he generates, rather than take a firm position in relation to him. They also tend to protect him from outside agencies, relatives, and other social systems. Rather than accept responsibility themselves, family members usually blame external systems, such as peers or the neighborhood, for the addict's problem. Should the parents take effective action, such as evicting him, they often undo their actions by overtly or covertly encouraging his return. They seem to be saying to him, in effect, "We will suffer almost anything, but please don't leave us." Thus it becomes nearly impossible for the addict to negotiate his way out of the family.

## CHOICE OF SYMPTOM

If one views opiate addiction not only as a physiological or biological predisposition but as a family phenomenon, one must ask how these families differ from others with problems. Questions also arise as to why this particular symptom is chosen, and what functions it serves.

### Comparison with Other Disorders

In some ways families of addicts appear to be similar to other severely dysfunctional families. Many types of problem families use a focus on the child's difficulties to avoid (1) conflicts between the parents, or

(2) other family problems.[63, 64, 65] However, families of addicts do seem to differ in a number of respects, as follows:

1. There is evidence for a higher frequency of multigenerational chemical dependency, particularly alcohol, among addicts' families, plus a propensity for other addiction-like behaviors such as gambling and television watching.[2, 4, 10, 16, 18, 43, 47, 70, 80, 105, 122, 123, 164, 179, 198] Such practices provide modeling for children and can also develop into family "traditions."

2. Addicts' parents' behavior is characterized as "conspicuously unschizophrenic" in quality.[2]

3. Related to the above, several of the authors (noted in the Preface) have been extensively involved in therapy research on both families of schizophrenics[66] and families in which an offspring has a severe psychosomatic disorder.[101, 104] Compared to these groups, addicts are more likely to form strong outside relationships and to retreat to them, even if only for a brief period, following family conflict. In other words, the illusion of independence is greater for addicts because, unlike the other symptom groups, they have a subculture to which they can relate.

4. Compared to families of schizophrenics and psychosomatic young people, addicts' families seem to be more primitive and direct in their expression of conflict.

5. Alliances among family members and within family subsystems (e.g., between an addict and his mother) are often quite explicit in addicts' families and may be confirmed verbally by members. Addicts' families often characterize themselves as "close," showing a good deal of nurturant (even infantilizing) behavior toward each other. On this point, Madanes et al.[95] compared the families of addicts, schizophrenics, and "normals" (high achievers) on a test in which members were required to indicate their closeness or attachment by moving cardboard figures representing themselves on a grid of family structure. Addicts' families were 6 times more likely than the other two groups to place the figures so that they touched or overlapped each other.

6. Mothers of addicts show greater "symbiotic" childrearing practices and needs than mothers of schizophrenics and normals. Attardo[6] compared these three kinds of mothers on a

symbiosis or separation–individuation scale that attempted to measure their tendency to use this kind of relating with their children. An intrapsychic scale was also administered. All three groups had similar symbiotic levels when relating to their offspring from birth to age 5. In age group 6 to 10, however, the mothers of drug addicts got significantly higher scores than the other two groups. In the 11 to 16 age group, the drug addicts' mothers were statistically higher than both groups, and the mothers of schizophrenics were higher than the normals. The intrapsychic scale showed addicts' mothers to have greater symbiotic needs than the other two groups of mothers. These findings imply that, relative to mothers of normals and schizophrenics, addicts' mothers get "stuck" at an earlier stage of childrearing, tending to hold on to their children and treat them as younger than they really are.

7. Addicts' families show a preponderance of death themes and premature, unexpected, or untimely deaths within the family. These aspects are discussed more extensively later in this chapter.

8. The symptom of addiction provides a form of "pseudo-individuation" at several levels (see below).

9. Acculturation and parent–child cultural disparity appear to play an important role in many cases of addiction. Vaillant[181, 182] raised this possibility based upon his data with heroin addicts. He discovered that the rate of addiction for *offspring* of people who immigrated either from another country or from a different section of the United States was 3 times higher than the rate for the *immigrants themselves.* In addition, he found that immigrants' offspring who were born in New York City were at greater risk for addiction than either their parents or immigrants' offspring born in the former culture. Rosenberg[122] also found higher rates of drug abuse among children of immigrants. Following this lead, Alexander and Dibb[2] determined that in a group of 12 families they were treating for drug addiction, the parents in 10 of them (83%) lived more than 200 miles from their place of birth; most were immigrants from Europe or the Canadian prairies. In another Canadian study, Smart et al.[139] found less inhalant use among children whose parents were born in North America versus children of parents from other continents. Finally, Scopetta et al.[133] compared acculturation scores between Cuban-

American parents and their problem offspring. Significantly greater parent–child acculturation gaps were found within drug users' families than within families of adolescents with nondrug problems; the drug users were more acculturated, and their parents less so, compared with the psychiatric group.

In an attempt to understand and explain this phenomenon, Vaillant[181] notes the abnormal dependence of addicted mothers on their children. He suggests that (1) immigrant parents are under the additional strain of having to cope with their new environment, (2) parental migration may be correlated with parental instability, and (3) "the immigrant mother, separated as she often is from her own family ties, may be less able to meet the needs of those dependent on her and yet experience greater than average difficulty in permitting her child mature independence" (p. 538). It might be added that immigrant parents are also faced both with the "loss" of the family they left in their original culture, plus their own possible feelings of guilt or disloyalty for having deserted these other members. Thus it is often worthwhile to examine issues in the extended family as well as interactions in the nuclear family. In any case, what appears to happen is that many immigrant parents tend to depend on their children for emotional and other kinds of support, clinging to them and becoming terrified when the offspring reach adolescence and start to individuate.

## Symptom Function

Stemming from earlier discussion of the interdependency and fear of separation that addicts' families show, we have concluded that opiate addiction has many adaptive, functional qualities in addition to its immediate pleasurable features. Our major conclusion is that it provides the addict and his family with a *paradoxical resolution* to their dilemma of maintaining or dissolving the family, that is, of his staying or leaving. Its pharmacological effects, and the context and implications of its use, furnish solutions to this dilemma at several different levels, stretching from individual psychopharmacology to the drug subculture. Some of these functions appear to be:

1. The individual–pharmacological level. Several writers have conceptualized the addict's experience of euphoria as analogous to a symbiotic attachment or fusion with the mother—a kind

of regressed, infantile satiation.[85, 128, 184] If so, then while he is in this state he can feel "close" to mother or family, and also in some ways appear to them much as he did when he was very young and clearly not autonomous. On the other hand, heroin blunts the anxiety accompanying separation and individuation,[195] often causes drowsiness,[26] and in effect allows the addict to be separate, distanced, and self-absorbed while physically present. Thus we hypothesize that he, and they, can "have it both ways" by means of the drug. Through the drug he can be both close or infantile and distanced at the same time.

2. Aggressive behavior. Because of the turmoil that ensues when he improves or succeeds, the family's covert message to the addict appears to be that he should remain incompetent and dependent. On the other hand, heroin, like alcohol,[99] has been noted to give a sense of new power, omnipotence, and "triumphant success."[115, 117, 124, 195] Perhaps more important is the point made by Ganger and Shugart,[51] however, that under the influence of heroin, addicts become aggressive and assertive toward their families, particularly parents. We note that in so doing they become autonomous, individuated, and "free." They appear to stand up for themselves, but not really. This is actually a *pseudo-individuation*, for their ravings and protestations are discounted. The drug is blamed. Without it they "really aren't that way." Through the drug cycle the whole family becomes engaged in a repetitive reenactment of leaving and returning in which the "leaving" phase is neutralized through denial of the possible implications of the addict's assertiveness. In short, the family is saying, "You don't really hate us—you're just high," and when he is not influenced by drugs the addict concurs with, "Yes, I don't really hate you, but when I'm on the drug I can't control myself."

3. Heterosexual relationships. Heroin may offer a compromise in the area of heterosexual relationships. Addicts have been noted not to have teenage crushes,[24] to be more likely than average to engage in homosexual activities,[54, 179, 200] or to be retreating from sexuality.[50] Scher[129] proposes that intense family ties serve to prevent the addict from developing appropriate relationships with spouses or offspring. It may be true that the drug produces a kind of sexual experience,[26, 116] which would partially explain the colorfully eroticized language and loving tenderness that addicts attach to various aspects of their habit[192, 195];

they seem to be addressing it as a love partner. Since it apparently reduces the sex drive also, it can in this way again provide a solution to the addict's dilemma. Through it he can have a quasi-sexual experience without being disloyal to his family,[19] and, most obviously, his mother. He does not have to form a heterosexual relationship but can relate sexually to the drug instead.

4. The drug subculture. Other aspects of drug addiction can help the addict out of his dilemma, especially those pertaining to extrafamilial systems. The addict forms relationships among members of the drug subculture. He "hustles" and makes a lot of money to support his habit. Thus he has friends or peers and is in this way grown-up, independent, and "successful." Paradoxically, however, this is not the case, for the more heroin he shoots the more helpless, dependent, and incompetent he is. In other words, he can be successful and competent only within the framework of an unsuccessful, incompetent subculture. It is a limited realm, restricted to people who need help and cannot really be expected to function adequately within society. Once again, through his addiction the addict almost has his cake and eats it, for he seems to be out of the family, but only in a way that is tolerable to them and keeps him within his assigned role.

5. Abstinence and the addict role. Previously we noted how the drug may serve as a problem that keeps the family together. In this way it transcends its pharmacological effect; it serves more as a symbol of the addict's incompetence and his consequent inability to leave the family or their inability to release him. Much has been made of the euphoria in drug addiction, but our experience indicates that this is of secondary importance to its function within the family. Given appropriate support, an opiate addict can, for example, tolerate large decreases in methadone levels. By far the greatest resistance is in the final step of going from 5 mg, or 1 mg, to nothing. It is an easy step to take, pharmacologically, and its real significance is *symbolic*. If he takes it, the addict is no longer an addict. He is making an assertion against the roles he has played and against his mantle of incompetence. Should the family still need him in the position of the addicted one, they can bring almost unbearable pressure to bear. If he cannot withstand it, he slips once again into the addictive cycle.

In sum, drug addiction serves in a number of ways to resolve the dilemma of whether or not the addict can become an independent adult. It is a paradoxical solution that allows a form of pseudo-individuation. By using drugs the addict is neither totally in nor totally out of the family. He is nurtured when he is "in" and the drug is blamed when he is "out." He is competent within a framework of incompetence.

## PRIMACY OF FAMILY OF ORIGIN VERSUS FAMILY OF PROCREATION

Male addicts who are married or living with a woman are involved in at least two intimate interpersonal systems—that of the marriage and that of the family of origin. Since more time is generally spent in the marital context, this system would appear to be the more influential one in maintaining the drug pattern. This idea made sense to us and our studies initially focused on the addict's marriage. It was also easier, because the addicts much more readily acknowledged a marital problem than difficulties with their parents. They tended to pronounce their independence from parents, saying they had outgrown the family, or the family had given up on them. Further, in looking at the marriage, it did indeed seem to contribute to symptom maintenance. However, as our work progressed and we began to make interventions, we found that this approach did not go far enough. Couples treatment appeared to stress the marriage so that, as Chein et al.[25] have noted, the addict would leave his spouse and return home to his parent(s). It sometimes seemed as if he were just waiting for an excuse to rebound back to them. It became evident that we could not deal with the spouse system alone and ignore the parental system if treatment were to succeed. (This is consonant with the findings of Eldred and Washington[42] that, in general, addicts believed the family of origin or the in-laws would be more helpful to them in their attempts to give up drugs than an opposite-sex partner.) Without getting ahead of ourselves, we noted, as did Scher,[129] that parental permission was often quite tentative for the addict to have a viable marriage.* There was a subtle pull for him to

---

*The senior author (Stanton) has asserted elsewhere[158] that the majority of all marriages that fail do so because one or both partners do not have parental permission for the marriage to succeed.

return. The conveyed message was, "Well, if you have trouble with your wife, you can always come back and stay with us." While this might have a noble, "caring" ring to it, covertly it is an instruction for him not to be too content with his spouse. A truly successful marriage would signify that his parents had "lost" him.

As a perhaps interesting sidelight, we observed three general types of relationships within one dyad of the system, that is, between the addict's spouse and his mother. In one type there was overt conflict and they rarely if ever spoke or came in contact. In the second, the daughter-in-law was tolerated, but mother frequently endeavored to undercut the marriage, usually through subtle means. For instance, on visits to the clinic she might make a point of sitting between her son and his wife, or she might mention how often he had been dropping by to visit her and tell her his troubles—visits of which the wife was unaware. She might, in addition, "let slip" information about his extramarital affairs or other transgressions that would upset the wife. The third type of relationship was somewhat different. Here the mother and the daughter-in-law joined in what can best be described as two sisters or young mothers responding to the addict much as they would if he were a baby in a playpen. They would fawn over him, chuckle when he stumbled or made a mistake, and rush to his aid if he hurt himself. They seemed to be happiest when his behavior was most child-like. Thus his incompetence brought them pleasure.

## DEATH AND MARTYRDOM

In perusing the literature on addict deaths,[31, 163] it is safe to conclude that this group shows high death rates, shorter than average life expectancies, and greater than normal incidence of sudden deaths. Addicts also tend to view death as more positive and potent than peers, and are more likely to express a wish for it than do other psychiatric patients. Much of this is indicative of a suicidal tendency, and a number of authors have likened addiction to chronic suicide (see references 31 and 163 for a more complete review of research on this topic and of the material to follow).

From a family viewpoint a number of studies have also documented the high incidence of parental loss due to death in the families of addicts. Most frequently these are of a traumatic, untimely, and unexpected nature. The rate of early death for paternal grandfathers is also higher than expected. Finally, there appears to be an association between the time of initial drug use by adolescents and the death of a parent or another significant person such as a peer.

From the above it seems fair to hypothesize that some sort of tie-in exists between addiction and death in these families. In an earlier paper[146] the case was made for a family basis to the addict's suicidal behavior. The addiction is part of a *continuum of self-destruction*[163] that is abetted, sanctioned, or at least not resisted by most or all family members (e.g., the case in Chapter 9). This may be related to the aforementioned separation issue in that many families state explicitly that they would rather see the addict dead than lost to people outside the family. There seems to be a contract within these families in which the addict's part is to die or come close to death. He becomes a martyr who sacrifices himself at their behest. It is as if they are saying, "If you have to separate, there is one way you can do it and that is by dying." Reilly[118] has noted that the addict's behavior might be viewed as part of an unresolved family mourning process. To this point, Coleman[29] observed that addicts' families vicariously reenact through the addict the premature or unresolved deaths of other family members, usually grandparents. In any case, we believe the family tolerates a solution in which the addict tempts death because the family mythology is such that death is an acceptable resolution to their dilemma. It is a desperate attempt to preserve the family in the face of escalating sociocultural pressures upon them to release their addicted member.

## A HOMEOSTATIC MODEL

While the aforementioned observations and studies may seem interesting and cogent, the need became apparent to us for them to be more adequately synthesized within a comprehensive model that also took into account repetitive family patterns and systemic thinking. Up to that point, of course, several attempts had been made to conceptualize drug abuse as a family phenomenon. For example, Alexander and Dibb[2] viewed addiction as stabilizing the family, while Noone and Reddig[108] regarded the family as "stuck" at a stage in the developmental life cycle as a result of unresolved family loyalties and grief.[19] Reilly[118] saw the issues of loss, mourning, and separation anxiety in the family as perpetuating the pattern of drug abuse. However, these conceptualizations tended to be linear in their view of causality, that is, to take the form "A leads to B," or "A and B lead to C." This contrasts with a nonlinear or "recursive"[11] notion of "A leads to B, B leads to C, and C leads back to A." In fact, the majority of theoreticians in this area, with the exception of Huberty,[70] regarded the addiction process in linear causal terms, rather than involving a complex set of feedback mechanisms within a repetitive cycle. For example, one can view a parent or even the whole family as "causing" the addiction and still be tied to a linear model. In the remainder of this chapter, the homeostatic aspects of addiction receive particular emphasis, and the previously described elements are incorporated as to their respective roles in the maintenance of behavior cycles.

The model presented here includes some concepts and ways of thinking about drug abuse–addiction and about people and their behavior that have not been a primary part of the epistemology in the drug-abuse field. In some ways they are discontinuous with traditional notions. They stem from a theoretical tradition extending at least from the earlier works on family homeostasis and triadic systems of Jackson[71, 72] and Haley.[60, 64] For those to whom they are unfamiliar, we ask that these ideas be approached with an open mind and, perhaps, with a sense of exploration.

## ADDICTION AND THE FAMILY CYCLE

We are proposing that drug addiction can be thought of as part of a *cyclical process* involving three or more individuals, commonly the addict and his two parents or parent surrogates. These people form an intimate, interdependent, interpersonal system. At times the equilibrium of this interpersonal system is threatened, such as when discord between the parents is amplified to the point of impending separation. When this happens the addict becomes activated, his behavior changes, and he creates a situation that dramatically *focuses attention upon himself.* This behavior can take a number of forms. For example, he may lose his temper, come home high, commit a serious crime, or overdose on drugs. Whatever its form, however, this action allows the parents to shift focus from their marital conflict to a parental overinvolvement with him. In effect, the movement is from an unstable dyadic interaction (e.g., parents alone) to a more stable triadic interaction (parents and addict). By focusing on the problems of the addict, no matter how severe or life-threatening, the parents choose a course that is apparently safer than dealing with long-standing marital conflicts. Consequently—after the marital crisis has been successfully avoided—the addict shifts to a less provocative stance and begins to behave more competently. This is a new step in the sequence. As the addict demonstrates increased competence, indicating that he can function independently of the family—for example, by getting a job, getting married, enrolling in a methadone program, or detoxifying—the parents are left to deal with their previously unresolved conflicts. At this point in the cycle marital tensions increase and the threat of separation arises. The addict then behaves in an attention-getting or self-destructive way, and the dysfunctional triadic cycle continues.

This cycle can vary in its intensity. It may occur in subdued form in treatment sessions or during day-to-day interactions and conversations around the home. For example, a parent hinting at vacationing without the spouse may trigger a spurt of loud talking by the addict. If the stakes are increased, the cycle becomes more explosive and the actions of all participants grow more serious and more dramatic; for example, the parents threatening divorce might well be followed by the addict's overdosing. Whatever the intensity level, however, we have observed such patterns so often that we have almost come to take them for granted. Viewed from this perspective, the behavior of the addict serves an important *protective* function and helps to maintain the *homeostatic balance* of the family system.

The onset of the addictive cycle appears in many cases to occur at the time of adolescence and is intensified as issues of the addict's leaving home come to the fore. This developmental stage heralds difficult times for most families and requires that the parents renegotiate their relationship—a relationship that will not include this child. However, since the parents of the addict are unable to relate to each other satisfactorily, the family reacts with panic when the integrity of the triadic relationship is threatened. Thus we find that most addicts' families become stabilized or stuck at this developmental stage in such a way that the addict remains intimately involved with them on a chronic basis. In addition to staying closely tied to the home, his failure to separate and become autonomous may take several other forms: (1) he may fail to develop stable, intimate (particularly heterosexual) relationships outside the family; (2) he may fail to become involved in a stable job, in school, or in another age-appropriate activity; (3) he may obtain work that is well below his capabilities; (4) he may become an addict.

## PSEUDOINDIVIDUATION

The drug addict is locked in a dilemma. On the one hand he is under great pressure to remain intensely involved in the family (it may fall apart without him), while on the other, sociocultural and psychobiological forces dictate that he establish intimate outside relationships. Addiction is the unique paradoxical solution to the addict and his family's dilemma of maintaining or dissolving the triadic interaction. On the systems level, the addiction cycle serves to give the appearance of dramatic movement within the family as the triad is dissolved, reestablished, dissolved, and reestablished again. In addition, the addict becomes involved in a homeostatic pattern of shuttling back and forth between his peers and his home. An interpersonal analysis of the system reveals, however, that the addict forms relationships with the drug culture that in effect *reinforce* his dependence on the family. Again, the outside relationships can be considered as the arena for pseudoindependent and pseudocompetent behavior by the addict while, paradoxically, the greater his involvement with the peer group, the more he becomes helpless, that is, addicted. This helplessness is redefined in a dependency-engendering way by the family, that is, as "sickness," and is therefore acceptable.

## SEPARATION AND DEATH

The fear that these families show of the addict's departure or development of outside relationships, that is, their fear of separation, has another paradoxical quality. At the same time that he is held back from attachments to others he is engaged in activity that can potentially end his life—for example, through drug overdose. Yet this ultimate separation—death—is not viewed with the same terror as are other types of separation. The family seems to feel that his demise will somehow preserve the family system or pattern. In the short run this may be so. Upon the addict's death, the triadic interaction is ostensibly dissolved, but in fact the parents are united in grief and, once again, can focus their attention on their child. Unlike addiction, however, this solution is only temporary. We have observed that the parents eventually find that marital conflicts once again lead to either (1) the formation of a new triad (e.g., another child becomes addicted, suicidal, or in other ways troublesome), or (2) the dissolution of their marital relationship.

## SINGLE-PARENT FAMILIES

In many addicts' families of origin one parent (usually the father) is absent. In such cases, one would think that a triadic model (as above) would not apply, and that a dyadic framework (e.g., one encompassing mother and son) would be more fitting. It would also appear to be more parsimonious and less complicated. Nonetheless, we have found that when the matter is pursued closely, a third important member generally pops up as an active participant in the interaction. Usually the triadic system is of a less obvious form, such as a covert disagreement between mother and grandmother, or mother and ex-husband. This is consonant with a point made emphatically by Haley that at least two adults are usually involved in an offspring's problem and that clinicians should look for a triangle consisting of an over-involved parent–child dyad and a more peripheral parent or grand-parent.[63, 65] Thus it has been our experience that in addition to the addict and his overinvolved parent, the triad may include the parent's paramour, an estranged parent, a grandparent, or some other relative. These alternative systems appear to exhibit patterns and cycles similar to those in which both parents are present and, again, revolve around interruption by the addict of conflicts between adult members. However, achieving separation and independence is even more of an issue in single-parent families, since the parent may be left alone with few psychological resources if the addict departs.

## THE MARITAL–PARENTAL SYSTEM INTERFACE

Earlier we noted how events in the marital system, while symptom-maintaining in themselves, were also being modulated by the addict's relation to the parental system. If the addict has not "checked in" at the home recently or the parents have some other reason to fear they are "losing" him, a crisis may occur in their home—often a fight between them—and he will be alerted to it. At this point he is apt to start a fight with his wife—a move that serves two purposes. It shows the parents that they have not lost him to marital bliss, and it gives him an excuse to return home to help, since he has "no place else to go." He will usually succeed in diverting attention from the problem in the parental home and once again function to reduce conflicts between adults.

At other times the precipitating event(s) will be less obvious and he and his wife will fall into a cycle of periodic altercations. Their temporal regularity may seem almost servocontrolled.* These appear to be maintenance cycles. They may not result in his moving out, but instead he will show up with some regularity at his parents' home to complain about connubial problems. He seems to be saying, "I just dropped by to let you know that things aren't going well and you haven't lost me." (In one case, every time the addict's mother called him, he would tell her he had just had a fight with his wife, even if this was not true—a rather ingenious way of keeping both systems simultaneously intact and pacified.) Marital battles thus become a functional part of the intergenerational homeostatic system, possessing both adaptive and sacrificial qualities. There are ways, however, in which the cycle can be broken. One of these is for the addict to substitute another person for himself, such as by giving his parents a newborn or other child to raise as a replacement (such as in the case in Chapter 10). If this alternative is acceptable, the child becomes a member of the key triad and the addict is released to his family of procreation.[19] In other words, issues between spouses, while real, cannot be viewed apart from the relationship between the addict and his parents—the two subsystems are often highly interdependent.

## EXTRAFAMILIAL SYSTEMS

A variety of extrafamilial factors also can threaten the family system and trigger the addictive cycle. These might include the father losing his job or facing retirement, a family member becoming seriously ill, or a sibling marrying and leaving home. Social systems, including peers, social agencies, and legal institutions, can affect the addict directly, and through him, the family. However, without denying the importance of extrafamilial systems, we believe that the family's influence is primary, and in fact accentuates or attenuates the impact of such external forces.

---

*In this case, "servocontrolled" refers to an automatic return to a prior behavioral state, once a specified limit is reached, such as the end of a time period.

## DISCUSSION

The model presented does not deal extensively with the historical etiology of drug addiction, but rather with current family functioning. Like most research, these studies examine families after the drug-abuse pattern is well established, without necessarily attempting to predict which families will produce an addicted offspring. We have also not dealt at length with factors affecting the onset of addiction, although the life cycle stages of adolescence and leaving home—especially when there is parent–child cross-cultural disparity—do appear to be of critical importance. Other factors also may influence the initial addiction experience, such as prevalence of addiction in the neighborhood, the prescribing of morphine during hospitalization, occurrence of deaths or losses in the family, genetic factors, and military service in Vietnam. Further, it is not clear how our model would apply to addicts raised without families, including those who grow up in institutions and become state wards for their entire lives. Whatever the variables affecting onset, however, in cases with exis-tent families it is our position that the family is a crucial factor in determining whether someone *remains* addicted. To this point, it would be interesting to study people who become addicted but do not manifest the family patterns and structures we have described. Would it be easier for them to get off drugs? This issue and others, such as the variables contributing to symptom choice, await further explora-tion.

Most of our discussion has concerned male addicts. We have had experience with only a few families in which the primary addicted member was a female. However, it is our impression that most of the principles set forth also apply to women addicts. Further, several studies mentioned earlier[36, 43, 78, 190] indicate that the relationship between the female addict and her parents, particularly her father, resembles the male addict–mother pattern. This is a client popula-tion that is receiving increased attention, and it is our hope that investigators will not neglect the family variables extant in the treat-ment of female addicts.

It is generally accepted that the addict who "cleans up" is sub-jected to pressure from peers, pushers, and acquaintances in the drug subculture to return to his habit. Conditioning to the paraphernalia and setting itself can also occur.[191] These influences can be very strong. We do not see our model as being inconsistent with conditioning theories, but rather that most such theories are not constructed to encompass family and interpersonal systems behaviors. Conditioning paradigms sit at a different level of integration, and therefore would not readily predict such phenomena as the behavioral sequences within the family homeostatic cycle, or the occurrence of symptoms or crises with other family members when the addict abstains. Further, our experience dictates that if change has been effected in the family system, the pull from conditioning factors can be resisted. With effective treatment the family can be a source of strength in helping the addict stay off drugs.[42, 92, 94, 152, 157] We have seen parents take charge of intercepting calls from "junkie" contacts and actively work to support their sons and shield them from their old ways. This sort of turnaround can fortify the "withstanding" process long enough for the old relationships and learned patterns of behavior to lose their potency.

Considering the role of the family may help to understand the successes and failures of other treatment approaches. For instance, individual therapy places the addict in a position of having to reconcile opposing loyalties.[19] The therapist becomes another outsider competing for him, and the addict usually returns to his primary relationships (i.e., his family) when pressures mount. Furthermore, it is possible that pharmacological substitution (e.g., the continued administration of methadone) may actually serve to perpetuate the family cycle because, at least initially, it tends to promote acceptance of the addict in his role as "sick" and unable to be drug-free.[130] In some ways it recreates the family system.[131, 132] We observe that these families show great tolerance for any treatment program that continues to keep the "patient" label on the addict. This may even occur in a tightly structured drug-free community, where the addict is treated as a "junkie" even when he is off drugs. In some families the addict's mere presence in such a program is sufficient to keep the family stable (e.g., the case in Chapter 7). For others this is not enough and the addict drops out of the program when a crisis develops among other subsystems in the family. We suspect this to be a major factor accounting for the unfortunately high dropout rates that occur in so many methadone and therapeutic community programs.

A fruitful direction for future research would be to identify the contribution of family factors to those situations in which drug-treatment programs succeed in producing long-term drug-free states in their clients. Can family considerations help to predict which clients will remain in a methadone program or in a drug-free community? Perhaps the oft-cited phenomenon of "maturing out" of addiction[193] also reflects changes in the family life cycle.

The emphasis here may appear to be on families with a member addicted only to opiates. However, we want to underscore that we consider the patterns we have described, and the conceptualizations we have offered, to be of a much more generic nature than this. As noted earlier, our combined experience includes many kinds of drug abusers' families. While we concede that the use of certain drugs may denote certain "psychodynamic" differences among abusers at different times, we would nonetheless posit that (1) such preferences are also greatly influenced by a complexity of external, nonindividual factors, such as availability and costliness of drugs, and (2) the processes and the model described would still apply to most of them, no matter what particular substance they compulsively abuse. Indeed, cut-and-dried opiate addicts may be on the wane, as the majority of chronic abusers in the United States appear to have grown more catholic in their tastes. (In fact, many of the AFP cases showed such polydrug use.) Consequently, we view the proposed model—especially in its more general form—as applicable to most families who have a young person compulsively using drugs.

Not all of the problems that we have ascribed to addicts' families must be present in a given case. For instance, many addicts are successful at work or school but live isolated lives in the homes of their parents. Conversely, it is not impossible to find an addict hundreds of miles from home, but having an unstable marriage, no secure job, and living in a deviant subculture. Even in these distanced cases, however, the addict may still be intimately involved in the family, as his physical presence is not necessarily required in order for him to maintain his function within it. He can simply check in with them by phone or letter on a periodic basis, or a social or rehabilitative agency (hospital, police, drug program) can communicate with the family about him. Nonetheless, whatever the configuration of problems, it is necessary for all of them to be overcome as part of the successful negotiation of this family developmental stage. Specifically, the addict must (1) cease his dependence on drugs; (2) achieve some measure of separation from his parents, typically by leaving home; (3) be seen by parents, himself, and the community as successful in some activity, such as work or school; (4) achieve stable, non-drug-related relationships outside the family.

## SUMMARY

The chronic relapsing nature of drug addiction can be explained from a family systems viewpoint. The addiction cycle is part of a family pattern involving a complex homeostatic system of interlocking feedback mechanisms, which serve to maintain the addiction and, consequently, the overall family stability. The pattern usually involves at least three people and follows a sequence in which, when the addict improves, the parental figures start to separate; when he again becomes problematic, they shift focus from their own conflict and join in directing their attention to him—at least until he again starts to improve, bringing the process full circle.

Drug taking usually starts at adolescence. It is related to an intense fear of separation experienced by the family in response to the addict's attempts at individuation. The family becomes stuck at this developmental stage. The drug provides a solution at several levels to the dilemma of whether or not to allow him independence. Paradoxically, it permits him to simultaneously be both close and distant, "in" and "out," competent and incompetent, relative to his family of origin. This is *pseudoindividuation*. An understanding of these concepts, and their integration into a homeostatic model, can provide the basis for effective treatment.

# 2

# CONTEXT:
## *PROGRAMMATIC AND*
## *RESEARCH SETTING*

M. DUNCAN STANTON
CHARLES P. O'BRIEN

MUCH OF THE MATERIAL in this book stems from a collaborative clinical research program carried out jointly at the Philadelphia Child Guidance Clinic (PCGC) and the Drug Dependence Treatment Center (DDTC) of the Philadelphia Veterans Administration (VA) Hospital. One of us (Stanton) served as Director of the family program and as Principal Investigator, with Thomas C. Todd as Co-Principal Investigator and later as consultant. The other chapter author (O'Brien) was director of the DDTC and also served as a consultant to the program. As noted in the Preface and in Chapter 1, several of the staff members had had experience in working with families of drug abusers within a variety of different kinds of institutions prior to the inception of this program, and observations from these other kinds of cases are sprinkled throughout the book. However, aside from the material on families of adolescent drug abusers (such as in Chapter 13), the main body of the text derives from work within what came to be known as the Addicts and Families Program (AFP).

This chapter briefly describes the two parent agencies (PCGC and DDTC) and the overall AFP study design. The final section covers aspects of the "marriage" between the agencies as it pertained to the carrying out of the work.


INSTITUTIONAL CONTEXT

PCGC is a family-oriented clinic treating children, adolescents, and young people. The clinic's general philosophy has been to view "psychiatric" problems as indicative of problems in and between the interpersonal *systems* in which they are embedded, particularly the family system. The "structural" approach to family therapy was developed at PCGC under the leadership of Salvador Minuchin, Braulio Montalvo, and Jay Haley.

The DDTC is a research-oriented, multimodal drug-treatment program within the VA system. Like PCGC, it is affiliated with the University of Pennsylvania School of Medicine. Methadone maintenance is the central form of treatment. The majority of patients are male veterans averaging 26 to 27 years of age. Approximately 60% of them are Black, with 40% being White. A more complete description of both the DDTC and PCGC is provided in Appendix B.


## DESIGN OF THE RESEARCH

This section will briefly outline the AFP research design. The reader interested in greater detail is referred to Appendix C or to an earlier publication.[171]

The adult addict cases described in this book came from a larger group of 118 DDTC patients. All were male opiate addicts, under age 36, in regular contact with their families of origin or parent surrogates.* All were on methadone, at least initially. A preliminary study showed that, relative to the overall DDTC patient population, they tended to be "poor prognosis" patients who were more likely to terminate treatment prematurely and maintain "dirty" urines while in the program.

Nine male therapists (of whom four were working at any given time) were involved in recruiting and treating families for the project.† Their academic credentials were modest and ranged widely (see Appendix C). In the initial stages of their cases they had two responsibilities: one was to oversee the patient's drug-treatment plan, such as

---

*Males were treated exclusively in this research partly because only 1% of the DDTC patient population was female, but mainly for purposes of research design. Including females would have required that the number of cases in the sample be increased twofold and funding was not available from the granting agency to double the size and scope of the study.

†The primary reason for using only male therapists was that this procedure allowed for control of sex of therapist in the research design, making the design "tighter." We do not wish to imply that female therapists could not do the job, although they might have been in a more difficult position given the safety factors inherent in visiting neighborhoods, as noted in Chapter 5.

adjusting methadone dosage, and the other was to bring in the family for treatment (Chapters 3, 4, and 5). The goal was to have both parents or parent surrogates, as well as any siblings age 12 or older living nearby, come in with the patient for a Family Evaluation Session—a nontherapy research exercise for which they were reimbursed. Families were randomly assigned to one of the three family-treatment conditions (see below) following this Family Evaluation Session.

## TREATMENT CONDITIONS

Four treatment conditions were employed, three of which included the families of the addicts during treatment. The treatment period (intake to termination) for the three family conditions averaged 4½ to 5 months in length. The treatment conditions were:

1. Paid Family Therapy ( $n = 21$). At the end of the Family Evaluation Session a contract was made with the family to attend 10 family therapy sessions (brief family therapy) and treatment commenced from that point. In this condition each family member age 12 and over got $5.00 for attending a session, with a chance to increase the earnings if the addict had been clean that week (see Appendix C for details on the payment procedures). Such payment raised the incentive for members to come to sessions. It also mobilized all family members to put pressure on each other to attend and to put specific pressure on the addict to attend and to abstain from drug use.

2. Unpaid Family Therapy ($n = 25$). Procedures for this group were identical to those for the Paid group except that no money was provided to the family (aside from that given for attending the Family Evaluation Session).

3. Family Movie Treatment ($n = 19$). This program required the family to come in once a week for 10 weeks to view 10 different, noncontroversial anthropology movies about people in various foreign cultures. These families were paid and got urinalysis reports in the same manner as the Paid Family Therapy group. The Movie condition thus served as a comparison or control for the effects of reimbursement per se and also for the effect on the family of attending weekly sessions together at the clinic.

4. Nonfamily (methadone and individual counseling) Treatment ($n = 53$). These were addicts in the DDTC who met all

of our criteria for inclusion in the study but were not selected for one of the three family-treatment groups. Nothing was said to them about family treatment. Instead they underwent the usual DDTC treatment procedures and received methadone maintenance, individual counseling, and other services. To be included in the study they had to remain in the methadone program at least 30 days. In comparison with other family-treatment patients, this group provides us with a baseline estimate of the treatment outcomes that can be expected with similar, fairly motivated subjects in an ongoing "standard" multimodal methadone program.

## PATIENT CHARACTERISTICS: FAMILY THERAPY GROUPS

The essential thrust of this book is to deal with clinical events and techniques for those cases actually involved in family therapy. While Chapter 5 discusses recruitment principles that also apply to the Family Movie cases and to treatment "refusers," and Chapter 17 presents outcomes for all four treatment conditions, the major concern is with family therapy. Thus attention will be given here to the 46 cases (21 and 25, respectively) in the combined Paid and Unpaid Family Therapy groups (although two Unpaid cases never did, in fact, attend a family therapy session). This gives a more accurate picture of the patient population with which the treatment principles have been developed. Demographics for the other groups are, of course, quite similar, and are presented elsewhere.[171]

Of the 46 family therapy patients, 48% were Black and 52% White. Among the Whites, 40% were of Italian, and 25% of Irish extraction. The mean age at intake was 24.7 years and ranged from age 20 to age 34. Some 24% were married and another 11% had been previously married but were unmarried at intake. All had been away from home in military service for at least a brief period in their lives; 32% had served in Vietnam and 5% had been dishonorably discharged from the military for drug use. Of the 46 patients, 61% still lived with their parent(s). Most had completed high school or an equivalency examination, 4% were in school or a training program, and 41% were employed at intake. The average length of time during which they had used opiates was 6.7 years, while 94% had been previously treated for drug abuse (i.e., they were "repeaters"). The socioeconomic composition of this (urban) group, as defined by Hollingshead and Redlich's Two-Factor Index of Social Position,[69] was Class III, 8%; Class IV, 66%; Class V, 26%.

Aside from their somewhat worse prognosis (mentioned above and in Appendix C), the major differences between this group and the overall DDTC patient population are probably that this group (1) was slightly younger; (2) had a slightly higher ratio of Whites to Blacks; (3) included fewer patients who had ever been married; and (4) included a somewhat lower percentage of patients in a school or training program (4% vs. 18%).

## THE COLLABORATIVE RELATIONSHIP

As happens in a marriage, when two institutions join or collaborate in a common endeavor, each brings to the relationship (1) its own philosophy or set of values; (2) its preferred modus operandi; and (3) a unique history or, perhaps, tradition. This was of course true of PCGC and DDTC as they interlinked within the Addicts and Families Program. An important task we faced was to reconcile these differences so as to allow the AFP to meet its goals and to function efficiently. The dialogue that evolved during this process took several interesting turns.

### MEANS AND GOALS FOR TREATMENT

The DDTC considered complete abstinence from both illegal drugs and legally prescribed opioids (e.g., methadone) to be a desirable goal of treatment. However, based both upon the literature in the field and their own experience, DDTC staff members were skeptical of this as a realistic goal with most drug addicts, particularly in the short run. Instead, the preference was to approach such a goal gradually, under planned conditions, and with the necessary "supports" intact. The main idea was that the addict should be in a stable situation before abstinence—including detoxification—was attempted, since failure was so prevalent with such attempts.

The AFP staff also suffered no illusions, at the outset, as to the difficulty of this endeavor. In fact, relative to some others in the family field, the AFP standards might not even be considered rigorous—especially at the outset—because detoxification was not necessarily espoused as a goal. Rather than labor under the pretense that "cure" was possible, the idea instead was to see whether significant change could be effected in the extent to which patients stayed off legal and illegal drugs over a given time period—the percentage of "days free," as described in Chapter 17. There was awareness that we were experimenting—trying to find out what worked with these families—and that some recognition should be given to the lore that existed in the drug-abuse field up to that time.

On the other hand, the PCGC contingent saw addiction as (primarily) part of a *family process* in which the addict was only one of a number of actors (Chapter 1). The view was that this process must be interrupted and a new process set in motion, one that did not include addictive behavior. Further, it was held that stopping the drug taking might require that a crisis be induced in the family (see Chapters 6, 8, and 9) as a way to, in a sense, "get them out of a rut." This contrasted starkly with the notion of a gradual, careful detoxification regimen. The therapy model also dictated that goals be clearly defined and that pressure be put on the addict (within a family context) to get off drugs.

How were these differences resolved? As the work progressed several confluential processes evolved. First, partly to obtain cooperation from DDTC staff and partly because it seemed to have merit, the family clinicians did tentatively embrace the DDTC idea of having "all the ducks in line" before detoxification. A reluctance developed toward prematurely rushing headlong into detoxification.

On the other hand, as the family therapists grew more experienced, and the techniques began to be identified and refined, confidence increased to move more rapidly in family treatment. This practice was also dictated by the urgency of having to accomplish something within 10 sessions. Eventually, it became more commonplace for a therapist to pose to the family the question, "When is he going to detoxify?" in the first or second session, whereas in early cases therapists tended to sidestep this issue initially. Interestingly, as a treatment paradigm emerged, and some successes were achieved, DDTC personnel grew more amenable to rapid action, moving somewhat from their previous cautionary posture. They began to accept that working with the family to pressure the addict against drug taking was a viable and feasible procedure, especially when there were no indications of a possible suicidal reaction. The eventual outcome was a paradigm that drew from the philosophies and practices of both camps.

## MONITORING OF PROGRESS AND PROCEDURES

There were at least two areas in which the AFP had interesting effects on the DDTC. The first of these concerned the monitoring of urine reports. Progress and changes in drug taking were a key part of family therapy. Clear contingencies were established for "dirty" urines given by family (and movie) therapy cases—especially in the two "paid" conditions. The treatment was sharply focused on this behavior. Thus it was essential that the urinalysis results processed at DDTC be obtained and recorded accurately and efficiently. In the early stages of the program, however, it was discovered that the DDTC was going through a "slippage phase" regarding strict adherence to urine test results: records were sometimes "lost," patients were able to get away with denying that dirty urines were their own, and (previously firm) established rules preventing clients with dirty urines from obtaining certain privileges, or even remaining in the program, were not being strictly followed. The AFP attention to, and insistance on, (1) clarity and efficiency of urinalysis results, and (2) adherance to program strictures based on urine results highlighted areas where slack had set in. As a result, the DDTC tightened up its urine-monitoring procedure and the total urine-reporting system was improved.*

Paralleling the above, a number of areas were uncovered by the AFP in which patients were finding it easy to manipulate the DDTC system. These included ways of getting around program rules, tricks for obtaining permission from staff for higher methadone dosages, methods for triangulating staff members and instigating or exacerbating conflicts between them, and so forth. Some of these are described in Chapter 16. As they came to light with AFP cases, or within AFP team meetings, they were responded to and corrected by DDTC staff, thus allowing improvement in the overall drug-treatment program.

## THE RESEARCH ETHIC

It is important to mention some significant aspects of the DDTC that contributed immeasurably to the success of this work. Because the DDTC (1) was established partly as a research center, (2) was

---

*This sequence of clinical research impacting positively on clinical procedures had happened before the AFP and has recurred since. It presents an interesting example of the interplay between treatment and research.

somewhat less vulnerable to severe viscissitudes of funding (compared to many other agencies), and (3) incorporated many treatment modalities within its walls, it was (and is) a very result-oriented institution. The treatment philosophy was not rigid, and there was a sincere interest in alternatives to methadone (in contrast to the total commitment to various forms of pharmacological substitution—mentioned in Chapters 1 and 6—that sometimes occurs in drug-abuse programs). This pragmatism fostered a kind of "live and let live" attitude toward new kinds of treatment, resulting in an atmosphere in which competitiveness between different modalities could be minimized. It is conceivable that a program such as the AFP, had it been established within a different context, might have encountered much greater difficulty and that resistance could even have increased as it began to demonstrate effectiveness. This did not occur in the present case.

## CONCLUSION

Given the inherent problems that occur when two separate institutions collaborate, we feel that the relationship and cooperation that developed around this work was closer to optimal than one can normally expect. Our task was certainly facilitated by common experiences shared (prior to the study) by several of the principal figures, and also by the shared institutional affiliations and research interests. On the other hand, some of the problems we faced would not occur in situations where all programmatic components exist within the same administrative, physical, and institutional structure. No doubt there are areas in which the PCGC and DDTC philosophies may never reach assimilation. Nonetheless the marriage seems to have "worked," and divorce has never been necessary.

# 3

## GETTING THE ADDICT
## TO AGREE TO INVOLVE
## HIS FAMILY OF ORIGIN:
## *THE INITIAL CONTACT*

JOHN M. VAN DEUSEN/M. DUNCAN STANTON/
SAMUEL M. SCOTT/THOMAS C. TODD/DAVID T. MOWATT

IN CONTRAST to the analysis presented thus far concerning the functional value of addiction in families,[67, 80, 134, 150, 152, 154, 170] a number of investigators have given evidence that the family can also be important in the rehabilitation of the addict. When family members are involved in the treatment process, the system can be changed toward helping the abusing member *overcome* his addiction rather than serving as a force that maintains it. To this point, Eldred and Washington[42] found in interviews with 158 heroin addicts that the people who the patients thought would be most helpful to them in their attempts to give up drugs were the members of their families of origin or their in-laws; second and third choices were an opposite-sex partner and the patient himself. A group of 462 heroin addicts interviewed by MACRO Systems researchers[94] reported that the family was second only to treatment (70.9% vs. 79.6%) as the influence they perceived as most important in changing their lives. Finally, a 5-year follow-up study of narcotics addicts by Levy[92] found that patients who successfully overcame their drug habits most often had family support.

Studies of the effectiveness of family treatment have shown this to be a promising approach with alcoholism and many other symptoms, and family therapies for drug problems have been gaining

This chapter is an expansion and revision of a paper by the first four authors entitled "Engaging 'Resistant' Families in Treatment: I. Getting the Drug Addict to Recruit His Family Members" and is reprinted with permission from the *International Journal of the Addictions*, 1980, *15*, 1069–1089. © Marcel Dekker, Inc.

momentum in recent years.[152] In fact, a 1976 national survey of 2012 drug programs by Coleman and Davis[30] indicated that 93% were providing some kind of family services for at least a portion of their clients—in many cases, family therapy. Consequently, if there is a validity to such efforts, it is important to be able to induct family members into the treatment program. This chapter presents techniques pertaining to the initial facet of this process, that is, dealing with the addict in recruiting his family.*

As noted in the literature review in Chapter 5, authors who have dealt with this matter have noted how difficult it can be to bring family members of compulsive drug abusers into treatment. Most family members, especially parents, generally refuse to become involved. This is particularly interesting in view of the aforementioned evidence that the majority of drug addicts—especially those who use opiates—maintain close ties to their families of origin. If they do not live with one or both parents they may reside nearby and be in frequent contact (see Appendix A for a review of these studies). Thus it becomes all the more important that methods for effectively involving members of addicts' families in the treatment process be developed.

The AFP research design called for a Family Evaluation Session (see Appendix C), which included at least the addict, both his parents or parent surrogates (e.g., stepmother, mother's boyfriend), and any siblings living nearby. This session was required before treatment could proceed. (Although not included in the Family Evaluation Session, spouses of married addicts were usually involved in the therapy that followed it.) Obviously, this put considerable pressure on us to succeed in our recruiting efforts. The general procedure was for the person responsible for inducting the family to function as both drug counselor and family therapist. In approximately 80% of the cases we were able to obtain cooperation from the addict toward including his family, and in 88% of these we were able to get the family—including *both* parents or parent surrogates—to physically appear at the treatment site together. In other words, *two-thirds of the subset of families we were unable to recruit occurred because the addict*

---

*It should be noted that the primary emphasis of this chapter is upon young adult addicts. Adolescents may also manifest resistance to family involvement. However, the way the therapist handles the process may differ when encountering an adolescent versus a young adult. Some pointers and strategies for getting adolescents to agree to having their families become involved in therapy are presented in Chapter 13.

*would not allow us to contact his family,* which underscores the emphasis given to the initial patient interview in this chapter.


## OVERALL RATIONALE

When a family orientation is to be used in treatment, it is advantageous for the therapist to present this idea to the "identified" patient (IP), that is, the addict, at the outset. This avoids the confusion and possible conflict inherent in forming a therapeutic relationship with an individual patient, which may compete with a later relationship with his family. The structuring of the initial interview with the patient therefore becomes crucial in determining whether he and the rest of the family can be recruited for treatment. If a therapist is aware of the behaviors the patient may use to resist involving his family—and counters these with appropriate tactics—chances are increased for successful induction of the family, whatever the patient's initial response to this idea.

It is certainly helpful in recruiting families to have strong pressure from the treatment program for family involvement, but in many programs this pressure is either nonexistent or unenforceable. In programs such as the methadone maintenance program with which the AFP was associated—a Veterans Administration (VA) program in which veterans could not be denied treatment if they refused to involve their families—it is usually necessary to receive the addict's permission before contacting the rest of the family.[119]

At this point we should state unequivocally that seeing the IP alone at the outset is *always* second best to having the whole family present at the initial contact. This is so, even if the therapist later decides to engage in individual sessions with the IP. However, given the infrequency with which whole families of drug abusers appear at intake, the therapist may use the initial (individual) session to advantage in several ways. First, the individual meeting can be used to convey to the addict the message that he is an adult—that although his individuation from his family is a tenuous one, he has amassed a complexity of interpersonal skills associated with his habit that need to be respected. Second, the intake interview provides an opportunity for the addict to admit that his efforts to stand alone are not working, in view of his habit and the unspoken family problems around the addiction.

## THE INITIAL SESSION

### SETTING THE APPOINTMENT

In arranging for the session, the therapist should do as little work as possible over the telephone (or via letter). A purpose for the meeting needs to be presented—usually that of getting the patient's history and setting up the appropriate treatment schedule for him. In some programs such a meeting is required before treatment can proceed. The patient should be informed that this will involve about 1 hour's time.

The time for the session should be set no later than 2 or 3 days from the telephone contact, preferably sooner. This adds to the urgency of the situation, and is a sign to the patient that the therapist is sensitive to his need for help. In fact, we have observed that a kind of *imprinting* process occurs during the intake period, whereby the patient attaches strongly to the first person (or persons) offering him help; this person appears to have much more leverage with him than those who deal with him later. Consequently, a delay of more than 3 days markedly increases the chances of either a cancellation or a no-show by the patient.

In the initial telephone contact, the therapist should also inquire (when appropriate) as to how the patient expects to travel to the clinic, and confirm that he is sure of directions. He should be given the therapist's phone number, and instructed to call if he is going to be late or if he should get lost.

Finally, the IP is told that it would ease the therapist's burden if the patient could bring in another family member—or the whole family—to this session. This can be framed as "helpful in setting things up more quickly." The patient's response gives some indication of how much the family knows about the drug problem, especially if the patient is reluctant to bring anyone with him.

### INTERVIEW RATIONALE

Since the initial interview is the first major contact between patient and therapist, many transactional rules will be instituted in the session. The therapist needs to know which aspects of the interview should be emphasized early and which should be postponed until later. With the family approach it is not necessary that the patient be familiar with the therapist's orientation at the outset. Nor are the conditions under which the patient comes in (voluntary or involuntary referral) key at this time. The patient may have been through a similar process before, and have expectations about the course and outcome of the interview. He may even arrive prepared to control the session, since most addicts recycle through the system frequently enough to have "memorized" the particulars.

What is primary in this session is that the therapist obtain some indication from the patient that he wants to get out of his drug habit. The indication may be either stated or implied, and should occur early in the session. This may require prompting by the therapist. Veracity of the statement is not essential at this point, however. The declaration may be presented merely as a move in the game of gaining entrée to the treatment program or system.

The statement that one wants to be drug-free and its acknowledgment by the therapist are important because such an exchange provides a basis for this and for all future sessions. Any work the therapist intends to do with the family derives its public rationale from this transaction. Occasionally, a patient will not declare a readiness to break his habit, so the therapist may have to do some preliminary work in this area. If the patient wants to be maintained on a prescribed drug, such as methadone, the therapist may point out that this requires becoming abstinent from street drugs. If the patient admits he does not feel he can stop using street drugs, the therapist might discuss with him the pros and cons of this, working toward an agreement that the use of illegal drugs is in some way detrimental to his welfare. Once a concession is made by the patient, it is easier to obtain later agreement on the more global objective of becoming completely drug-free.

## PROTOCOL

The protocol for the remainder of the interview depends largely on the scope of the clinician's responsibilities. If he is to act strictly as a therapist, he may focus immediately on the matter of getting the family recruited. If, on the other hand, his role includes that of drug counselor, the intake strategy may require more complex structuring. Here, the therapist should be prepared for a variety of secondary issues that could come up in the session, including requests for dosage increases, program privileges, and so forth. Since the present chapter is directed at the major issue of getting the patient to recruit his family, drug-counseling strategy will be dealt with in summary fashion, that is, only where it is directly relevant to the recruiting task.

## THINGS SAID AND THINGS DONE

In conducting the initial session, the therapist may find that he is getting minimal resistance to his ideas from the patient. This is surprisingly common. The therapist should think carefully about the possibilities underlying this situation, and prepare to deal with any contingency. On the positive end of a continuum, compliance could signal a true readiness to detoxify from drugs; the therapist's guidance is all that has been needed to get things started. Some people *do* get off drugs without considerable prodding. Tactics can in this instance be centered around getting the family organized to assist with the process.

A more difficult situation arises when the patient is simply "jiving" the therapist, or stringing him along, with no intention of carrying out the plans he is agreeing to. Here, the compliance is wholly fictitious. When this occurs, avoiding entrapment in an undesirable position requires that the therapist focus his maneuvers and make immediate use of the verbal compliance. It may be as easy to get the patient into action at this time as it is to exact promises from him. For example, a parent might be telephoned on the spot in order to set up an appointment for the family interview—a technique that Coleman[28] has also used. Even where a call cannot be worked out during the session, the therapist can set the conditions at this time for later contact with the family. This includes collecting names, addresses, and phone numbers, and instructing the patient to inform his parents that the therapist will be calling them. As a quid pro quo and demonstration of good faith or commitment, it may be helpful for the therapist to give the patient his own phone number in return.

## STRUCTURING THE INTERVIEW

What happens when things do not go smoothly in the initial session? The therapist should expect some kind of resistance from most patients, especially longtime users, who know the usual ins and outs of the drug-treatment system. Obstacles are easier to handle when the therapist applies a standard structure to this first interview, segmenting it to deal separately with drug history, the patient's interests, and relations with the family. This structure allows the therapist to begin the discussion with a topic that the patient expects to discuss, joining with him as his problems and ambitions are brought out. This precedes talk about family matters, the domain of central importance here. At the same time, information is accumulating in a way that will provide the therapist with reasons for suggesting a family approach. He also obtains clues about which paths the patient's objections to this approach may take.

### Opening: Drugs

First inquiries in the session should concern the patient's history of drug use and treatment. Typical queries by the therapist include, "Tell me a little about your habit," or, "Have you ever tried to kick it before?" The therapist should show here that he is properly concerned about the patient's present condition, which might very well include the first stages of withdrawal.

If the patient concedes that he is in a "bad way," or gives a history of prior, unsuccessful treatment, the therapist can later use these in his arguments for a family approach to the problem. It works best if the therapist implies knowledge and authority in the area of drugs, then moves on, since getting caught up in details is a game that the patient will play as long as the therapist permits.

It is not unusual for a drug-dependent individual to spend from 1 to 3 hours setting up a situation so that it is favorable to him, no matter how small the nature of his request. This is routine behavior in pursuit of a change in medication or other treatment benefits. He could, for example, wait around the treatment premises until the staff is obviously rushed before making his request, hoping to slip it through without being checked. Or it could involve relating a long and complex story—some addicts are prodigious storytellers—in a manner meant to inform the therapist that there is no option left but to give the patient what he needs. As soon as the therapist anticipates that a story is about to unfold he can counter it by cutting the tale short with a question or statement that leads the discussion onto another track. This tactic should be repeated until the patient has been engaged in an appropriate topic. Incidentally, this is least difficult to accomplish when the patient is "high"—his persistance is generally much lower in that state.

## Personal Interests, Goals

Discussion moves from the area of drug problems into that of the patient's interests and future plans. Employment and educational status are the key topics, since these may be shaped into concrete goals that are agreeable to everyone who is to be involved in the family therapy. The therapist can start by asking whether the patient is presently working, and if so, in what kind of job, with what hours and pay. If the patient is not working, the therapist can turn to job history. When a patient discusses a job he has enjoyed, his conversation will change to a more positive note. The therapist can then switch tactics, and encourage him to dwell upon the positive areas. What the therapist should be searching for in this discussion is alternatives—kinds of activities that can be shaped into reasonable goals.

The talk becomes less formal, more relaxed, in this segment. The patient should next be asked about plans and desires for the future. If he is unclear about what he wants, the therapist can provide cues, using the job or school information already given, or asking about other matters ("Have you got a girl?" or, "Do you work out at all, engage in any sports?").

Altogether, the discussion of personal interests should have two results. First, the patient should come away from this session with a better idea about what he would like to do after he gets off drugs. Second, he should feel that the therapist is interested in him as an individual, and in helping him to work toward his goals. Ordinarily, patient goals will require some assistance from outside. It should be made clear in this segment of the interview whether help is needed and who is best able to supply it.

## Family Matters

Discussion should move to the patient's family of origin only when the therapist is ready to raise the matter of involving them in the treatment. Of first importance is information about (1) the composition of the family, and (2) the amount of contact between members. This will aid the therapist in deciding who is central in the family, which will vary from patient to patient. Both parents are important in most cases. Parent substitutes are acceptable only where they have played, or are presently playing, a major role in the patient's life. Initial questions to pick up this information can include, "Do you live with your folks?" "Who raised you?" "How often do you see them?" "Who else lives at home?" and "Who do you spend the most time with in the family?"

The patient's spouse or girlfriend and children may also be relevant to treating the drug problem, and should be considered for inclusion. However, it is our own (Chapters 1, 4, and 6) and others'[42,92] experience that the family of origin and marital systems are highly interdependent, and that treatment initially must include the family of origin. The marital relationship should be dealt with later, if it is dealt with at all. If spouse and parents do not get along, the therapist might, for the present, contract for two separate sessions, with a goal of bringing the two subsystems together later in treatment.

While the patient is talking about his family, the therapist should be mapping its configuration in his own mind, deciding which members he will want to bring in. Any family member attending this initial session should be included and called upon here for his opinion about who in the family knows the patient best. With enough suggestions on the floor, the therapist will be able to work toward consensus with the patient on the few crucial family members, while compromising with him about others.

After ascertaining the composition of the family, but *prior to suggesting that they be brought in*, the therapist must inquire how much they know about the drug problem. If the patient says they do not know anything, he should be made to elaborate on this statement (e.g., "You mean they don't know you're using now, or that they don't know you've ever used?"). Getting this information straight is crucial, since the patient has a legal right to confidentiality, which cannot be violated without his consent.[119, 152] If he continues to claim that no one in the family knows he uses drugs, and that he wants it kept that way, the therapist will have to work on this matter before going any further in the interview. The best approach is, again, to force him to elaborate by acting as if this situation were incredible ("Surely *someone* must know something?"). We feel the therapist can ask this with some confidence, as we have yet to see an addict over age 20 whose family was not aware of his drug involvement at least to some extent. An alternative tactic is to suggest that maybe not bringing the family in to help before is one reason his prior attempts to get off drugs have been unsuccessful.

*Introducing Family Therapy*

This is where the therapist should begin to discuss his own orientation. The general aim is to set up the situation so the patient can admit to the value of getting his family's help "this time around." Depending on the amount and type of resistance encountered, the therapist can go in one of several directions. However, before deciding which tack to take, the therapist should first find out where the family members are at this exact moment, especially the parents. This is a preventive step that disallows the patient from stating later—should he be looking for ways to resist—that he does not know their whereabouts. For example, when the therapist subsequently informs the patient that he wishes to telephone the father, it will be less easy for the patient to deny knowing Dad's location if he has already told the therapist that his father is at work.

Assuming that family members know the patient is using drugs, the most common type of "excuse" given for their nonparticipation is that they are unable or unwilling to come in for a session with the therapist. If the patient indicates that his father or mother is sick, disabled, working long hours, or too poor to come in, the therapist should explain either that he would like to contact them anyway, or that he will need to confirm this by contacting them. His best move is to find out from the patient which member(s) can be reached by telephone *at this moment.* Or, the therapist can ask the patient to make a "bridge" for him with the parents, by telling them that he will be calling at a specific time later.

When a patient says that his family is unwilling to help, this may prove to be genuine. The therapist needs to know, in that event, if it is a result of their being excluded from prior treatments (which is usually the case). Again, he needs to talk to them directly to verify this. If he cannot call one of them during the session, he should set up a later contact. It is important for this reason to gather several telephone numbers (home and work numbers of patient, parents, and siblings), and, again, to make sure the patient has the therapist's telephone number.

The patient may state that his family has known about the problem and was included in dealing with it before. However, it is unlikely that the kind of family treatment the therapist has in mind has been attempted previously. It is important for the therapist to learn the details of this earlier family involvement so he can differentiate between what has happened before and what is being proposed in the present. Usually, nothing akin to family *therapy* has been experienced. More likely, the patient's mother drove him to the clinic each day to pick up his medicine. In other words, family involvement was minimal.

When the patient has his mind set on "doing it alone," it is worth discussing his strategy in detail, right in the initial session. While he may be sincere in his desires, his plans may be hazy or nonexistent. The therapist can join with him on the importance of "doing it right this time." The patient should be encouraged to talk about his plans with the therapist.

As the discussion proceeds, the therapist should take control by asking primary questions: "How are you going to get off of drugs?" "What are you going to do with your time when you don't have to spend it copping?" "What will you say when your buddies want you to cop with them?" "How many times in your life are you going to go through this again?" If he has not planned for such contingencies as these, the patient is already becoming dependent on the therapist's guidance, whether he knows it or not, as the issues are brought to light.

What the therapist is doing here is gradually maneuvering the discussion so that the patient agrees with him that his parents know and are concerned about his problems (i.e., "Don't you think they know that you use drugs?" or, "Hasn't there been a cloud there, between you and them, all the time you've been using?"). Another tack is to note that the family has known and been close to the patient for a long time and it would help the therapist to get some background or history from them. Having to explain his denials or support them with evidence may prove more tiring for the patient than placing the family in the therapist's hands. From here, work can start on how to bring the parents in, and what to discuss when they come.

In some cases it may be possible to short-cut the interview process. For instance, going directly from drugs to family talk may be possible if the patient offers that he feels "bad" because his parents have been greatly concerned about his drug problem.

## REHEARSING

We have found the technique of contacting one or more family members by telephone during the initial interview with the addict to be highly successful. At times, however, it may seem clinically contraindicated or may not be feasible. Scheduling problems may inter-fere, it may be putting too much pressure on the addict, or it may be preferable to let the addict approach his family first, if only to "prep" them for a subsequent call from the therapist.

When the latter strategy is employed, it is useful to rehearse with the addict in the session the task of contacting family members for the initial family interview. This not only solidifies the relation-ship between the addict and the therapist, but also provides the latter with more information about the present family crisis and how to approach it in the first family interview. The following segment is from the intake interview of a 24-year-old heroin addict who lived with his mother and father and had a long history of drug abuse. His enrollment in the AFP was concurrent with his mother's loss of employment due to the closing of a store where she had been a longtime employee. The therapist, Samuel M. Scott, rehearsed with the addict in how to engage mother, underlining the crisis of mother's unemployment and associating it with the problem of addiction. This technique gives both the addict and the therapist an understanding of where the initial session with the family needs to go.

*SCOTT:* If you were going to tell your parents that you were in this program, this detox program, and you were going to kick it once and for all, how would you tell them?

*ADDICT:* Mmmm.

*SCOTT:* I just put you on the biggest spot of your life right now. I know that.

*ADDICT:* That's very hard for me.

*SCOTT:* I hear ya.

*ADDICT:* You see, she's had too many hurts in her life, and this would hurt her. You see, I don't want to hurt her because she's had too many hurts in her life.

*SCOTT:* (*emphatically*) Yeah, I hear ya.

*ADDICT:* I'd rather just get off of it, then after, then I would tell her.

*SCOTT:* But that's not the question I asked you.

*ADDICT:* You asked how would I tell her.

*SCOTT:* How would you tell her *now*?

*ADDICT:* (*after a pause*) Well.

*SCOTT:* Just project yourself.

*ADDICT:* I believe I'd just have to say, "Mom, I'm sorry, I'm trying to do something . . ."

*SCOTT:* OK, you'd apologize for the past, obviously.

*ADDICT:* Right.

*SCOTT:* And then you'd say, "But I'm trying."

*ADDICT:* Right.

*SCOTT:* How about if you took a more positive approach?

*ADDICT:* So what you're saying is you want me to just tell her, right?

*SCOTT:* Well, no, I'm not saying that, not at all, not at all. . . . If you tell her, and how you tell her, is important.

*ADDICT:* Yeah, right.

*SCOTT:* And what's a more positive way of telling your mother? Would you tell your mother or your father first?

*ADDICT:* My mother.

*SCOTT:* You wouldn't tell your father first?

*ADDICT:* No.

*SCOTT:* Why?

*ADDICT:* See, because my mother has very strong emotions.

*SCOTT:* Yeah, sure, I hear it—so you would not tell your father . . .

*ADDICT:* (*emphatically*) I'll tell him after I tell *her.*

*SCOTT:* Would you tell them both together?

*ADDICT:* Yeah, I could. (*quietly and more cooperatively*) But I'd rather just talk to her first, because then I can express, I don't know why, myself a little bit more toward her, 'cause I just want to talk to her personally.

*SCOTT:* I hear ya.

*ADDICT:* Because, ya see, that's the only friend I really have.

*SCOTT:* Woo, woo, woo! . . . How about your girlfriend?

*ADDICT:* That's on a different level.

*SCOTT:* I hear ya.

Rehearsing the recruitment of family members focuses on the nature of the immediate crisis as well as enabling the therapist to identify structural characteristics within the family that maintain the addiction. Usually those members who are described by the addict as the most unapproachable are the most important in resolving the crisis at hand. This is particularly obvious where the addict is overinvolved with mother, while father maintains a distant role, as in the case above. Mothers in these families are frequently easy to engage, as they have an investment in being involved in their sons' problems, although there is usually resistance to involving mother and father together (see Chapter 5). Addicts from these families tend to describe their fathers as totally disinterested, or they protect their fathers by claiming that they are too busy and are not to be disturbed. Sometimes a discussion around engaging the more difficult parent provides an opportunity for the addict to inadvertently tell the therapist how this parent needs to be involved if the crisis is to be resolved.

In other families, it is obvious that the way to approach difficult members is through another family member. For example, the best way to reach father may be through mother. What is critical in this aspect of the interview is that the therapist have an understanding of which family members are most involved with the addiction and that an alliance be established with the IP toward involving these members in treatment. In cases where this does not happen, the recruitment effort is more difficult and treatment frequently fails. For example, one addict stressed that it was very important to him that his uncle be included in the therapy. The AFP research design dictated that the initial (nontherapy) research session involve only the nuclear family. It developed that the crisis in the family was around disagreement between the addict's parents concerning this uncle. The failure of the therapist to include the uncle in the initial research session was received by the parents as a message that the therapist was insensitive to the issues at hand. The family withdrew from treatment and the case foundered.

## HANDLING "STALEMATES"

Ideally, the initial interview should end on a positive and hopeful note, with a clear strategy defined with the addict on how to contact the family for the first family interview. The therapist works out a time with the addict to contact his family, preferably when all members of the family (including the addict) will be present. It is also important to allow the addict sufficient time to discuss his knowledge of the family-treatment program with them.

There will, of course, be situations where this ideal outcome cannot be achieved and the therapist cannot get the patient to budge in the initial session. "Stalemate" encounters are usually the result of the patient denying the therapist access to information needed to construct the framework for placing the drug problem in a family context. The interview structure presented may not elicit all relevant facts in any area, but its application does ensure that the questions of major importance are discussed without prematurely "turning the patient off" to therapy.

If these strategies are not effective, the therapist can postpone further discussion, possibly even for a week or two, while the patient "thinks things over." Or, the patient might be told to return "when he's ready to make a move." This last tactic is most workable when the therapist has some form of leverage with the patient, such as control over medication or liaison with the physician who has this control. In such instances he can withhold small changes or privileges until the patient complies. However, it is best to reserve use of this tactic, making it a last resort when all else fails to work. It should not be used more than once, and care must be taken that it does not fall into the category of denying the patient treatment to which he is entitled.

## CONCLUSION

In conducting an initial interview with a drug-dependent individual, a therapist must deal with three major concerns. First, he must demonstrate his understanding of drug dependency in general, and this patient's drug problem in particular. Second, he must show a willingness to help the patient formulate and realize concrete plans for a better future. Third, and most important, he must be able to convey throughout the course of the interview a sense that he is competent in this work. Unwillingness by the patient to involve his family in the task of getting him drug-free is minimized when these concerns have been dealt with in the context of the initial session. The general structure of the interview process is schematized in Table 1.

The model described here structures the contents of the session in a manner that maximizes the likelihood that these concerns will be brought out and discussed. It should be noted, however, that all the model actually provides is a form of technical assistance. We are not suggesting that it supplies answers in itself, or that it in any way reduces the responsibilities of the therapist. Each patient will have unique aspects to his problem. He will discuss these in unique ways, and the therapist should respond uniquely.

We have used this model successfully throughout the life of the AFP in recruiting families through the IP. Although it was developed with heroin addicts, there is no reason why the procedures described could not be applied to other kinds of family problems. In fact, adult

Table 1. Working with the Drug Abuser toward Involving His Family in Treatment: Schema for the Initial Session

| FOCUS | ACTIVITIES | POSSIBLE ISSUES | POSSIBLE TECHNIQUES |
|---|---|---|---|
| Setting the appointment | Therapist describes purpose, schedules appointment. If possible, gets other family members in. | Client does not contact therapist to set up appointment. | Therapist contacts patient by telephone, at home or at the treatment center. |
| | | Client objects to need for a session. | Session is described as an integral, necessary part of treatment. |
| | | Client does not want other family members involved. | Usefulness of other members as sources of information about the client, or the problem, is explained. (Patient has a right to confidentiality and this must be respected.) |
| Resetting (no-show) | | Client does not show for appointment. | Prevented by (1) scheduling the appointment within 2 or 3 days of setting it; (2) confirming on day of appointment, via telephone; (3) reviewing travel directions; (4) having client call therapist if he is late or lost. A final tactic is to restrain privileges at treatment center, if allowable. |

| Topic | Therapist | Client | Therapist response |
|---|---|---|---|
| Opening: Drugs | Therapist probes (1) history of drug use and treatment; (2) previous attempts to get off drugs; (3) current problems. | Client questions therapist's expertise. | Therapist uses an objective, authoritative style, avoiding discussion of particulars or credentials; cites general experience and success, if necessary. |
| | | Client digresses or nods. | Therapist repeats directives, reorients client to appropriate topics. |
| | | Client focuses on demand for current medication. | Therapist explains that he requires a fuller picture before he can assess how to best help the client (stresses "This way works best"). |
| Personal interests and goals | Therapist determines (1) range of current interests and activities, especially job and/or school status; (2) future plans. | Client questions need for discussing this area. | Therapist frames interests and plans as areas of past or present success and/or areas where concrete treatment goals can be instituted. |
| | | Client not working or not in school. | Therapist directs inquiries to job or school history to assess client's experience, skills, and preferences. |

*(Continued)*

*Table 1. (Continued)*

| FOCUS | ACTIVITIES | POSSIBLE ISSUES | POSSIBLE TECHNIQUES |
|---|---|---|---|
| Family history and present contact | Therapist determines (1) client's present living situation (where, with whom, etc.); (2) contacts with family members (frequency and quality of relationships); (3) family's knowledge of past and present drug problems and treatment. | Client does not divulge specifics or details. | Therapist begins either with indirect queries regarding the family (e.g., "Where are you living now?"), or by branching from previous mention of family by the client (e.g., "You said your dad wants you to go back to school; what kind of work does he do?"). |
| | | Client questions need for discussing this area. | Therapist repeats description of the need for a fuller picture of the client's experience, to work successfully. |
| | | Regarding family members' knowledge of drug use, client says they have no knowledge. | Therapist asks for clarification (e.g., "They don't know about *this* time, or at all?" "Who doesn't know?" "They don't know you're using drugs, but they must sense that something is going on"). |
| Orientation to family therapy | Therapist describes this approach as involving the whole family and as very effective. Two objectives are central: (1) getting the client's trust, and authorization to contact his family; (2) completing the arrangements needed to bring the family in for the first session. | Client does not want to involve his family; reasons include: | Therapist repeats his explanation of need to work with the family; cites effectiveness. |
| | | (1) "Won't (can't) ask them." | Has client ever asked them to help before? What happened? Therapist may enact a scenario via role play, to help client practice for this. Or, therapist will call and explain treatment to parents. |

| | | |
|---|---|---|
| The therapist should aim to telephone or otherwise contact at least one family member (father or mother) during the session, to recruit for therapy. | (2) "They aren't willing." | Have they been involved in treatment before? What happened? This is a different approach. Who is not willing? What are their reasons?" Therapist will call them to explain. |
| | (3) Family members cannot be called right now. | Therapist reviews times, day or evening, when they can be called; gets complete list of phone numbers. The client is directed to tell them to expect a call from the therapist (optimally, the same day). |
| Rehearsal | Therapist rehearses with client how client could approach family members. | Client verbalizes desire to protect family members from pain, unnecessary hassles, and so forth. | Therapist discusses the family members involved—their needs, their hopes for the client, their wishes to help. |
| | Client describes particular family member as "unapproachable." | Therapist explores working through another family member to reach the "unapproachable" member. |
| | Client indicates unwillingness to approach family. | Therapist returns to alternative strategy of contacting family himself. |

(Continued)

*Table 1. (Continued)*

| FOCUS | ACTIVITIES | POSSIBLE ISSUES | POSSIBLE TECHNIQUES |
|---|---|---|---|
| Stalemate | In instances where the therapist has not obtained permission to induct family, or has not completed arrangements with them, further sessions with the client may be necessary. (*Note:* The client usually retains his rights to confidentiality and to treatment, within limits; the therapist should know and use these to advantage, negotiating privileges without infringements of basic rights.) | Client still refuses to allow contact. | Therapist's strategy depends on rapport already established. He may either postpone further contact with the client indefinitely, or for a set period, allowing him to make up his mind on this (leaving the issue open); or, he may demand another session immediately, to continue the discussion. |
| | | Client wants to "Do it alone" (expresses confidence in ability to do so). | Therapist asks if client has done this before, with what success? If done previously, it certainly was not completely successful, or client would not be here now; perhaps family is needed. Another approach is to review the client's plans for detoxing, and point out where and how family needs to be involved to ensure that it works (even if only to steer clear of the client). |

male addicts constitute an extremely taxing test population for the techniques, since drug dependency is seen by most addicts and parents as a social or individual problem rather than a family matter.

We have dealt, here, with the first interview and have not discussed the next step of actually contacting and personally recruiting family members; this is covered in Chapter 5. When the therapist is allowed to contact the family, the question of why they need to be involved in treatment will become an important issue. The initial, individual contact is crucial, however, in helping the patient to shift from perceiving his problem solely within the traditional treatment setting to viewing it as part of a family context.

# 4

## USING THE INITIAL CONTACT
## TO ASSESS THE FAMILY SYSTEM

DAVID T. MOWATT

MOVEMENT BY AN ADDICT toward becoming an independent person is usually accompanied by an unspoken threat of crisis within the family that is felt to be potentially more destructive to the family than the addiction itself. The addict's enrollment in a methadone maintenance program can be seen as a sign that the addict's detouring behavior has failed and the family is in a state of crisis. Many investigators view enrollment in a program as influenced predominantly by such factors as the availability of street drugs and changes within the drug subculture; although these factors may influence the addict's decisions, the position taken in the present volume is that the addict's behavior can best be understood within the context of the family addiction cycle. One way of understanding the failure of many treatment programs is that the treatment facility becomes the arena for the addict's detouring behavior, rather than the family. Consequently, the emerging family crisis is never addressed and the addiction is maintained. The decision to maintain a young adult on methadone and work out his problems "in the program" may thus unwittingly become a form of collusion with the family to keep the family problem "out there" and to maintain the addict as a handicapped person.

An alternative to this is to use the addict's entry into a program as an opportunity to intervene in the family in such a way that the crisis can be contained within the family. Implicit in this approach is the assumption that the crisis associated with the addict's movement toward individuation needs to be resolved within the family, if any lasting change is to take place. Although the initial stages of treatment typically focus on the addiction and the behavior of the addict (see Chapter 6), the therapist needs to assess the family structures maintaining the addiction and the crisis that must be negotiated if the addict is to improve.

This chapter discusses the initial encounters with the addict and his family, noting ways in which such encounters can provide a basis for identifying critical family issues and set the initial direction for their resolution. The ideas presented here are based on a retrospective analysis of successful and unsuccessful treatment of addicts' families when the approach described in this text was in its formative stages. Intake interviews with families showing successful outcome were compared for similarities of content and process. These ideas are also a result of group discussions concerning the design of the initial family interview among the author, Paul Riley, Jay Lappin, MSW, and Kilian Fritsch, MSW.

The focus here is on two sources of information about the underlying family crisis, which are available during the pretherapy contacts with the addict and family members. The first source is initial contact with particular subgroups of the family, which can provide useful clues about family coalitions and important inter-personal issues. The second source is indirect data obtained from the initial interview with the addict alone.

## WHO SHOWS UP FOR THE INTAKE INTERVIEW

One way of assessing the nature of the family's crisis is to examine why the addict brings particular family members to the intake inter-view. Although in the majority of cases the addict appears alone, when another person is brought to the session this is usually an unspoken statement on the part of the addict about important issues to be addressed during treatment. Most typically, if the addict does not appear alone, he will appear with one other person; it is ex-tremely rare for him to bring his entire family to the intake interview.

Our retrospective analysis of the initial stages of therapy vis-à-vis outcome has taught us that the appearance of certain dyads early in treatment provides information about the crisis at hand, and also alerts us to the direction in which treatment needs to go. What follows is a review of the possibilities that have been encountered in our work with this patient population.

## UNMARRIED ADDICT AND
## OVERINVOLVED GIRLFRIEND

In such cases the (male) addict is accompanied to the intake interview by a girlfriend who is usually not an addict, but frequently has problems of low self-esteem and difficulty in separating from her own family. Usually this girlfriend is in alliance with the mother of the addict and is frequently a carbon copy of the mother. In such a case, the therapeutic issue is to focus on the overinvolvement between the addict and his mother, rather than on the relationship presented. In one case, the addict came to the intake interview with a girlfriend who bore a striking resemblance to his mother, both in physical appearance and in her overprotective attitude toward the addict. The addict improved when issues of separation were negotiated with his parents and he became involved with a woman, whom he eventually married, who was very much unlike mother.

## ADDICT AND ADDICTED (OR TROUBLED) PARTNER

When an addict appears for the intake interview with a girlfriend or wife who is also an addict or who has apparent psychiatric problems, it is probable that both of them are coping with issues of separation from their families of origin and are maintaining a sense of pseudoindividuation through their mutual relationship and/or their symptoms. Here the therapist must immediately decide which person in the relationship is to be the focus of treatment. In our research project, the male addict was always the identified patient (IP). In programs without such constraints, it is probably best if the addict whose family appears to be more in crisis is worked with first. As treatment with the IP and his family progresses and the IP improves, issues between the spouse or girlfriend and her own family usually emerge. At this point, the nature of their dyadic relationship is renegotiated and the issues between the addict and this woman are less complicated by issues of separation from his own family of origin.

## MARRIED ADDICT AND GIRLFRIEND

The appearance for the intake interview of a married addict with a girlfriend can be seen as a statement on the part of the addict that his marriage is in trouble. Usually the marriage has not provided the addict with the opportunity to separate appropriately from his family of origin; the spouse is in some way allied with the addict's over-involved parent (usually mother) and during times of crisis tends to side with the parents against the addict, or takes the place of the addict while the addict takes off. The appearance of a married addict with a girlfriend should be seen as a message that such a crisis is present and the addict is seeking an ally. For example, one addict appeared for an intake interview badly shaken after a car accident and a fight in a neighborhood bar and accompanied by a young woman he had met the day before. The addict attributed his self-destructive behavior to his heavy usage of heroin ("When I'm on heroin I have no idea of what I'm doing"). Further inquiry with the addict alone indicated that he and his wife had fought and that his wife had moved in with his parents. The addict took off, and the wife became depressed, being hospitalized for suicidal ideation. During the course of therapy it became obvious that there was considerable blurring between difficulties in the addict's marriage and difficulties between the addict's parents. When either of the couples began to experience problems, there was considerable spillover to the other couple. In this particular crisis, mother and father had fought, threatening separation, which precipitated trouble in the addict's marriage. The addict's absence from home was in response to trouble between his parents, while the wife, feeling abandoned, moved in with the addict's parents. She became depressed and suicidal, suggesting that problems between her husband's parents were detoured by "protecting" her, fulfilling the same function that the addict had previously served during a time of crisis. The thera-peutic effort in this situation required creating a boundary between the two couples.

## ADDICT AND COMPETENT BROTHER OR SISTER

The addict will often appear for the intake interview with a sibling who is functioning noticeably better than he. For example, the addict might be accompanied by a sister who is 2 or 3 years older than he is, but is married and very successful in her profession, so that chrono-logically she appears to be a great deal older than the addict. The difference in functioning is often an indication that the sister has somehow managed to achieve some distance from the family's prob-lems. This is usually accompanied by a certain amount of guilt that it has been done at the addict's expense. The appearance of the addict with a competent sibling is also a statement that a crisis is at hand, and that the brother or sister is in some way asking for professional help for the family. It is important for the therapist to form an alliance with the sibling, but to make it clear that it is his job to deal with the family problem. He respects the sibling's concern while helping that person to maintain some distance from the family crisis. The therapist in a sense joins with the sibling much as he would with another professional who has been involved with the problem, requesting that the sibling remain available and provide any useful knowledge concerning the problem. The therapist also needs to assess how the sibling is involved in the current crisis, and to respond accordingly. This takes the form of questioning why this person is involved with the addict now and how this person relates to the entire family. For example, one addict appeared with his older sister after an unsuccessful attempt at detoxing from methadone. After further inquiry about the situation, it became clear that the addict's parents had fought and the addict had attempted an unsuccessful detoxification at his sister's house. His actions could thus be viewed, at least in part, as a way of detouring conflict between the parents. In this particular family, the sister tended to side with the mother in these differences, so it also became critical, therapeutically, to involve the addict's older brother, who tended to side with the father. This had the effect of balancing and stabilizing the crisis, so that the issue could be contained between the parents and the addict, and therapy could progress around issues of separation between the parents and the addict. In this family the addict began to improve when the mother and father were reunited around making decisions about detoxifying their son from methadone.

## ADDICT AND ADDICTED BROTHER OR SISTER

In cases where more than one member of the family is addicted to heroin, the therapeutic strategy is to join with the parents in a way that supports their authority and establishes a clearer hierarchical boundary around parental decisions in the family (see Chapter 6). Such families are particularly heavily invested in avoiding issues of separation and individuation and are the most difficult to treat. Frequently, the improvement of one of the identified patients is experienced as a real threat to the homeostatic balance of the family, which then results in more destructive acting out on the part of other members of the family. It is critical that these families be treated as a whole unit and that parental competency be supported (see Chapter 12).

## INDIRECT ASSESSMENT OF THE FAMILY SYSTEM

The majority of addicts appear alone for the initial interview. Whether or not others attend, however, the content of the session will primarily be focused on the addiction problem, with much of the data about interpersonal factors coming indirectly. As discussed in Chapter 3, the drug problem is addressed in three segments: (1) present drug status; (2) a history of drug usage and former involvement with treatment programs; and (3) a discussion of the family issues surrounding the drug problem. Each segment of the interview can provide the therapist with more information concerning the family crisis at hand and the structures maintaining the addiction. This section will describe how to elicit and assess such information in each stage of the interview.

### PRESENT DRUG STATUS

The first stage of the interview typically begins with a general discussion of drug usage, level of methadone dosage, and the like. Statements about the level of addiction and the dosage of methadone required to stablilize an addict often can usefully be considered as indirect statements of the intensity of the family conflict at hand. For example, one addict who requested an unusually high level of methadone to "hold" him tended to use large amounts of heroin and behave self-destructively when his family was in crisis. Another addict was unable to come for the first session because he was homesick and because his current methadone level did not sufficiently hold him, forcing, in his words, a "premature detox." In this case the family was in crisis in response to the addict's plan to marry. The crisis around the "premature detox" served to detour the family from the mother's drinking problem, which had exacerbated at this time, and to put off issues of separation that the upcoming wedding had forced the family to deal with "prematurely." It was also evident that the addict was "homesick for Mom," and vice versa.

It is critical not to get drawn into a discussion of the details of drug usage, since the addict has considerable expertise in manipulating others around the specifics of drug treatment as a way of warding off interpersonal issues. Instead, one should present the goal of engaging the *family* around detoxification, thereby addressing interpersonal issues in which the *therapist* is the expert. When pressured by the addict for an increase or change in his medication, it is wise to define these as issues to be dealt with by the family.

## HISTORY

### Drug Usage

The second stage of the initial interview involves an inquiry about the addict's history of drug usage. It is important to note not only when the addict began using drugs, but also to be clear about what was happening in the family life cycle at that time. In cases where the addict started using heroin at an early age, the addiction is usually in response to long-standing family problems and involves more than the family's inability to negotiate the leaving-home stage. For example, one addict started using drugs when his father lost union privileges as an electrician and had frequent and long periods of unemployment. The problem with the father's status in the home was a chronic, repetitive one, as was a triadic sequence in which the mother became disappointed and critical of father, father withdrew, and mother became overinvolved with the IP. Although prior to the addiction the addict had problems at school and tended to act out family problems outside of the home, the emergence of heroin addiction as a symptom suggested the emergence of problems in the parental marriage serious enough to threaten marital separation. In this family the initial stage of treatment involved improving father's status in the home, so that marital problems could be contained within the parental dyad and the binding interaction between the mother and the addict could be challenged. Issues concerning the addict's separation from the family could only be addressed following this restructuring.

In cases where the addict started using drugs in later adolescence, the problem is usually associated with the addict's leaving home. For example, several veterans' families interviewed suggested that their son was doing fine until he joined the service and "got hooked on drugs." In these families, further inquiries indicated that the addiction accompanied the addict's first separation from the home, and that the parents were in disagreement about the addict joining the service as a way of separating from the family. Usually one parent felt abandoned and sabotaged the other's attempts to help the son. The addiction became a real problem when the son returned home and the family problems remained unresolved. In these families, the process of separation needs to be renegotiated without drugs. In some families, heroin addiction began at a time when a grandparent or a member of the extended family became sick, died, or in some way changed. In these families, differences between the couple concerning the extended family member, such as whether or not to take care of grandmother, threatened the parental marriage, and the addiction served to detour this conflict. Again, therapy needs to address the differences between the parental couple in a way that does not involve addiction.

## Previous Involvement in Treatment Programs

A history of the addict's involvement in treatment programs indicates the degree of chronicity of the problem and the immediacy of the family crisis as a viable therapeutic focus. Addicts who have a long history of methadone maintenance—with few efforts at detoxification—and an allegiance to a particular drug program are the most difficult to treat from a family perspective. Addicts with such a history are particularly resistant to having the family involved, suggesting that the addict is intent on protecting the family and in making the best of his drug difficulties by finding a substitute "family" in the treatment facility. In such families the parents are also content with such a compromise, and are equally determined to maintain it. One addict who was a member in good standing with the Drug Dependence Treatment Center (DDTC) was especially skillful at keeping his parents away from the therapist. In this family the addict's enrollment in the methadone program occurred simultaneously with the parents' decision to buy a home in the mountains and live in semiretirement. The addict's involvement in the program served as a base for the mother in the city, providing an excuse for her to return religiously to see if her son was getting his methadone appropriately. After 6 months of unsuccessful attempts at engaging the family for an initial session, it became quite clear that the parents were intent on their semiretirement house in the mountains and that the addict was equally intent on his semiretirement status in the community. What was also clear was that mother and father had a strong need to avoid discussing differences between them about the house in the mountains. Cases such as this can be particularly frustrating to engage in treatment.

Addicts who have a history of only sporadic involvement with methadone treatment programs and frequent failures at detoxification are more receptive to family intervention and offer a more hopeful prognosis. Here the family crisis has not reached a static compromise in which the addict accepts a more chronic, marginal lifestyle. The frequency of failure in treatment is often indicative of the failure of the family to divert and maintain the crisis outside of the family. In such cases, it is important to point to the omission of family members in treatment as the major reason for previous failures. If the family has previously been included in treatment, the therapist needs to stress that the family was not involved in the "right way." Describing past failures as an error in involving the family appropriately establishes a working alliance with the addict by (1) directly challenging the addiction cycle, but placing the blame elsewhere; (2) increasing the parents' authority, thereby reestablishing clearer hierarchical boundaries around the problem of addiction; (3) communicating to the addict that the problem of addiction is to be resolved within the family; (4) suggesting that the family has the resources to resolve interpersonal differences surrounding the addiction. In the following transcript of a session it becomes clear that such an intervention dramatically reduces the addict's resistance and allows him to discuss in more detail the nature of the family problem, giving the therapist a sense of the necessary direction for treatment.

*MOWATT:* I guess by now you know we work with the family.

*ADDICT:* There's no way I want my parents involved in this. They've been up the pike, down the pike, trying to help, and they're through helping.

*MOWATT:* Were they involved in therapy before?

*ADDICT:* Yeah, of course they're involved. They know I've been a junkie for nine years, and it's been nothing to them but heartbreak, man. . . . I've been nothing but a heartbreak.

*MOWATT:* That's not what I mean.

*ADDICT:* My parents have done everything they can to help, and they're through helping; believe me, they're done helping.

*MOWATT:* What I mean is, did anyone bother to ask them about your habit and work with them to help you get off this stuff?

*ADDICT:* What do you mean?

*MOWATT:* I mean, you're a guy who's been in and out of treatment programs for the past nine years and no one's bothered to give your parents a chance to help. Don't you think they'd like to see you get yourself together?

*ADDICT:* To be honest, I think they're the kind of people who rush in when someone's going up the pike, but when someone's going down the pike, they can't be bothered.

*MOWATT:* Yeah, tell me some more.

*ADDICT:* I mean, my old man drives a cab and it's rough. . . . He's too tired to handle. . . . They've got enough to take care of themselves to worry about taking care of me.

*MOWATT:* Well, one of the reasons this program is successful is that we realize your parents know you better than anyone—I mean, you and I will go through some rough times together, but your parents watched you grow up and they know you better than I or any professionals will ever know you.

*ADDICT:* I hadn't thought of it that way.

*MOWATT:* The reason things failed in the past is that they weren't included in the right way. The only way we can do it right this time is for you to get them in. I need you to get them in.

*ADDICT:* Is that the only way?

*MOWATT:* It's the only way.

*ADDICT:* OK, I'll do my best.

In this case, the addict and his family were genuinely demoralized by past treatment failures, although a more important therapeutic issue is the addict's suggestion that his parents, and particularly his father, are in distress in a more general way now. Recruiting the family around starting things afresh and differently served as an important intervention within a more general strategy of emphasizing the parents' competencies, so that issues of separation could be negotiated at a later point in treatment.

A history of attempted detoxification is frequently a good indication that the addict and his family are interested in resolving issues without addiction, although this is not always true. Frequently the addict will stage a detox as a way of detouring more significant family issues. We have seen addicts "rush" to detoxify in order to avoid having their families engaged, thus preventing larger family issues from emerging (see Chapter 8). In other cases, addicts might detoxify on their own thousands of miles from home, only to become re-addicted upon reengagement with the family system; thus, the extent to which the detoxification "takes hold" is contingent upon a total family process. These examples underscore the importance of containing the detoxification within the context of the family (see Chapter 6).

## THE SHIFT TO A FAMILY CONCEPTUALIZATION

A discussion of the addict's drug history and previous treatment failures flows quite naturally into the discussion of the family crisis at hand. There is a gradual shift in authority from the addict to the therapist as the problem is reframed from an individual problem in the addict to an interpersonal problem that can be resolved within the family and without drugs. The problem no longer seems as unsolvable as new, alternative views of the addiction are considered. When the therapist has made this shift successfully with the addict, he will usually note a marked reduction of tension in the room and a shared consensus with the client that the thrust of treatment is in the right direction. In part, such a change stems from the addict's relief in sensing that the therapist will be able to handle his parents in a nonblaming way.

For the therapist to achieve this shift, he must develop some understanding of (1) the family addiction cycle, (2) the therapeutic interventions that have failed, and (3) at least a general idea about the family structure and the present crisis in need of attention. Hypotheses the therapist might have concerning the addiction cycle and the crisis at hand need to be tested (but not shared uncritically with the addict) as the family engagement process unfolds. Since these hypotheses are derived primarily from information provided by the IP, they should, of course, remain tentative working hypotheses until the therapist is able to deal directly with the whole family.

# 5

# PRINCIPLES AND TECHNIQUES FOR GETTING "RESISTANT" FAMILIES INTO TREATMENT

M. DUNCAN STANTON
THOMAS C. TODD

IT DOES NOT SEEM untoward at this time to state that family approaches to treating symptoms have "come of age." In a recent literature review, Gurman and Kniskern[57] found over 200 family- and marital-treatment studies that present outcome data—to say nothing of the hundreds of other related papers on theory and technique of family treatment.[53] Of the outcome research in which nonbehavioral family therapy was directly compared with other modes of treatment, the former emerged with superior results in two-thirds of the studies and equal results in the remainder.[57] Given that family approaches have attained a position of viability and credibility, it is appropriate to ask about specific applicabilities and limitations. One such potential limitation pertains to the extent to which clients can actually be engaged in family treatment. This issue is hardly new to the field of psychotherapy, and has occupied many pages of the literature on individual therapies. However, the task for family therapy seems greater, as it frequently requires that a number of people be directly involved in treatment. This chapter addresses many of the problems that arise in engaging families. Principles and techniques for getting them into treatment are presented, most of which apply both to families of addicts and other "resistant" families.

This chapter is a revised and expanded version of a paper by the authors entitled "Engaging 'Resistant' Families in Treatment: II. Principles and Techniques in Recruitment" and is reprinted with permission from *Family Process*, 1981, *20*, 261–293.

Considerable credit for creative development of the techniques discussed herein goes to the nine Addicts and Families Program therapists cited in the Preface to this book.

## RELEVANT LITERATURE

### GENERAL FINDINGS

The general literature on engaging families in treatment is not very extensive. Much of it appeared as the importance of the father in the treatment process became more obvious.[14, 46, 86, 91, 137, 138] Investigators began looking at treatment results with and without fathers and also at the means for recruiting and retaining fathers. Fathers have been noted to be the most difficult family members to engage,[46] especially among lower classes,[138] yet they are pivotal both in the recruitment[14] and continuation aspects of therapy.[14, 137, 138] Berg and Rosenblum[14] make the point that if the therapist is not insistent and does not underscore how necessary the father is for treatment, the latter will feel confirmed in his supposition that he is not important. Shapiro and Budman[137] found that engaging the father is particularly difficult for inexperienced therapists, who tend to be less successful at it than their more seasoned colleagues. L'Abate[86] has proffered a number of ways for countering the father's resistance, including (1) reassuring him of his importance, (2) pointing out that changes depend upon his participation, (3) making him aware that he has the power to sabotage therapy, (4) noting that he has choices, such as transferring to another therapist who will work only with an individual, (5) placing responsibility for changes squarely on his shoulders, and (6) getting him to consider realignment of his priorities (e.g., his family's happiness vs. acquisition of more material goods).

More generally, however, both parents or spouses can be responsible for nonengagement in family therapy. Either can show the tendencies noted for therapy refusers, that is, giving vague rationalizations for not becoming involved, or denying that a problem exists.[14,137] In fact, refusers tend to be resistant to any mode of therapy, whether family- or individual-oriented.[137] Sager and associates[126] note, as we have,[183] that identified or "index" patients (IPs) often tend to have expectations that are not consonant with family therapy and may grow anxious or angry when the subject is broached. Thus the therapist needs to stimulate motivation,[126] and the IP's experience of him in this effort becomes all-important.[137] Sometimes the process can be aided through an involuntary influence. For example, Johnson[75] found that family intervention ordered by a juvenile court made it less difficult to involve families in a three-session family "evaluation" program. Through a restructuring of the family therapy intake process, Sager et al.[126] were able to get 75% of their families to come in; they did this by (1) streamlining the screening interview so that an overly intense relationship did not develop between client and intake interviewer; (2) reducing the emphasis given to family involvement within the screening interview; (3) occasionally waiting until the first individual therapy session before broaching the issue of family therapy; and (4) taking one or more therapy sessions, as needed, to work through differences between the expectations of client and agency as to involving the family. Slipp et al.[138] also recruited 75% of their clients in a maritally oriented program, partly because attendance by all family members was required at the initial interview; the rate was lower (65%) for cases with a severely disturbed IP than for those diagnosed as moderately or mildly disturbed (85%). Finally, Berg and Rosenblum[14] found that the success with which therapists were able to recruit whole families was positively correlated with the number of family therapy training experiences (workshops, courses, etc.) they had had, implying that therapist variables may be as important as family and IP characteristics.

## FINDINGS WITH ADDICTS' FAMILIES

If one accepts that the family can be an important focal point for intervention, it is obvious that family members must be brought to treatment. The task, however, is particularly difficult with addicts' families. They often abdicate responsibility for the IP's problem and place the blame entirely on external systems and agencies such as peers, schools, courts, the neighborhood, or the treatment program.[44, 152, 170, 180] Most of those who have written on the subject have lamented the difficulty involved. Seldin[134] has called it a "monumentally discouraging task," Salmon and Salmon[127] note that such attempts have met with "little success," Vaglum[180] states that making family contact and getting members' cooperation is the therapist's "greatest problem and challenge," and Davis[37] identifies addicts' families as "among the most difficult of all psychotherapy patients to get into the office" (p. 198). Mason's[98] experience in trying to get addicts' mothers involved in their sons' inpatient program proved "uneconomical," "time consuming," and "disappointing," and he observed that of 1000 eligible parents, only 30 or 40 would appear at monthly parent–staff meetings and almost none of these attended more than three times. Alexander and Dibb[2] reported that with the majority of addicts' families they contacted for outpatient treatment, either the IP or one or both parents refused to participate (even though these were cases in which the IP either lived in the parents' home or visited twice a week or more). Kaufman and Kaufmann[78] describe a program in which only 25% of addicts' families were recruited for multiple family therapy. Entin and Schumann[44] tried to engage six families of drug-using adolescents in Bowenian family therapy; their paper is a retrospective analysis as to why, after a few exploratory contacts, they were unable to get any of them in. As part of a therapeutic community, Ziegler-Driscoll[197] reported a success rate of approximately 71% in trying to get addicts' families in for a family research interview that preceeded family therapy: 48% of the total group with which attempts were made continued for at least one therapy session. Ziegler-Driscoll also observed that the percentage of Whites recruited was nearly twice as high as that for Blacks. The only exception to this trend is described by Fram and Hoffman[48] for a large, private, mental health center. They do not give statistics, but note that families were "most interested in becoming involved with the treatment" and often "welcomed it with delight" (p. 610). They do note that (1) their patients' socioeconomic status (White, middle-class) and (2) the nature of their program dictate that their patients be considered an "unrepresentative sample" of the addict population, especially since there was enough cohesiveness in these families to seek and find private care for the IP. In sum, then, the experience of those in the field indicates that, with the possible exception of highly selected samples, the difficulty in engaging addicts' families in treatment cannot be overestimated.


## TREATMENT CONTEXT

The research design and the various family-treatment modalities of the Addicts and Families Program(AFP) have been described in Chapter 2 and Appendix C and are not germane to this chapter. Rather, our concern here is with the means used for getting the families actually involved in treatment. Again, the study demanded that (1) the addict, (2) both parents or parent surrogates,* and, whenever possible, (3) siblings, attend an (initial) Family Evaluation Session before being assigned to a family-treatment group. For theoretical reasons (Chapters 1 and 6) and purposes of research design,[171] wives, while usually included in treatment, were not required to attend the evaluation exercise. This session included videotaped family interaction tasks and family perceptions tests. Each member age 12 or over was paid $10.00 for participating. The therapists did not know beforehand to which treatment group the families they were recruiting would be (randomly) assigned. These stipulations, while perhaps more stringent than those of most clinical programs, had their benefits. Although they made our job more difficult, they also prohibited us from either taking the easy way out and settling for partial family representation, or excluding family members who we later determined were crucial for the success of treatment. Further, we *had* to recruit a high percentage of families in order both (1) to meet the requirements for a certain number of cases within the grant period, and (2) to avoid the criticism that our sample was nonrepresentative because we had skimmed off the "easy," "compliant" families.

Initial recruitment efforts were made with 125 families. Of these, 33 were deemed ineligible for the study, usually because the IP was not addicted at intake. This left 92 families with which full engagement attempts were made.

At the outset of the study we anticipated that our biggest problem would be in retaining these families beyond one or two family sessions—the dropout issue. In this we were wrong. First, 94% of those who attended the Family Evaluation Session continued with treatment. Second, once they were "hooked," the majority of families tended to be fairly conscientious in their attendance, especially when compared with results reported elsewhere in the literature. Even the treatment group with the least optimal retention potential averaged six sessions, that is, 64% of their prescribed number of sessions[165,171]; attendance rates for the other two treatment groups were 88% and 94%. What we did not foresee was the inordinate amount of difficulty we would have in simply getting the family members in for the initial Family Evaluation Session (since, at the time, almost none of the

---

*This requirement was based partly on the knowledge that the IP was in contact with these parents and partly on the theoretical tenet that most severely symptomatic people are involved in a triadic relationship that is serving to maintain the symptom.

literature on engaging addicts' families had been published). Recruitment became one of the most demanding aspects of our work. This unexpected hurdle forced us to reconsider our situation and attempt to be innovative. The substance of this chapter is derived from our responses and experiences in the face of this dilemma.

## PRINCIPLES AND TECHNIQUES

While engaging families in treatment is a major problem in the addiction field, there is almost no literature on how to do this in practice. Aside from an occasional pointer in a few articles,[14, 28, 37, 86, 126, 180] the therapist trying to recruit addicts' families—or even difficult "nondrug" families—is essentially without published guidelines. This chapter will attempt, at least partially, to fill that void and provide therapists with material aimed at optimizing the recruitment effort.

The material in this section is subdivided into various content areas. Within each of these, one or more principles are set forth, followed by explanation and discussion. The reader may note an air of finality in these principles. This is not altogether unintentional. While every rule has exceptions, these tenets have been arrived at through the pain of multiple failures, so we feel we can state them with a certain degree of confidence.

### INITIAL CONTACTS WITH THE INDEX PATIENT

Unless they enter the treatment program with the expectation that their families will be involved, it is our experience that most addicts are extremely resistant to including other members. This resistance stems to a great extent from the treatment modes that have historically prevailed in the drug-abuse field—mainly the therapeutic community and methadone maintenance methods. In the former, the family is usually seen as an undesirable influence to be shunned, while the latter simply does not take families into account. In any event, many of these clients would attempt to brush us off with a "don't bug me" attitude. They knew, in our case, that continuation on the methadone program could not be made contingent upon family participation, so we were sometimes seen as introducing another hassle in their regimen. In some cases they lied to us about who was in the family, how often they saw family members, or even whether these people were alive or not. Since our experience and our data led us to believe otherwise, we rarely accepted these ploys at face value (although we did not get caught in challenging them outright). Rather, we saw them as protective moves. Sometimes it was self-protection, because the addict did not want his cover blown by people who would come in and tell stories about him that differed from his own. Also, the IP appeared to fear that his family might be criticized or blamed by the therapist, and then get on his back for getting them in trouble; he then would not only feel beleaguered but also guilty, disloyal, and traitorous to what was usually a very enmeshed family system. We found it most useful to see his actions as *protective of the whole family*, especially his parent(s). Since his role in the family was often as one who served to divert fighting among others (Chapter 1), his attempt to buffer the system from potential challengers from outside was both natural and functional.

In Chapter 3 a number of techniques are described for working with the addicted member toward recruiting his family for therapy. Details are given on the structuring of the initial recruiting interview (with the IP, alone)—what points need to be covered, what sequence of topics seems to work best, how to parry or neutralize resistant moves, and so forth. The process usually requires that the therapist obtain as much information as possible about the IP's family and interpersonal system before "showing his cards," that is, before stating that he would like the family to come in. Such questions as, "Do you live with your folks?" "How often do you see them?" "Who else lives at home?" and "Who do you spend the most time with in the family?" are appropriate. The therapist also wants to learn how much the family knows about the drug problem before he suggests including them. Using this information, the therapist then can decide who he wants in attendance at the first session.

*Principle 1: The therapist should decide which family members need to be included, and not leave this decision to the index patient.* We have found that when this rule is not followed, the tendency is for only certain family coalitions to show up. The common ones include the IP plus (1) a sister, (2) his mother and sister, (3) his mother, or (4) his wife or girlfriend.* Often other members were not even informed that the meeting was to take place.

---

*Chapter 4 presents a discussion of the clinical significance and treatment implications of having particular coalitions appear.

*Principle 2: Whenever possible, one or more family members should be encouraged to attend the initial or intake interview.* This is a variation on the above theme. We discovered, in a few early cases, that if another member was present at the intake interview (before family treatment had ever been mentioned) the amount of time and effort required to get the whole family in for a session was greatly reduced. Sager *et al.*[126] also noted this phenomenon for non-drug-using families. Whether such an event helped to lessen anxiety or to spread the blame, or whether it was indicative of a less resistant or more "healthy" family, is not known. One way to facilitate this phenomenon is to make it standard procedure for program intake staff to request attendance of family members when they receive a call for an admission interview.

*Principle 3: Do not expect the index patient to bring in the family on his own.* If we have a cardinal rule, this is it. Innumerable times we got ostensible cooperation from a client, but no results. We got promises and guarantees, but if the task was left to the IP, the family simply did not show. He either would not, or could not, bring them in. In fact, expecting the patient to bring in his family failed so often that we eventually abandoned it entirely.

*Principle 4: Obtain permission from the index patient to contact his family, and then get in touch with them, whenever possible, right in the interview.* This evolved into our primary goal for the initial interview, as was noted in Chapter 3. An effective technique, employed by others also,[14, 28] is to find out where family members are located at the moment, and telephone them directly from the session. This allows the therapist a proper introduction, and does not put the IP in a position of advocating a program about which he himself is unsure or unconvinced.

A number of other techniques were used during the initial contact period. Since they were applied selectively, rather than to most or all cases, they do not qualify as principles. Whether they were chosen or not depended on the particular context, the idiosyncracies of a certain client or family, and the style of the therapist. Some therapists engaged in heavy, informal personal contact with the addict, such as playing ping pong with him during the "interview," and the like. Others employed the telephone extensively in making frequent contact with the IP and inviting him to call back whenever he felt the need. In at least one case (seen by Peter Urquhart, Family Counselor) this took an interesting twist. Urquhart had been "chasing" the client by calling fairly constantly (four or five times a week) for several weeks, and getting very little reciprocation. Eventually he cut down to one call a week. The client then became curious as to why the calls had tapered off, and began to contact Urquhart. This paved the way for an agreement to have the family come in.

Less commonly employed was the use of veiled pressure to induce cooperation. Unlike some programs,[31] ours did not allow therapists to refuse methadone if a client was adamant about excluding his family.* The client obtained methadone and other treatments in the drug program, as desired, during the whole recruitment process. If he objected strongly and persistently enough, the family issue would be dropped. However, in a few cases the therapists tried to get around this by (1) simply "waiting the client out" for a week or so; (2) stating confidently, "We have found that this treatment works best," or, "The people who know you best and are best able to help us both lick this problem are your family members"; (3) giving the addict no (ostensible) choice by stating firmly, and without irritation, that this was "the way it is done" and that he had to do it; (4) as a last resort, threatening not to increase his methadone dosage until the family came in. We did not use the last two tactics very often, because we really could not back them up. The particular technique applied to avoid refusal depended on the therapist's sense of where the client was "coming from" and how close he seemed to be to acquiescence.

Overall, when we were unable to succeed at this point it was because the IP either would not permit his family to be contacted, or would not participate in the family evaluation session or treatment himself. Nonetheless, use of the above techniques resulted in the addicts' permission to contact their families in 80% of the cases with which attempts were made.

## IMMEDIACY AND PRIMACY OF CONTACT

One of the difficulties encountered in engaging addicts' families in a program described by Ziegler-Driscoll[197] was that family treatment could not begin until the IP had completed a therapeutic community

---

*In this respect our program might be seen as one with special problems. Because the clients were, first of all, Veterans Administration (VA) patients, we did not have the option of refusing therapy, since, by law, the VA is required to provide treatment to all who are eligible.

(inpatient) program. This had the double disadvantage of starting "treatment" when the client was supposed to be "cured," and also of reinforcing the idea that the problem was the patient's, not the family's. Another hindrance, noted with nonaddicts' families by Sager and associates,[126] and others, was the frequency with which clients were passed from one agency or treater to another. This reduced the chances for family engagement. We ran into these problems also, albeit to a lesser degree. Of central importance is the immediacy with which both the IP and family are engaged.

*Principle 5: The closer the family therapist's first contact with the index patient is to the time of intake, the greater are the chances for recruiting the family.* We discovered early that this was a critical variable. If the family therapist cannot see the client on the day of intake, he should set an appointment for no later than 2 or 3 days afterward. At the very least he should be able to manage a brief telephone conversation with the client prior to the actual meeting. We were sensitive enough to this issue to eventually equip therapists with beepers. In this way we increased the chances of contacting them immediately and having them talk to the IP over the phone, should they have been unable to come to the drug-treatment clinic that day. This procedure added to the urgency of the situation and was a sign to the client that the therapist was sensitive to his need for help.

*Principle 6: The earlier the family therapist enters the chain of "treaters" encountered by the client, the better are chances for family recruitment.* As noted in Chapter 3, we observed that a kind of "imprinting" process occurs during the intake period, whereby the client attaches strongly to the first person (or persons) offering him help; this person appears to have much more leverage with him than do those who deal with him later. Consequently, if the therapist does not want his influence diluted, he should try to be among the first in the line of treaters with whom the client will come in contact.

*Principle 7: The sooner the family is contacted, the more likely they are to be engaged.* This conclusion is obvious from the above discussion, and has also been emphasized by Davis.[37] In addition, it speaks to the possibility that the family may be in crisis (see below, and also Chapter 4) and more amenable to help at the time of intake than later on; the therapist has greater leverage because defenses are most vulnerable and the family is more in a posture of requiring help. This is the best time to expect everyone to come in.

## CRISIS ASPECTS

When the addict enters a treatment program it may either be at a time of crisis,[28] or, if his entry is a step toward growth or individuation, a family crisis may soon ensure (Chapters 1, 4, and 6). In addition, the very fact that the family is asked to participate in therapy can produce a crisis.

*Principle 8: Viewing the family recruitment effort as crisis-inducing can help the therapist in his engagement efforts.* With these families, the very mention of their involvement can lead to a crisis. The message given is not one usually received in conventional drug-treatment programs, which tend to view the IP and the problem more individually. Nor is it a message that the family expects. The whole recruitment process, then, is an intervention that shifts responsibility for the problem to the total system of intimate others. These people are told that they are important—if not in generating the problem, then in helping to alleviate it. There is an implicit statement to the parents that "you have not resolved something with your son." Carl Whitaker has noted that just getting the family to consider who is to come—who belongs—is itself a major intervention. Furthermore, the act of coming to treatment may be the first time the family has organized itself to do something together as a family.* If the therapist recognizes this, it will help him make appropriate joining and supportive moves. Also, if he conveys a sense of calm and confidence, he may help reduce the inevitable tension that the family will feel in the face of this crisis.

## CONTACTING THE FAMILY

It should be noted that not every family fought bitterly against being involved in treatment. Some of them were pleasantly surprised to be asked, and glad to participate. They may have resented being excluded when their son had been enrolled previously in a treatment program. These families were obviously not difficult to enlist, so the remainder of this discussion will deal with resistant families. It should be kept in mind that the therapist was working toward involving both parents and any siblings living in the home or nearby. A problem unique to

---

*We are indebted to Jay Haley for this notion.

our research program was that he could not sell family *therapy* per se, because, once inducted, the family members might have been assigned to another kind of family treatment.

*Principle 9: The therapist must get past the index patient and directly contact each family member, or at least both parents; if, prior to the first session, he can obtain from them an agreement to participate, the chances of their actually attending are increased markedly.* This is an extension of Principles 3 and 4 and is our other cardinal rule. We cannot emphasize enough the importance of getting the IP out of the middle in this task, so that the therapist can obtain individual contracts with each member. This takes pressure off the IP for anything that (it is feared) might happen later in therapy. The family members cannot charge him as readily with, "You got us into this," because each of them shares responsibility for agreeing to participate. In other words, it allows the therapist to deal with, and counter, their fears firsthand, rather than leaving this task to the IP. Also, the IP is not put in a position of indirectly blaming them by stating that *he* wants them involved in treatment.

The two major vehicles for contact we have employed are heavy use of the telephone and home visits. Once the therapist gets past the IP, he should make as many calls as necessary to other family members. This might entail calling parents at home or work, in the day or evening. If there are two telephones in the home, it is advisable for him to set up a conference call involving both parents.

Upon making telephone contact, the therapist can introduce himself to the family in a friendly way by saying, "I guess by this time your son has had an opportunity to tell you a bit about our program." It is best not to get into therapeutic issues over the phone, but if they are presented, to emphasize the importance of a family meeting around the problem. Where there is a difficult member to engage, it is wise to ascertain which family member is crucial in excluding this member and to find a way to put the responsibility for recruitment on the member who is supporting the exclusion. For example, where the mother has an interest in excluding father, it may be advisable to approach father through mother. One way of doing this is to say to the mother, "I would like to discuss the program with your husband, but I would like you to discuss it with him first." This has the effect of respecting mother's authority, but at the same time placing some responsibility for father's inclusion or exclusion on her. It also provides the therapist with a clear understanding of how differences between the couple are maintained. In cases where there is a member of the extended family about whom the parents differ, the therapist can approach the spouse who is allied with this person and then negotiate this with the couple. For example, when mother and father are divided about the maternal grandmother, it is helpful to say to the mother (in the father's presence), "Well, she is your mother, and you know her best, so why don't you try to contact her first? If this doesn't work, the three of us will try another approach." This has the effect of hinting at the marital difference, while at the same time developing an atmosphere in which these differences can eventually be worked out between the parental couple and the therapist.

Since it is quite easy to become involved in major therapeutic issues over the telephone, this should be avoided whenever possible. This is more difficult when a family is in acute crisis—for example, when the mother cannot come to a meeting because the grandmother is in the hospital due to a heart attack. The therapist needs to be seen not only as collaborating with the parents in organizing session attendance, but also as clearly in charge of the timing and content of such sessions. The resolution of issues that maintain the presenting problem should be orchestrated by the therapist, utilizing the developing alliance between himself and important members of the family. As the therapist contracts with the family for the initial session, other family issues may be acknowledged, although, as noted in Principle 11, the primary focus should remain on the presenting problem, usually the addiction, which is the reason for bringing the family together.*

In about a quarter of our cases, home visits were made. Usually this was done when the parents were particularly resistant or hard to get in touch with. Sometimes the therapist would visit the home if he felt he was getting "stalled in the front office," for example, if he sensed the parent(s) might be home, but the person answering the phone said they were not. The home visit has the advantages of conveying the therapist's true concern and interest and also in allowing direct, person-to-person contact. If the family meets him and finds him to be personally acceptable, accepting, and nonjudgmental, they might be more willing to attend. Fear of the unknown is assuaged. They can be more assured that the therapist is not out to "get" them.

---

*Appreciation is extended to David T. Mowatt, EdD, for the material in this and the preceding paragraph.

*Approaches to Parents and Family*

In line with the experience of Vaglum[180] and others, the therapist needs to take special pains not to ally with the IP against the parents or family. His approach in therapy will be to join them so that the three of them (the therapist and both parents) can work together to straighten their young person out. He should stress to them that this treatment is different from others because the family is involved.* The therapist needs to be convinced, and convincing, that it will help.

In addition to the general rationale described, specific approaches were preferred by particular therapists or were tailored to certain families. They are presented below as vignettes. They are not necessarily "typical," as some of them depict more extreme therapist efforts, but they do give a picture of what can be done, and how. Additional vignettes that pertain to the rationale for family treatment also follow under sections on "The Nonblaming Message" and "Therapist Factors."

*Vignette 1.* Paul Riley, Family Counselor, frequently took the tack that he needed to get the family in to know more about the *history* of the client. Only the parents could give him the information about their son necessary for him to do the best job. He asked them, "Please come in so I can get more background."

*Vignette 2.* David Mowatt, EdD, had the highest rate of recruitment success among our therapists (100%). This example stems from an interview with the IP, but the content is also applicable in talking with the family. Mowatt broached the family involvement issue by stating, "One reason we do well in this program is that we involve families to help you get off this stuff." A minute later, he said, "One of the reasons the programs you were in before failed is that they didn't understand that your parents know you better than anyone. I am going to know you really well, and will go through some tough times with you, but you know your parents know you best. They saw you as a kid, they knew you when you were doing well; the way they see you will be valuable information for me in helping to get you off the stuff. So, the first thing I need is for them to come in."

---

*Jay Haley has stressed the need to provide a rationale for why this treatment is different and should succeed where others have failed.

*Vignette 3.* Jerry I. Kleiman, PhD, routinely made home visits, using a number of approaches. First, he tended to ally with parents by telling them that they had the "right" to work with him to straighten their son out. He gave them hope that they could succeed. He offered them the opportunity to be more involved than they had been up until now, noting that this was their last chance and they had to bail their son out. He told them that this time treatment would be different because, "This time you will know everything that is going on and be a part of it."

*Vignette 4.* In one difficult case, Alexander Scott, MSW, made 4 contacts with the IP, 24 contacts with other family members, at least 5 failed attempts to reach the IP and family members, and 15 talks with the drug counselor and project staff. The process took 30 days. This family probably showed up for no other reason except that Scott "wore them down." It was easier just to come in and get him off their backs than to continue to resist. Cases such as this were more the exception than the rule, since in only 7 of 92 families did the engagement process involve more than 25 contacts with family and counselor. Also, in only four cases did the process take 3 or more months. Most families required much less effort than this.

## Approaches to Fathers

As might be expected, fathers were the most difficult family members to recruit. However, the lore in the field may be exaggerated on this point. We have heard other therapists complain, "We can't get the fathers in," when they never contacted these men directly and left the recruiting to someone else. What these therapists may really mean is they cannot get *other family members* to bring fathers in. As other authors have stated,[14, 86] contacting fathers directly can make a difference.

Even granting the above, however, the fathers in our sample presented special problems. At least 72% of them had drinking problems[164] and did not want this brought to light in a therapeutic situation. Some were rarely at home, and asleep when they were. Still more common was a family pattern in which the father was shut out from communications about the IP or his treatment. The family structure was tight and rigidly channeled. It was not unusual for the rest of the family to agree to participate and then come in without telling the father where and when they were going, or for what reason. On more than one occasion a therapist called a father to confirm an appointment, only to get a "What are you talking about?" response. Again, preappointment contact with fathers became a necessity.

Engaging fathers was one of our more demanding tasks and often one requiring the most creativity. At one time or another we used all of the guidelines (summarized earlier) that L'Abate[86] has presented for enlisting fathers. The following vignettes give some idea of the latitude and innovation that can be applied to this endeavor.

*Vignette 5.* The therapist (Paul Riley) tried numerous times to reach a father at home, but to no avail. Finally, he made a visit to the father at his place of work in order to foster trust and explain the treatment program.

*Vignette 6.* Three home visits were made. On the first, the therapist (Jerry I. Kleiman) commiserated with the mother while she cried and talked about how things were. The next night he returned to the home and sat with the father in the den, where he had numerous pictures on the wall of his son as a Marine. The father lamented about what his son "could have been." The two of them talked and drank beer together. The following morning Kleiman went over and brought the family in for treatment.

*Vignette 7.* In this case the therapist (Paul Riley) sensed that the father was suspicious and jealous because this strange man (Riley) had come to his house to talk to his wife. Consequently, Riley brought his own wife along for the next visit. This reduced the threat, because now Riley had *his* woman and the father had *his*.

*Vignette 8.* In a case seen by Sam Kirschner, PhD, the father was adamantly against coming and said his son didn't deserve the effort. Drawing upon his clinical knowledge and experience, Kirschner sized up this situation as one in which, unless change occurred, the addict was in danger of "going off the deep end." He sensed that the young man was feeling desperate and that something had to be done to avert a tragedy. It became clear that a harsh reality was being ignored and that the father's (and family's) denial had to be confronted directly. Because the stakes were so high he decided to take a gamble, which required two steps. First, he moved to counter the father's resistance by referring to a pattern that is typically seen in addicts' families and one that was suspected in this particular family: he made a joining pitch by connoting positively that the father really cared more about his son than he let on, and that if something happened to the son, father would be the first to help him out. The second move was to confront the denial. Kirschner left the father with the prediction that if he did not come into treatment, his son would either be dead or in jail within 2 weeks. The son obliged by getting arrested 3 days later, and the father took out a second mortgage on his home to raise the bail money. These events obviously gave Kirschner considerable power from that point on.

While Kirschner's prediction might seem extreme, or even absurd, it should not be mistaken for a paradoxical intervention. Rather, he was rubbing in a harsh *reality*. The probability for disaster *was* high, and this was not being recognized by the father. It needs to be emphasized that these addicted young men die or become imprisoned at rates that are many times higher than for similar men in their age group (see Chapter 1). From our own data[171] (see also Chapter 17) 10% of a matched group of clients (who were not assigned to family therapy) died over an 18- to 48-month follow-up period (average 31 months). This mortality rate was five times higher than the 2% of deaths that occurred during the same period for cases that engaged in family therapy. Our therapists were aware of the threat to life or other dangers extant when the addictive process was allowed to continue unchecked, and Vignette 8 presents one response to this exigency. In this context a sense of "mission" was hardly inappropriate.

*Vignette 9.* Therapist Samuel M. Scott encountered a case where the father worked two full jobs and was only at home and awake for 15 minutes of each day. Father's routine was to arrive home, wolf down a meal, and go immediately to bed. Scott made several telephone attempts and missed the father by 5 or 10 minutes. When he finally did catch him, he opened by being *extremely* contrite, recognizing how busy the father was and how hard he worked, and apologizing for interrupting his schedule. He was so apologetic that the father's curiosity was aroused, and the conversation turned into one with the father asking Scott questions about his son's program and about how he and the family could help.

An important ingredient of this vignette was the way Scott intuitively responded to signals from the father about the latter's personal space. He let the father know immediately that he was sensitive to issues of "turf," in a sense saying, "I respect your boundaries and your privacy." Establishing such respect early allowed rapid joining and a smooth transition into the matters of treatment.

*Vignette 10.* This was a situation in which the mother and siblings agreed to participate, but they claimed that there was no way the father would become involved. Mother said she had petitioned her husband about it several times without results. She conveyed to Sam Kirschner, the therapist, the pain and frustration she felt at her husband's intransigence—she could not move him. She noted how badly things were going, both in general and with her husband. It was clear to Kirschner that she hoped he would do whatever was necessary to budge her husband from his position, and that the information she conveyed might provide Kirschner with momentum. After several attempts, he finally reached the father by the telephone. The following is a reconstruction of that conversation.

*KIRSCHNER:* Hello, Mr. Jones. I'm Sam Kirschner, Joe's counselor at the drug clinic. I've been talking to your family about our treatment program, in which we have the family come in and help out. Did your wife mention this to you?
*FATHER:* (*grudgingly*) Yeah, she said something about it.
*KIRSCHNER:* Well, I'm calling because I'd like you to come in and join us if you would. Joe needs all the help he can get, and I think it would be a much better program if you could give me a hand. Whatta you think, could you maybe come in?
*FATHER:* Naw, I don't want no part of it. I got enough to do.
*KIRSCHNER:* Yeah, your wife told me you might be hesitant, so maybe you'll want to change your mind later on. Anyway, there's another thing I wanted to talk to you about also. I've been talking to your wife and she tells me that things aren't going so well lately between you and her.
*FATHER:* (*more intense, slightly irritated*) She told you that? What'd she say?

KIRSCHNER: You know, that you two haven't been getting along as well as you could, and that she's not happy with the way things are.

FATHER: So what?

KIRSCHNER: Well, it's all right that you don't want to come in. That's OK. It's just that I've heard *her* side of the story, but that's just one side. I thought maybe I should hear what *your* view is so I could get a better picture of what's going on . . .

FATHER: Yeah, well, maybe . . .

KIRSCHNER: (interrupting) Anyway, there's something that I think you should know—that I want you to know so you won't get confused later on. Your wife and your family are going to be coming in here and there are going to be some changes taking place. Your wife is going to be changing. She will be a different woman, in some ways, from the woman you know.

FATHER: What do you mean?

KIRSCHNER: Well, just that things are going to be different from now on. She will be different. And I wanted to let you know this ahead of time, so that you aren't surprised when it happens.

FATHER: Yeah, well, I don't know . . .

KIRSCHNER: Anyway, I feel I have an obligation to let you know these things. By the way, if you happen to think it over and you do change your mind, you're welcome to come in and clarify things and help keep me on the right course. But that's up to you. Either way is OK.

Several days after this interchange, Kirschner talked to the addict's mother about arranging the first meeting. At that time she told him her husband had reconsidered and would probably come (which he did).

This telephone conversation provides an example of the kind of ongoing feedback process often required in engaging a family member. During the dialogue Kirschner was constantly hinting in one direction, sensing the resistance, backing off, and trying a new tack. He respected the father's space by not pushing too hard, moving to another topic in order to (1) avoid confrontation and (2) find an area for connection and leverage.

A major factor in success here was the skillful way in which Kirschner aroused the father's curiosity, irritation, and fear of changes in his wife. Also, the prospect of his marital troubles being exposed without him having a chance to defend himself probably raised his motivation. The fact that this was going to be done by a male outsider only heightened the intensity. Even these factors, however, might not have done the trick if the therapist had not structured the conversation in such a way as to (1) make it clear to the father that he had a choice and was not being coerced in either direction, (2) let him know the therapist was at least impartial and might even see things his way, and (3) give him the option of changing his mind without losing face (e.g., "Maybe you'll want to change your mind later on," and "If you happen to think it over and you do change your mind, you're welcome to come in and clarify things").

## Approaches to Mothers

Compared to fathers, there seemed to be more variability in the difficulty entailed in engaging mothers. More mothers than fathers responded positively to the opportunity to become involved in their son's treatment. Some appeared to want to control what happened to their sons, especially if the sons were improving. They wanted to know what was going on, so they could take charge of it. This was fine with us. We could "fly" with it. Our main concern was to get them in, no matter what their motivation.

On the other hand, there were mothers whose resistance equaled or exceeded that of their husbands. They might not oppose the idea openly, but instead would use the intransigence of their husbands as an excuse for not participating. Some techniques that could be used for recruiting mothers have been described. Others are discussed in the next section. Only one vignette will be presented here, partly due to its uniqueness.

*Vignette 11.* In this case the addict had a 6-year history of drug problems. He started heavy drug use at age 16, injecting amphetamines and taking barbiturates regularly. By age 19 he was addicted to heroin. He had failed two prior treatment attempts and at intake was still addicted to heroin (10 bags per day), supplementing this with regular use of barbiturates and marijuana. It also appeared that the family had many problems and was clearly making the situation impossible for the addict to improve. Samuel M. Scott, the therapist, determined from his conversations with the addict that the family members were downplaying their importance for therapy. The addict was about to drop out or be pulled out of treatment and the family was scared. The sense that they were slipping away and had lost any notion of urgency prompted Scott to give it his best—and perhaps last—shot.

The family was a large one, with seven children. For such a sizeable group, the payment for participating in the evaluation session gained salience. This unusual aspect provided the therapist with a means for (1) gaining attention, (2) downplaying the possible negative implications of family involvement in treatment, and (3) underscoring the urgency of the situation. The following is a reconstruction of Scott's first phone call to the mother.

*SCOTT:* (*urgently*) Hello, Mrs. Smith. This is Sam Scott, Ron's counselor.

*MOTHER:* Yes?

*SCOTT:* I had to call you right away to tell you about the *ninety dollars!*

*MOTHER:* What?

*SCOTT:* The *ninety dollars!*

*MOTHER:* What are you talking about?

*SCOTT:* The *ninety dollars* that you are supposed to get.

*MOTHER:* What ninety dollars?

*SCOTT:* Oh, didn't Ron tell you?

*MOTHER:* No. What ninety dollars are you talking about?

*SCOTT:* The ninety dollars that you are supposed to get from the program.

*MOTHER:* I don't know anything about it.

*SCOTT:* You and your family are supposed to get ninety dollars for coming in to the program. I was *afraid* that you hadn't heard about it.

*MOTHER:* No, I hadn't heard anything. What is this all about?

*SCOTT:* Your family gets *ninety dollars* for coming in for an interview. But we have to act fast. Can you get them in right away?

*MOTHER:* I guess so, but . . .

*SCOTT:* (*interrupting*) Everybody has to come in: you, your husband, the kids. Everybody, or they won't pay it.

*MOTHER:* When do we have to do this?

SCOTT: I think they need you within the next week. But everybody has to come in. I've got to tell the people here when to set it up. I'd hate to see you lose the money.

MOTHER: Well, I guess . . . I'll have to talk to them.

SCOTT: OK! When can you let me know?

MOTHER: I guess later on tonight.

SCOTT: OK. Here's my number. Call me as soon as you can.

MOTHER: OK. Thanks for letting me know.

When the mother called later, she was given more details about the evaluation session. By that time, the decision had been made to participate, however, so she was not looking for reasons to back out.

The humor in this vignette should not obscure the sound theoretical base underlying Scott's approach. It derived from his prior knowledge of the family. Scott was aware of their increasing reluctance. He attempted to create a sense of urgency and surprise in order to catch them off guard and cause them to focus on a positive aspect of their participation.

The money served as a convenient vehicle for taking the family's side against an "impersonal" institution. While financial incentive seemed important in this case, a similar tack could have been taken using a different source of leverage.* For instance, the therapist could have called with a different scenario, saying, "It's finally come *through*! They're gonna let us *do* it!" ["Do what?"] " They're finally gonna let the *family* help with the *treatment*! It's fantastic! We've been trying to convince them for years that they should let the *family* know what's going on. My God, let's get it set up before they change their minds. We can't lose this opportunity! I'm really *glad* for you," and so forth. This particular variation of the approach might be appropriate for a family who had previously experienced treatment for their son and had felt closed out. It should be recognized that the specific content chosen should be in response to a given family and its situation, rather than an indiscriminate application of a series of "pat" or "canned" phrases.

An important point in this handling of the recruitment process is that it reframes as positive an event that has the potential to be

---

*In general, money proved to be less influential in recruitment than we had initially anticipated (see following discussion).

viewed negatively by the family. Instead of presenting them with the prospect of having their dirty linen examined by a "bunch of shrinks," they are presented with an *opportunity*. This opportunity is portrayed as beneficial and no blame is attached to it. Consequently, the "reality" is shifted. The tone of urgency, enthusiasm, or concern only supports the importance and the positive features of the event, thereby fortifying the shift.

## Approaches to Wives

In our experience with this population, wives of the clients were perhaps the most willing participants of all family members. For the most part, if the IP would cooperate, his wife was easy to bring in. For whatever reasons, they just did not give us much trouble, and sometimes even helped us recruit their husbands' parents.* The only exceptions to this were cases in which the wife and the IP's family of origin were openly antagonistic toward each other. In such instances our research design dictated that we concentrate on involving the family of origin (since they, but not the wife, were required to attend the evaluation session), and bring the wife in after treatment began.

## THE NONBLAMING MESSAGE

When these families are approached they often feel frightened, defensive, and guilty. At some level they know they are to a great extent to blame for the problems of the IP. Thus they are *ready* to hear blaming from the therapist. They anticipate it, and often attempt to deny or avoid the blame they fear the therapist will place on them by diverting it to external influences such as peers, the neighborhood, or the treatment program. The therapist's task is to get beyond this stumbling block and reduce resistance arising from fear of blame.

*Principle 10: The therapist must approach the family with a rationale for treatment that is nonpejorative, nonjudgmental, and*

---

*If the interpersonal problems of which the addiction is a part are viewed as primarily seated in the larger family system that includes the addict's parents, the wife's willingness to come in could be seen as a decoy—as a means for drawing the therapist's attention away from the family of origin. It is, then, a homeostatic move, involving the collusion of wife, addict, and parents. The fact that treatment that initially centered on the addict's marriage usually failed (see Chapter 6) attests to the validity of this interpretation.

*which in no way blames them for the problem.* This requires skill. Some responsibility is being ascribed to the family by the very fact that they are being asked to become involved. There is an implicit message that the family has not resolved something with one of its members. Consequently, the therapist must approach them in a nonconfronting way, which gets them off the hook, thereby reducing resistance and making them more amenable to hearing what he has to say. Our experience is consonant with that of Vaglum[180] that family members should not be treated as "patients," but as "healthy" people who, themselves, are without problems. Under no circumstances should the therapist become involved in a struggle with the family over whether they are the problem or not. Instead, he should allow them to become acquainted with him in order to remove mystery and fear; if they sense that he is both genuinely concerned and not out to put them on the "hot seat," they will be more agreeable to his requests.

*Vignette 12.* In this case the therapist (Jerry I. Kleiman) underscored the parents' martyrdom, talking about all they had been through and how their son never listened to them. He emphasized repeatedly that the son did these things despite "all they had done so far." He empathized with the father's plight—nobody listened to him, people kept secrets from him—and told him it was time for this to stop. He talked to the parents as victims, telling them that there was a need for them to be in control of the situation.

*Principle 11: Primary focus should be on helping the index patient rather than the family.* This approach stems from the work of Haley, and is described in Chapter 6. It has also been applied by others with these families.[28, 180] Again, the emphasis is on joining the parents in helping their son to "be the kind of person he *can* be." To the extent that the therapist ever takes a blaming stance, it would be in this context. He might join the parents in mildly blaming the IP for the problem. Alternatively, he could state, "No one is to blame." Or, he might emphasize how difficult it is to get off drugs, and, "Your son needs all the help he can get." The family is then redefined as a group that can help the IP, rather than one that causes his problem.

*Vignette 13.* In this family the therapist (Jerry I. Kleiman) empathized and shared with them. He got them to admit that with all they had done so far, they had not been able to help. He suggested that maybe this was an opportunity for them to teach their son what the world is all about.

*Vignette 14.* The therapist (Jerry I. Kleiman) talked to the father about his goals for his son. The discussion had a kind of "reparenting" flavor, as the father talked about his lack of success both with his son and in general. Kleiman suggested that perhaps this program would give him a chance to succeed in a new way.

*Principle 12: The rationale for family treatment should be presented in such a way that, in order to oppose it, family members would have to state openly that they want the index patient to remain symptomatic.* While not necessarily easy to do, succeeding at this task can greatly facilitate the recruiting effort. If nothing else, the family may come in to disprove an implication that they do not want change. It sometimes helps to begin by "ascribing noble intentions" to the family (see Chapter 6): "Of course, your goal is to see him straighten out." In fact, the therapist ought to operate under the assumption that the family wants to help and desires to see the IP get better. He has to believe that, in the end, the parents really do not want a drug addict for a son. If he implies that they do want an addicted son, he will have a battle on his hands. If he is able to avoid such an altercation, the therapist can instead proceed with establishing his case for family treatment, using strategies of the sort described in other sections.

## GOAL TAILORING

Sometimes, upon encountering the family, the therapist found that their agenda for change differed somewhat from his own. They may have either had goals that were very specific, or had more goals than he did.

*Principle 13: The therapist should adopt the family's goals for the index patient as the primary ones for treatment.* Examples of this have been presented above. For instance, the therapist might learn that employment for the IP is paramount for the family. He should accept this and describe how the family-treatment program can lead toward job placement. Usually, then, the therapist wants to first find out what the *family* is interested in changing, because this is what they are motivated to come in to work on. The issue could be drug use, staying out of jail, taking "more responsibility," or whatever. The therapist's next move is to explain how a treatment program that includes them will allow progress toward this goal, and that such a goal is an integral part of the process. He explains that the treatment is tailored to their needs. In a sense, he says, "Whatever you want, we've got it." He then utilizes himself toward actually realizing their goals.

In discussing goals for coming in, the question arises whether the families were motivated by the money they would receive. Each member got $10.00 for participating in the Family Evaluation Session, a nontreatment research exercise. While the money was mentioned as an incentive in many of our cases (usually as "payment for your giving up your time, since I know you're very busy") we and our staff are convinced that it was not a very important variable—less important than we anticipated. Of the cases that were not to receive any money beyond what they got for the Family Evaluation Session, 92% continued past this session into family treatment. Only in rare instances did it appear to make a crucial difference. In fact, some families actually tried to refuse it, and these were not wealthy people. While reimbursement did help the *retention* of families in treatment (see Appendix C), we are not impressed with its importance in family *recruitment*. For the most part, we would advocate the use of money during recruitment as a helpful option mainly in cases when it is requested by the family to defray transportation expenses to the treatment or evaluation site.

## THERAPIST'S LEVERAGE

A number of factors can markedly increase or decrease the therapist's leverage during the recruitment effort.

*Principle 14: The chances for successful family recruitment are increased if the therapist does the recruiting.* There are several advantages to this. First, it avoids the problem of passing the family from one treater to another, with the accompanying increase in dropouts; the process is not diluted between an intake worker or recruiter and a therapist. Second, as mentioned earlier, by seeing the family during engagement the therapist can sell himself, helping to instill trust and assuage fears about being blamed and so forth.

It is probably an advantage if the therapist is of the same race as the family. Our research design dictated that, whenever logistically possible, therapist and family should be matched as to race. This was achieved in 84% of the cases. While we feel that such matching may be less important during the actual therapy, it did seem to help at the time of recruitment. In addition to getting around the barriers that can occur in many instances when people of different races interact, it facilitated the task of getting information. Often our therapists made visits to the home or neighborhood to locate the IP or his family, and being of similar race engendered more cooperation from relatives and neighbors. The safety factor also cannot be ignored. Many of the families lived in "rough" neighborhoods, and it could actually be dangerous for a Black man to be walking around at night in a White neighborhood, or vice versa.*

*Principle 15: The therapist should be the primary treater of the index patient and his family.* Below, in Chapters 6 and 16, we state that we believe family therapy will fail with these cases without this provision. It is likewise extremely important in the recruitment effort. In the early days of our project the IP had both a drug counselor and a therapist. The procedure was for the IP to become enrolled in the clinic and have his program and medications determined in conjunction with his drug counselor. Then the counselor would serve as a kind of middleman or "matchmaker" in introducing him to the family therapist. (In the meantime the counselor continued with the patient in monitoring therapeutic issues, providing individual counseling, and the like.) This procedure frequently fell on its face (see Chapter 16).

The decision was made for the therapist to also function as drug counselor for those cases selected for our program. This modification was crucial: wearing both hats, the therapist was brought into the treatment process immediately upon intake. As mentioned earlier in this chapter, he had the advantage of being the first treater encountered by the client. He had the added leverage of control over decisions about medications such as methadone. With the advent of the dual role model, a major recruiting hurdle was removed, leading

---

*We wish to make it clear that we are not endorsing a system in which only Black therapists treat Black families, and White therapists treat White patients. The material presented here refers to the recruitment, not the therapy, process.

to a marked decrease in the amount of effort needed to engage families, and an increase in the rate of recruitment success.[169]

## THERAPIST FACTORS

Frequently we are asked what therapist variables lead to success in recruiting. The following four principles are devoted to such factors.

*Principle 16: An important recruitment variable is the extent to which the therapist shows interest in the family through his willingness to expend considerable effort in engaging them.* From our experience, there are a number of therapist characteristics and attitudes that lead to more favorable recruitment rates. These include the following:

1. The therapist must be energetic. The recruitment process can be demanding in time and effort. Rather than expecting to sit in his office, the therapist should be willing to get out into the field and make home visits.

2. Enthusiasm for the work is obviously essential. Sager *et al.*[126] noted a reluctance by many of their therapists to work with "poorly motivated" families.

3. The therapist must be persistent and able to tolerate rebukes by family members.

4. Flexibility and lack of rigidity are necessary, since they allow therapists to adroitly counter family resistance moves.

5. The therapist must be convinced of the value of his endeavor and feel that it will be helpful to the family. This conviction will be conveyed to clients, and will help to change their negative "set."

*Principle 17: Providing incentives to therapists for each successfully recruited case increases the rate of success.* Early in the life of our project the therapists began to complain that they were paid to do therapy and the recruitment effort was demanding an inordinate amount of their time. If this objection had been allowed to dictate our procedures, we would have been left with an unacceptably small, select sample, composed of "easy" or highly motivated families. Thus we were forced to rearrange our priorities and shift incentives. We did this by making a portion of the therapists' pay contingent upon successfully recruiting families—a bonus system. This had the double advantage of (1) reordering therapists' priorities through tangibly demonstrating the importance we placed on enlisting families, while also (2) providing them with reimbursement for the time they spent in recruiting activities. They were, of course, paid in addition for the time they spent doing therapy. However, money need not be the only incentive, and other programs might be able to establish alternative, nonmonetary procedures (see Chapter 16).

*Principle 18: The program must be structured in a way that does not allow therapists to back down from enlisting whole families.* This is a crucial point. We are convinced that if we had not held firmly to our requirement that the total family—or at least the IP, both parents, and siblings living in the home—be involved, the therapists would have settled for less. Without this mandate, we estimate that one-third of our families would have arrived incomplete, and treatment would have commenced without one or more important members. It would have been too easy to proceed with only the most willing participants.

*Vignette 15.* Adherence to Principle 18 sometimes had unexpected benefits. In one interesting example (in a case seen by David B. Heard, PhD) the recruitment requirement prevented a potential problem from developing in our research and treatment design. The addict in this case was in trouble with the law (although we did not know it at the time) and had a court hearing pending. Heard devoted great energy, including seven individual interviews plus numerous telephone calls, toward getting the IP to agree to engage his family. As the situation developed, it appeared that all members except the stepfather would agree to participate (the natural father was deceased). However, Heard could not make direct contact with the stepfather. This process went on for approximately 2½ months with no results. Eventually the addict was caught selling drugs at the treatment center and was discharged for disciplinary reasons. He defected to another program and soon thereafter went to jail. We later learned from a counselor in that program that (1) the addict had been facing serious legal charges for some time, and (2) he *had* no "stepfather." The person the addict was trying to bring in as his stepfather was his *uncle.* Apparently the addict was trying to avoid prison by presenting a case to the judge that he was motivated to change, had entered a treatment program, and that his effort was earnest to the point where he could claim, "See, even my *family* is involved with me in treatment." However, he knew that we would not accept him in the family program without a father figure, so he tried to get the uncle to pose as stepfather. The plan failed because the uncle refused to take part in the masquerade. The point is, if Heard had not persisted in his demand for inclusion of the "stepfather," the rest of the family would have come in and treatment would have progressed under the false assumption (by the therapist) that the nonexistent stepfather would eventually participate.

*Principle 19: A mechanical approach to recruitment is insufficient to guarantee success—flexibility and skill are crucial if the therapist is to avoid getting deadlocked.* While the initial interview procedure described in Chapter 3 can probably be handled by most experienced clinical interviewers, recruitment of the whole family is more difficult. The latter demands a certain level of skill in dealing with families—essentially the kind of experience one gets in performing family therapy. Not only must one be able to show proper empathy and effective joining techniques, but one must also be able to respond to family interaction patterns.

The importance of recruiter skill cannot be overestimated. We do not agree that positive results are primarily due to "highly motivated therapists." Therapists must be able to adapt the basic principles of recruitment flexibly and creatively in order to meet the unique requirements of each case. Simply "plugging away" is insufficient. As in Vignettes 10 and 11, a skillfull recruiter can sometimes get results with a minimum of well-directed effort, much like the judo flip succeeds when direct overpowering will not.

## ADMINISTRATIVE SUPPORT

By now it is probably apparent that the activities described herein require substantial administrative support from the treatment facility. Many of the points below are enlarged upon in Chapter 16.

*Principle 20: The treatment agency must have flexible policies to allow therapist flexibility.* The most obvious example of this principle concerns therapists' working hours. Families, especially those with low incomes and/or multiple problems, cannot always get time off to engage in treatment during the 9 to 5 workday. In addition, the working member(s) are sometimes on an evening or night shift, further complicating the scheduling problem. Berg and

Rosenblum[14] found that the "work schedule" was the most frequently given reason for the father's failure to become engaged in treatment. These authors also obtained a positive correlation between the percentage of families successfully engaged and the lateness of the hour the therapist was able to see them. They state, "Family therapists must be more flexible in the hours that they see a family and the agency for which they work must accommodate this flexibility" (p. 91). We feel this is even more crucial for the recruitment effort. When trying to engage a family, there is even greater need to meet them on their turf, and be able to contact them when they are available, usually at night. Consequently, the agency must not only allow, but must *encourage* late, long, and irregular hours if family enlistment is a goal.

There are other ways in which the agency can be flexible. For instance, simply allowing therapists easy access to the telephone can be important, since this is such a crucial instrument in the recruitment effort. Regular consultation time from supervisors can be helpful, especially when a therapist has reached an impasse or is trying to figure out ways of obtaining leverage with a family. As before, permitting staff to function in the dual role of therapist–drug counselor may also be pivotal. Finally, flexibility in the kind of services offered, such as job counseling, may be necessary to allow the therapist to make commitments to the family during the goal-tailoring process.

*Principle 21: The treatment agency must be willing to back up the recruitment effort through commitment of tangible resources.* While related to Principle 20, this goes beyond flexibility, per se, and refers to the allocation of real monies and related resources for recruitment. It is not enough to tell a therapist to "do your thing," since his time also costs the agency money. The therapist must be given clear indication of the importance attached to recruiting, so that he is not, for example, penalized on his caseload quota while trying to engage a particularly resistant family. Nighttime hours must also be rewarded. A possible way of handling this is to count recruiting time as patient contact time, and unsuccessful attempts to reach family members as "treatment backup" time. Another option is to credit evening hours as compensatory time. In addition, coverage of travel expenses for home visits may be necessary. Other areas for commitment of agency resources have been mentioned earlier, such as the provision of incentives for successfully recruited cases, the use of beepers during the engagement process, and payment to families for parking expenses.

## DISCUSSION

### *EFFECTIVENESS OF ENGAGEMENT*

It is beyond the scope of this chapter to give data on the success of each of the recruiting principles. Only overall results will be presented. It is worth noting that Black families were more difficult to recruit, and that the recruitment effort—including those successfully and unsuccessfully engaged—required a median of 5.4 direct contacts (telephone or face-to-face) over a median of 20.5 days. A more detailed analysis of the factors leading to successful recruitment, and the cost-effectiveness of our efforts, has been published elsewhere.[169]

For the present purposes, the term "engager" will be used to denote those families who participated in the initial Family Evaluation Session. The term "refuser" will refer to families in which one or more family members refused to participate in such a session. Out of a total sample of 92 eligible families, we were able to recruit 71% (i.e., there were 65 engagers and 27 refusers). An important variable was whether the IP gave us permission to contact his family directly (Principle 4). As noted in Chapter 3, in the 74 cases where such permission was granted, 88% of the families were successfully engaged. Put another way, two-thirds of our failures occurred when we could not get past the IP. The reasons why we think this occurred have been presented earlier in this chapter. Sager *et al.*[126] experienced similar difficulty with single persons, and recommended spending "a great deal of time working through individual problems with the identified patient so that he does not experience family therapy as an attempt to return him to his original difficult family situation" (p. 720). These authors also noted that patients who had difficulty accepting the importance of their families in their problem were also more likely to drop out of treatment prematurely.

The dual role of having therapists also serve as drug counselors deserves special mention. Before this procedure was implemented our recruitment success rate was 56%. Afterward the rate rose to

77%. Under the dual role, therapists required fewer contacts (mean of 6.4 vs. 7.2), a shorter period of time (median of 17 days vs. 33 days),* and fewer home visits (11% vs. 48%) in order to get families into treatment. More important, our data[169] document that recruiting families under the dual role was *more than twice as cost-efficient* than when both a therapist and drug counselor were involved in the recruitment process.

The rate of success with which these families were engaged in treatment is considerably higher than other reports in the literature with similar clients. This is especially true considering (1) the clients' predominantly lower socioeconomic status,[126, 138] (2) the severity of their addictive problems, and (3) the fact that, unlike nearly all of the earlier studies, we considered a case to be successfully recruited only if *both* parents or parent surrogates appeared together at the treatment site; most other studies satisfied themselves with one parent or a spouse. These results, then, offer general support for the aforementioned principles, as well as for the effectiveness of the major effort applied to recruitment.

## CLINICAL ASPECTS

Some of the clinical vignettes presented earlier may appear to have an unusual, or even outlandish, flavor. This is a direct result of the tremendous difficulty encountered in engaging many of these families. They rarely responded to gentle urging or a "kind word." Often the therapist had to respond very quickly in order to keep from losing a family. It sometimes seemed as if he could not think of something fast enough to turn things around. Frequently the dangers of death or imprisonment of the addict, balanced against resistance or complacency on the part of the family, put additional pressure on him. Thus he responded with what came to mind, hoping it would work. The massive resistance shown by so many of these families, and the inadequacy of more standard techniques, dictated that the therapists develop new approaches.

Although the recruitment effort might be termed a "pretherapy" exercise, it is (as stated in Principle 8) a clear intervention. This is especially true in cases that require considerable effort to engage,

*These two time figures apply only to engagers, since such measures are not applicable to families who were not recruited.

bringing us to a point made by Jay Haley* about the difficult position that our therapists were in. Unlike many clinical situations where the family petitions the treatment program for help, we enjoyed no such luxury. These families neither expected nor, in most cases, wanted to be involved. The majority of them had already seen a drug-treatment program fail with their sons, and they may have been even less impressed this time. Instead, the impetus for their participation usually generated from the therapist. They knew he wanted them in, that he "needed" them in order to perform his job. Often this led to his working hard while they sat back and "played coy." Thus, in light of these handicaps, the percentage of families actually engaged could probably be considered quite credible.

Problems such as the above can be reduced considerably by program procedures. There are at least 40 drug-treatment programs in the United States in which family participation is mandatory.[31] This obviously reduces the amount of time and effort required for recruitment. We know of at least one multimodal methadone program that has established this condition, and 75% of its clients bring their families in† (although their requirements are less stringent than our own, in that any cluster of family members is acceptable for the first session, and both parents are not necessarily required to participate at the outset). However, even if only 25% of the families are resistant, the principles set forth herein would appear applicable for this select subgroup.

Treaters who might want to institute family recruitment programs in the future would want to keep in mind the characteristics of our patient population, that is, all the clients were male, between ages 20 and 35, in touch with two parents or parent surrogates, veterans with at least a brief military stint, from the lower socioeconomic classes, nearly equally divided between Blacks and Whites, and living within 1 hour's drive from the clinic. We also excluded a number of good-prognosis clients who were detoxifying from opiates and therefore on an immediate path toward nonaddiction. Further, since our clients were outpatients, they may have been more difficult to engage than those in the more "captive" status of inpatients. Many of these factors probably operated to make recruitment more difficult, and

---

*Jay Haley (personal communication, November 1976).

†Alexander Panio, Northwestern University Department of Psychiatry (personal communication, December 1977).

some of them might also serve to limit the applicability of our findings to other contexts.

On the other hand, we would posit that most of the principles we have presented can be generalized to other types of "difficult" and "unmotivated" families. Their application seems appropriate with other types of disorders and "tough" cases. We suspect that similar recruitment problems exist, in particular, with symptom groups in which there is a heavy focus on the IP or where there is considerable family "underorganization," such as is often found with low-income families. We are sensitive to the tendency to pass off our recruitment endeavor as "inapplicable" or "not do-able" simply because other programs have not been engaged in such activities, or because these activities would require the development of additional skills. Another common counterargument is to oversimplify family recruiting as primarily a function of "highly motivated therapists," followed by the disclaimer that one's own therapists are "not as motivated." While we recognize that recruitment is not a simple exercise, the difficulty of the task should not be used as an excuse for failing to make an earnest effort. Clinicians who claim to be interested in helping people should not be too quick to write off a significant number of families who could be reached if properly approached.

Looking to the future, it seems safe to predict that, as family therapy becomes more widespread and accepted within the general populace, the task of engaging families will become easier. The idea of family involvement will seem less alien or irrelevant to the layman. However, it is very doubtful that all resistance will dissipate, any more than it has with individual therapy. Thus we can expect that family therapy will be faced with engagement challenges, at least in certain cases, for some time to come.

## IS RECRUITMENT NECESSARY?

The question naturally arises as to whether the additional time and effort required for recruitment is worth the investment. The issue for treatment agencies may be as much one of policy as of resources. For instance, an agency might ask whether it is really necessary to establish procedures that maximize recruitment effectiveness, and, again, "Is it worth the effort?" Based upon our data, we feel such questions can be answered in the affirmative. In the 1-year posttreatment follow-up data from several modes of family and nonfamily treatment presented in Chapter 17, family therapy substantially increased the percentage of days free from a number of illegal drugs and methadone. If we address this issue in terms of dollars and cents, we might consider what the costs are to society for an untreated heroin addict. Estimates of these costs range up to $24,000 per year.* Taking a conservative approach, let us adopt a lesser figure of $12,000 per year. This, then, converts to a daily cost of $32.88. From our most expensive cost-efficiency estimate[169] of $152.63 for each successfully recruited family, family therapy would only have to make a difference of 5 more nonaddicted days, beyond the improvement needed to cover the costs of the therapy itself, to have paid for the recruitment effort. Our outcome data indicate that the number of such days produced by structural-strategic family therapy greatly exceeds this requirement, to say nothing of the preventive potential of this kind of intervention.[152, 157] While other agencies may want to adjust our cost analysis formulae to account for their own personnel and other costs, we doubt that their estimates would be substantially more expensive. These results imply that agencies that are resistant to a full-scale family recruitment effort cannot justify their resistance based on issues of cost-efficiency, especially if one considers the costs saved to society.

As a final note, it should be clear from the presented material that engagement of resistant families requires a rethinking or re-framing of the therapeutic enterprise. The traditional philosophy that therapy should be provided only for those who "ask" for it is being challenged, since such a view overlooks both the importance of the family in maintaining the disorder and the desperate situation in which these same families may find themselves. *The practice of sitting back and waiting for family members to show up under their own steam serves to neglect a major portion of those most sorely in need.* Instead, a new ethic is proposed, based on an "outreach" philosophy.[7, 15] In order for these families to be helped, emphasis must be placed on *seeking them out and engaging them.* Such a course demands a shift in the allocation of time, effort, and resources, and also calls for unconventional techniques. This field is wide open to exploration and innovation on several levels, extending from the ways in which personal contact is handled, to the educative employment of mass media. We hope that we may have communicated to the reader some of what we see as its exciting potential.

*While many estimates have been made of such costs, this upper figure comes from the *Addiction and Drug Abuse Report,* 1977, 8(1), 1.

# STRATEGIES AND TECHNIQUES OF TREATMENT

# 6

# THE THERAPY MODEL

M. DUNCAN STANTON
THOMAS C. TODD

THIS CHAPTER presents the background, rationale, and clinical principles that we have applied in developing a treatment model for working with families with a drug-abusing member.

## BACKGROUND

### FAMILY CHARACTERISTICS

The families we have treated exhibited many of the patterns described in the general literature reviewed in Chapter 1. There was usually a very close, dependent, mother–son relationship paired with an (ostensibly) distant, excluded father. (However, in line with the findings of Alexander and Dibb[2] and Kaufman and Kaufmann,[78] some families—approximately 5% in our sample—showed a reversal of these roles, with the father the parent most involved or "closest" to the addict.)* Approximately 80% of our cases had a parent with a drinking problem.† Furthermore, in most cases the fathers were observed to be most upset by their son's addiction, and the mothers tended to minimize it. This differs from typical child problems, where the mother is more likely to voice the complaint.

Much like the families of schizophrenics, there is usually a lack of constructive pressure for change in these families. The abuser is discounted as a person and the family feels powerless, often blaming

---

*Chapter 9 presents such a case.

†While this percentage may seem higher than most reports in the literature on alcoholism within such families, we have data[164] that indicate that the lower rates cited by others may be a result of protectiveness and guardedness on the part of the IP and family, and that 80% may be closer to the real incidence level.

outside causes (peers or the neighborhood) for his problem. In some families, the identified patient's (IP's) drug problem is the focus for all family problems. Further, the abuser is often overprotected by the family and treated as a helpless and incompetent person. In these families, drugs are viewed as an all-powerful force that he cannot resist.

## THE FAMILY LIFE CYCLE

As a contrast, or perhaps an adjunct, to more static notions of family patterns and structure, we have become increasingly impressed with the utility of the family life cycle as a paradigm for identifying variables surrounding the drug abuser's problem and dictating the direction for treatment (e.g., Chapters 1 and 4). Clinical use of the family life cycle was first accentuated by Haley in his analysis of Erickson's work,[64] and it has received increasing attention in recent years.[23]

Two life cycle stages appear particularly salient in the development of addiction in a young person. The first is the point at which he reaches adolescence. This is when drug taking—although not necessarily addiction—usually starts. As outlined in Chapter 1, it is the stage in which he becomes, or is under pressure to become, more oriented toward heterosexual activities. Whereas his previous actions tended to be seen as asexual, now he is developing "sexy" interests. This change toward relationships that are more adult in nature, and imply a growing up and individuation from the family, can herald parental panic, and set the stage for later addictive behavior.

The second life cycle stage of importance in addiction is the stage of *leaving home* emphasized by Haley.[64, 66] This stage brings issues of the individuation and adult competence of the IP to a head, becoming the hub around which the addiction commonly develops and revolves. Since it has been underscored earlier, and will be covered at greater length in subsequent chapters, it will receive no further discussion here.

Several other life cycle issues deserve mention. One of these concerns the occupational status of the abuser's parents—particularly the breadwinner(s). If a parent loses a job or reaches retirement (Chapter 11), the effect can be catastrophic on these families. The nonworking parent may become weak, ineffectual, depressed, and unable to appropriately discipline or control his offspring. Conflict between parents usually increases. In such cases, the IP may become increasingly incompetent and problematic, seeming at times to assume even lower status in the family hierarchy so that the unemployed parent is not relegated to the bottom of the totem pole.

Other life cycle events that often tie into the onset of drug abuse or the addiction cycle are (1) sudden deaths in the family and their accompanying bereavement; (2) severe illness in a member, particularly a parent; (3) impending illness or death, such as can occur subsequent to a heart attack in a parent in which he recovers but the family lives within a pall of gloom or is afraid to place any stress on him for fear that it will kill him; (4) the "empty-nest" syndrome (see Chapter 11), which is, of course, a special case of the leaving-home phenomenon. It is important both for diagnostic and therapeutic reasons for a therapist to assess whether a given family has encountered, or is presently coping with, one of these events before proceeding very far with treatment.

## STRUCTURAL AND STRATEGIC FAMILY THERAPY

The theoretical and operational facets of our therapy are derived primarily from structural family therapy and certain aspects of strategic therapy.* While there are differences between these approaches, they also share certain commonalities. As a rule, both schools subscribe to the following view of the family or couple:

1. People are seen as interacting within a context—both affecting it and being affected by it.

2. The family life cycle and developmental stage are important both in diagnosis and in defining therapy strategy—a problem family being seen as stuck at a particular stage in its development.

3. Symptoms are both system-maintained and system-maintaining.

4. The family or couple can change, allowing new behaviors to emerge, if the overall context is changed. Further, in order for individual change to occur, the interpersonal system itself must change. This would permit different aspects of such family members' (potential) "character" to come to the fore.

*This section on structural and strategic family therapy is adapted from two earlier publications by Stanton.[158, 161]

Both schools also regard therapy and the therapist in the following ways:

1. Treatment is viewed pragmatically, with an eye toward what "works."

2. Emphasis is on the present rather than the past.

3. Repetitive behavioral sequences are to be changed.

4. While structural therapists may not be as symptom-focused as strategic therapists, both are much more symptom-oriented than psychodynamic therapists.

5. Process is emphasized much more than content. This includes interventions that are nonverbal and noncognitive—in a sense, "doing away with words." Such interventions are derived from viewing the system from a "meta" level and recognizing that verbalizations, per se, by therapist or family are often not necessary for change.

6. The therapist should direct the therapy and take responsibility for change.

7. Diagnosis is obtained through hypothesizing, *intervening*, and examining feedback.

8. Therapeutic contracts, which relate to the problem and the goals of change, are negotiated with clients.

9. Interpretation is usually employed to "relabel" or "reframe" rather than to produce "insight."

10. Behavioral tasks (homework) are routinely assigned.

11. Considerable effort may go into "joining" the family positively and reducing apparent "guilt" or defensiveness. This is more than simply "establishing rapport," as it is often done selectively with particular family members and in line with specific therapeutic goals.

12. Therapy cannot usually progress from the initial dysfunctional stage to a "cure" stage without one or more intermediate stages, which, on the surface, may appear dysfunctional also. For instance, a therapist may have to take sides with a spouse, thereby "unbalancing" the couple in a way opposite from which it entered treatment, in order to restabilize at a point of equality.

13. Therapy tends to be brief and typically does not exceed 6 months.

It may be apparent that some of these points are shared by other, more active interpersonal therapies also, such as the behavioral and "communications training" approaches. However, most of them are distinctive of structural and strategic therapy.

## Structural Therapy

The structural approach to family therapy is most closely identified with Salvador Minuchin, Braulio Montalvo, and associates. Its literature has been covered by at least two reviews[5, 155] and the principles and techniques appear in four books.[100, 103, 104]* It has demonstrated its utility and efficacy with a variety of different kinds of symptoms and problem groups. It has also been applied with a range of therapist types—a prime example being the important and effective work with psychosomatic families by Minuchin et al.[101, 104] in which their 53 cases were seen by 16 therapists who differed greatly in levels of experience and who came from four different disciplines.

The coverage of structural therapy here will necessarily be brief. However, while there are specific features of structural therapy that distinguish it from other modalities, it is important to note that a structural aspect of treatment applies to all therapies and to therapists of all persuasions, as follows: *Any therapeutic intervention made by any therapist necessarily includes a structural component.* For example, by choosing to talk to or interact with one family member or another, or with two parents together, the therapist makes a structural decision, whether or not he is aware of it; not to do so would mean that the therapist acts at random with the participants. In focusing his attention on, or making a statement about, a given member (or subsystem) at a particular point, he is, by nature of the power and status vested in him as a therapist, elevating that person and separating him from the other(s). He shares his power by his attention, so that, as Haley[65] states, "A comment by the therapist is not merely a comment but also a coalition with one spouse in relation to the other or with the unit against a larger group" (p. 160). The therapist cannot (and probably should not) avoid doing this in most treatment contexts, so the important point is that he should do it with some plan in mind and remain consistent with his plan. In other words, does his (structural) intervention lead the family toward the change that he would like to implement? Ignoring this notion handicaps the therapist and can even prove detrimental to treatment.

*The fourth book is *Family Therapy Techniques*, by S. Minuchin and H. C. Fishman. Cambridge, Mass.: Harvard University Press, 1981.

Relative to, for example, certain strategic approaches that emphasize change and, on the average, are more likely to treat individuals,[159] in structural therapy the focus is less on theory of change than on theory of family.[155] The model is not particularly complex, theoretically. Some of the primary concepts are:

1. Attention is paid to *proximity and distance* between family members and subsystems and these are defined through *boundaries*, that is, the rules that determine "who participates and how" in the family.[100, p. 53]

2. The extremes of the proximity and distance continuum are *enmeshment* and *disengagement*, with most (i.e., "normal") families and subsystems lying at intermediate points between the two poles.

3. A family is described or schematized spatially, in terms of its hierarchies and its alliances or coalitions.

4. Problems result from a rigid, dysfunctional family structure.

Some of the basic structural therapeutic techniques are as follows:

1. The primary goal is to induce a more adequate family organization of the sort that will maximize growth and potential in each of its members.[100]

2. The thrust of the therapy is toward "restructuring" the system, such as establishing or loosening boundaries, differentiating enmeshed members, and increasing the involvement of disengaged members.

3. The therapeutic plan is gauged against a model of what is normal for a family at a given stage in its development, with due consideration of its cultural and socioeconomic context.

4. The desired interactional change must take place *within the actual session* (enactment), with the family sitting in the room.[68, 103]

5. Techniques such as *unbalancing* a system and *intensifying* an interaction are part of the therapy.

6. The therapist "joins" and accommodates to the system in a sort of blending experience, but retains enough independence both to resist the family's pull and to challenge (restructure) it at various points. He thus actively uses *himself* as a boundary-maker, intensifier, and general change agent in the session.

7. Treatment is usually limited to include those members of a family who live within a household or have regular contact with the immediate family. This might involve grandparents living nearby, or even an employer, if the problem is work-related.

8. The function of assigning tasks and homework is usually to consolidate changes made during sessions and extend them to the real world.

9. The practice is to bring a family to a level of "health" or "complexity" and then stand ready to be called in the future, if necessary. Such a model is seen to combine the advantages of short- and long-term therapy.

*Strategic Therapy*

Haley[64] has defined the strategic approach as one in which the clinician initiates what happens during treatment and designs a particular approach for each problem. Strategic therapists take responsibility for directly influencing people. They want to enhance, at least temporarily, their influence over the interpersonal system at hand in order to bring about beneficial change. In fact, they are not as concerned about family theory as they are with the theory and means for inducing change.

The strategic approach has been used with innumerable kinds of problems and several outcome studies attest to its efficacy.[155, 159] A number of people and groups are considered representative of this school, such as Milton Erickson, Jay Haley, the Mental Research Institute (MRI) group, Gerald Zuk, the Institute for Family Study group in Milan, Italy, Lynn Hoffman, Richard Rabkin, Peggy Papp, Olga Silverstein, Cloé Madanes, and others. All of these therapists do not operate in exactly the same way, but rather than devote space to their individual contributions, styles, and differences, we will instead present some of the concepts, principles, and practices that apply to most of them, and conclude with an overview of Haley's particular approach.*

Strategic therapists see symptoms as the resultants or concomitants of misguided attempts to changing an existing difficulty.[186] However, such symptoms usually succeed only in making things worse, while attempts by the family to alleviate the problem often

*The reader interested in greater detail is referred to their various published works or to several synopses that have emerged in the literature.[96, 155, 159]

exacerbate it. A symptom is regarded as a communicative act, with message qualities, which serves as a sort of contract between two or more members and has a function within the interpersonal network.[185] It is a label for a nonlinear or "recursive" sequence of behaviors within a social organization.[11,65] A symptom usually appears when a person is "in an impossible situation and is trying to break out of it."[64, p. 44] He is locked into a sequence or pattern with his significant other(s) and cannot see a way to alter it through nonsymptomatic means. The symptom is thus a homeostatic mechanism regulating marital or family transactions.[71]

A basic tenet of strategic therapy is that therapeutic change comes about through the "interactional processes set off when a therapist intervenes actively and directively in particular ways" in a family or marital system.[61, p. 7] The therapist works to substitute new behavior patterns or sequences for the vicious, positive feedback circles already existing.[188] In other words, his goal is to *change the dysfunctional sequence of behaviors* shown by the family appearing for treatment. Some primary techniques are listed.

1. The main therapeutic tools are *tasks and directives.* In fact, this emphasis on directives is the cornerstone of the approach.

2. The problem must be put in solvable form. It should be something that can be objectively agreed upon, that is, counted, observed, or measured, so that one can assess if it has actually been influenced.

3. Considerable emphasis is placed in *extrasession change*—altering the processes occurring outside of the session.

4. Power struggles with the family are generally avoided, the tendency being to take the path of least resistance and use implicit or indirect ways of turning the family's investment to positive use.[188] In fact, the development of techniques for dealing with resistance constitutes one of the foremost contributions of the strategic approach.

5. "Paradoxical" interventions are common and may be directed toward the whole family or to certain members. This category encompasses more than simply "prescribing the symptom," and may also include strategies outlined by Rohrbaugh *et al.*[121] such as "restraining" (discouraging or denying the possibility of change), and "positioning" (i.e., exaggerating a family's

position, for instance by becoming more pessimistic than they are). In a sense, the therapist becomes more homeostatic than the family and "turns their resistance back on itself."[159, 162]

The strategic approach developed by Jay Haley is the one most germane to our work with addicts. It was originally developed with families of young schizophrenics. However, we felt that of the various symptom groups, schizophrenics' families came closest to addicts' families (but not necessarily families of adolescent drug abusers) in the ways that they functioned and in the skill that they applied in resisting change. Thus, in scanning the approaches that were in use when we began our work, Haley's model came closer to meeting our needs than most others.

Of the various strategic approaches, Haley's model shares the greatest number of common elements with structural therapy. This is not surprising, since Haley worked with Minuchin and they influenced each other in the development of structural family therapy. In particular, both approaches place considerable emphasis on hierarchical family organization, noting that aberrant hierarchies (such as cross-generational coalitions) are frequently diagnostic of family dysfunction.

In an earlier publication[167, pp. 58-60] we presented a synopsis, by Haley, of his approach with disturbed young people. It is condensed from his book *Leaving Home*[66] and is reprinted here.*

> There are certain assumptions that improve the chance of success with young adults who exhibit mad and bizarre behavior, or continually take illegal drugs, or who waste their lives and cause community concern. For therapy, it is best to assume that the problem is not the young person but a problem of a family and young person disengaging from one another. Ordinarily, an offspring leaves home by succeeding in work or school and forming intimate relationships outside the family. In some families, when a son or daughter begins to leave home, the family becomes unstable and in distress. If at that point the young person fails by becoming incapacitated, the family stablizes as if the offspring has not left home. This can happen even if the young person is living away from home, as long as he or she regularly lets the family know that failure continues. It can also exist even if the family is angry at the offspring and appears to have rejected him. Family stability continues as long as the young person is involved with the family by behaving in some abnormal way.

*Reprinted with permission from Gardner Press.

A therapist should assume that, if the family organization does not change, the young person will continue to fail year after year, despite therapy efforts. The unit with the problem is not the young person, but at least two other people: these might be two parents, or a mother and boyfriend or sibling, or a mother and grandmother. It is assumed that two adults in a family communicate with each other by way of the young person and they enter severe conflict if the young person is not available to be that communication vehicle. The therapy goal is to free the young adult from that triangle so that he or she lives like other normal young people and the family is stable without the problem child.

This therapy and its premises have no relation to a therapy based on the theory of repression where an individual is the problem. Therefore, there is no concern with insight or awareness and there is no encouragement of people to express their feelings with the idea that this will cause change. Therapists accustomed to experiential groups or psychodynamic therapy have difficulty with this approach.

The therapy should occur in the following stages.

1. When the young person comes to community attention, the experts must organize themselves in such a way that one therapist takes responsibility for the case. It is better not to have a team or a number of separate therapists or modes of therapy. The one therapist must be in charge of whether the young person is to be in or out of an institution and what medication is to be given, and when. Only if the therapist is in charge of the case can he put the parents in charge within the family.

2. The therapist needs to gather the family for a first interview. If the young person is living separately, even with a wife, he should be brought together with the family of origin so that everyone significant to him is there. The goal is to move the young person to more independence, either alone or with a wife, but the first step to that end is to take him back to his family.

There should be no blame of the parents, but instead, the parents (or parent and grandmother, or whomever it might be) should be put in charge of solving the problem of the young person. They must be persuaded that they are really the best therapists for the problem offspring (despite past failures in trying to help him). It is assumed that the members of the family are in conflict and the problem offspring is expressing that. By requiring the family to take charge and set the rules for the young person, they are communicating about the young person, as usual, but in a positive way. Certain issues need to be clear.

a. The focus should be on the problem person and his

behavior, not on a discussion of family relations. If the offspring is an addict, the family should focus on what is to happen if he ever takes drugs again; if mad and misbehaving, what they will do if he acts bizarrely in the way that got him in the hospital before. If anorectic, how much weight she is to gain per day, and how that is to be accomplished.

b. The past, and past causes of the problem, are ignored and not explored. The focus is what to do now.

c. The therapist should join the parents against the problem young person, even if this seems to be depriving him of individual choices and rights, and even if he seems too old to be made that dependent. After the person is behaving normally, his rights can be considered. It is assumed that the hierarchy of the family is in confusion. Should the therapist step down from his status as expert and join the problem young person against the parents, there will be worse confusion and the therapy will fail.

d. Conflicts between the parents or other family members are ignored and minimized even if they bring them up, until the young person is back to normal. If the parents say they have problems and need help too, the therapist should say the first problem is the son, and their problems can be dealt with after the son is back to normal.

e. Everyone should expect the problem person to become normal, with no suggestion that the goal is a handicapped person. Therefore, the young person should not be in a halfway house, a day hospital, kept on medication or on maintenance methadone. Normal work or school should be expected immediately, not later. Work should be self-supporting and real, not volunteer.

3. As the problem young person becomes normal (by achieving self-support, or successfully going to school, or by making close friends) the family will become unstable. This is an important stage in the therapy and the reason for pushing the young person toward normality. The parents will threaten separation or divorce or one or both will be disturbed. At that point, a relapse of the young person is part of the usual pattern, since that will stabilize the family. If the therapist has sided with the parents earlier, they will lean upon him at this stage and the young adult will not need to relapse to save them. The therapist must either resolve the parental conflict, or move the problem young person out of it while it continues more directly. At that point, the young person can continue to be normal.

4. The therapy should be an intense involvement and a rapid

disengagement, not regular interviews over years. As soon as positive change occurs, the therapist can begin to recess and plan termination. The task is not to resolve all family problems but the ones around the problem young person, unless the family wants to make a new contract for other problems.

5. Regular follow-ups should be done to ensure that positive change continues.


## A STRUCTURAL–STRATEGIC APPROACH TO DRUG ABUSE

This section covers the principal elements of our model.* We use the term "structural–strategic" because we drew from the predominent practices of both these approaches, in addition to introducing some distinctive features of our own.† The general thrust is strategic, but many of the moment-to-moment or "micromoves" within sessions are of a more structural nature. In other words, the broad strokes tend to be strategic and the brushwork structural, with the single exception of the regular use throughout of "noble ascriptions" (a description of which follows). More specifically, the procedure is to (1) apply Minuchin's structural theory as a guiding paradigm; (2) work structurally within sessions through the actual enactment of new patterns, and the application of structural techniques such as joining, accommodating, testing boundaries, restructuring, and so forth; (3) apply Haley's strategic model in terms of its emphasis on a specific plan, extrasession events, change in the symptom, collaboration among treatment systems, and the like.‡

This therapy is goal-oriented and short-term. One advantage of a brief therapy model is that it catalyzes and compresses into a time

---

*Portions of the remainder of this chapter are excerpted from an earlier publication by the authors entitled "Structural Family Therapy with Drug Addicts," in E. Kaufman and P. Kaufmann (Eds.), *Family Therapy of Drug and Alcohol Abuse.* New York: Gardner Press, 1979. Reprinted with permission.

†Subsequent to this work, a more systematic and generic structural–strategic model has been developed by Stanton. Its clinical features[158, 161] and theoretical underpinnings[162] are presented elsewhere.

‡With families of typical adolescent drug abusers the structural–strategic mix is somewhat different, with a greater emphasis on structural techniques (see Chapter 13).

span of 3 to 5 months a process that may otherwise be prolonged with no attendant increase in effectiveness. The short-term, contractural arrangement forces more rapid change. If the therapist can maintain the family as an ally in this process, the approach can be quite effective.

Unlike prevalent practices in the drug-abuse field, we put heavy and continual emphasis on *actively involving the addict's family of origin in therapy*, even if he is not living with them. Part of the rationale for this rests on a developmental framework. As discussed earlier, these families have commonly gotten stuck at the stage when it is appropriate for the IP to leave home. They have not been able to traverse this stage and instead become fixed in a cycle in which the addict either moves out and then back in, or remains inappropriately and overly tied to the family in other ways. By convening the whole family, the therapist can more easily help them to go through this correctly. In a sense, the family is being asked to return to an earlier stage that was not successfully negotiated, and to do it "right" this time. Thus parental control is reinstated and then gradually and appropriately relaxed. It should be noted that this process frequently intensifies the whole experience for the family, as members are brought closer together. Sometimes the result of this "compression"[162] is a counterreaction in which family members begin to insist on separation with much less of their previous ambivalence. During this period the therapist should attempt to prevent the process from running its usual course by slowing it down and planning the IP's departure carefully; an example of such a strategy is given in Chapter 7.

It has become clear to us that family treatment must first deal with the triad composed of addict and both parents (or parent surrogates) before proceeding further. It is our experience, and that of some others,[152] that if this step is skipped, therapy will falter and possibly fail. In some cases with married addicts we started with the marital pair and found that it only served to stress or dissolve the marriage; thus, the addict would end up back with his parents. However, families differ in the ease with which the transition from family of origin to family of procreation can be made. Sometimes the parents can be eased out of the picture (or, as in Chapter 10, their involvement reduced) within a few sessions, while other cases may require that they be involved throughout treatment. The key is to *start with the parent–addict triad and to move away from it in accordance with the parents' readiness to release the addict.*

We attempt to include all siblings living at home or in the immediate vicinity. The rule of thumb is to see how family members interact before concluding that any member is not needed in the sessions. Certainly absent siblings can behave homeostatically and undercut in-session accomplishments, and we consider it important both to get direct input from them and to gain some control over their interferences. For example, it is not uncommon for a male addict to have a powerful older sister who acts as a kind of mother surrogate. Agreements or contracts negotiated in the session, but without her concurrence, probably would stand a slim chance of success.

On the other hand, siblings may serve a number of functions in the sessions. They may act as allies to the addict and help to get him to assert himself more appropriately. Or, as in Chapter 9, they can be rallied to strengthen the position of a parent who is taking an appropriate stand. Often they provide a useful alternative focus and prevent exclusive attention from being given to the addict. It is not unusual to find siblings who are also addicted or have problems as severe as those of the addict (e.g., the case in Chapter 12). Finally, siblings always provide additional data on family interactions, which the therapist may use to advantage.

From the above it may be clear why we place such inordinate emphasis on family recruitment and engaging members in therapy, as outlined in Chapter 3, 4, and 5. Because the drug taking of the IP is so intimately a part of the interactional behavior of the whole family, a therapist who does not have direct access to other family members operates at a severe disadvantage. In addition, efforts by members to control session attendance are usually attempts to resist change,[140] so decisions as to who should or should not attend therapy are best made by the therapist, not the family.

It would not be accurate to view our treatment approach as always limited just to the addict and his immediate family. This may be the primary system involved, but other interpersonal systems are also engaged, as appropriate. We deal with them if they are particularly relevant to the case and can serve to facilitate or hinder therapeutic progress. Such systems might include friends, important relatives, vocational counselors, employers, school or legal authorities, and, of course, the staff of the drug-treatment program itself. The interfaces among these systems are discussed at greater length later in the chapter.

## DRUG ISSUES

There are, of course, distinctive aspects to undertaking therapy within the addiction field. Dependency on chemicals—either physiological or "psychological"—is the prime one, along with the "craving" that is frequently reported to accompany it. Further, addicts are commonly involved in a drug subculture with their peers and use a unique language, much like the subcultures that develop in street gangs. In addition, because they use substances that are normally illegal, addicts often become involved in criminal behavior, in many cases spending periods of their lives incarcerated.*

Our general tendency in addressing the above features of addiction is to respect them as valid. They are both true—at least at some level of interpretation—and an integral part of the addiction tradition. On the other hand, we consider it prudent not to be too easily seduced by these notions, because they can readily be embraced by clients and families as reasons not to change. For instance, one of the favorite (mythical) arguments for not detoxifying rapidly from narcotics is the supposedly hellish experience it engenders, a notion that has been fostered by the media. From this view, only a sadistic therapist would suggest such a course of action. On the other hand, Milton Erickson noted years ago that heroin addicts undergoing detoxification only complained when someone else was nearby who could provide an audience. The truth of the matter is that, while rapid detoxification from barbiturates and some other drugs may indeed be life-threatening, detoxification from most levels of opioids is an uncomfortable experience—much like influenza—but hardly hellish.[73] Consequently, while we tend not to engage in direct controversy with a family on such issues, we do try to keep such notions in perspective and to note when they are possibly being used as ploys of resistance.

While the bulk of the material in this volume deals with narcotics addicts, we do not believe that the principles set forth are necessarily limited only to this group. Many of them apply to abusers of other psychotropic substances and, as Haley[66] emphasizes, even to other symptom groups at similar life cycle stages. Also, they may have utility with other families with a young substance abuser who has not progressed to the point of narcotic addiction, but would eventually

---

*Appreciation is extended to John M. Van Deusen for outlining the factors presented in this paragraph.

end up that way if the process were not interrupted (see Chapter 13). Finally, while opiate addicts are perhaps the most intractable of drug abusers, we believe that if a therapist can develop competence in effectively treating *these* cases, families with other, less entrenched drug problems will be comparatively easy.

## NOBLE ASCRIPTIONS

Anyone working with addicts' families for the first time is impressed with the tremendous defensiveness that most of them show. It sometimes seems as if they are just waiting for the therapist to cast even a minor aspersion so they can protest (or perhaps abort therapy prematurely). Consequently, the kinds of confrontation techniques that may be useful in group therapy with drug abusers generally do not work with their families. Instead, such approaches tend to foster massive family resistance and counterattack, rendering the therapist impotent and denying him control of the therapy.

The tendency of therapists who treat families strategically is generally to ascribe positive motives to clients. Again, this is primarily because blaming, criticism, and negative terms tend to mobilize resistance, as family members muster their energies to disown the pejorative label. This applies both in therapy and in recruiting members for therapy (Chapter 5). Consequently, the therapist might, for example, relabel "hostile" behavior as "concerned interest"[88] or as "a desire to get the best care possible" for the IP. This approach has a paradoxical flavor, as the family finds that its efforts to fight are redefined.[59] It is also a form of reframing[141] and of joining.[100] Another facet of this approach is that simply defining problems as interactional or familial stumbling blocks serves to have them viewed as *shared*, rather than loading the blame entirely on one or two members—that is a "we're all in this together" phenomenon.[187]

In his initial work with addicts' families in the early 1970s, the first author (Stanton) noted their tendency toward defensiveness and decided to develop ways to counter it. He was partly influenced in this effort by Ivan Boszormenyi-Nagy. Boszormenyi-Nagy often succeeds in defusing families by pointing out to them that their behavior is adaptive for the family group across generations; members are thus, in a sense, fulfilling a script and are absolved of blame. They are functioning as loyal family members. However, Boszormenyi-Nagy does not use such ascriptions for effect, but because he truly believes them. Our own position is less focused on the validity of the interpretation (although we do not deny it), as much as it is focused on pragmatic effectiveness—whether or not it reduces defensiveness and resistance and paves the way for other, more direct interventions.

The use of a nonblaming stance, that is the avoidance of pejoratives, is not a new addition to the field of family therapy. Erickson, Haley, the MRI group, Minuchin, L'Abate,[87] and others have been applying it for some time. However, we are referring here to the practice of taking it a step further and assuming—or at least conveying to the family—that "everything that everybody does is for good reason and is understandable." This applies to even the most "destructive" of their behaviors.[146] We have termed such therapeutic moves as *ascribing noble intentions*," or "*noble ascriptions*."* This is not to say that we do not challenge families, but that we often try to express our points in nonpejorative ways that allow therapy to proceed more smoothly and rapidly.

The ascription of noble intentions is an effective way for the therapist to enlist parents as his allies. This is important, because parents seem to be among the most sensitive of family members to being blamed for the addict's problems. We might tell a mother, "You are just being a good mother," or, "*Nobody* could care more about their son than you do—more parents should feel this way," or "You didn't tell your husband about your son's stealing because you cared about him and didn't want to upset him." A father might be praised with, "People probably don't realize how concerned you are about your son, that you really care about him," or, "You got angry with your son because you truly want him to grow up right and you know he needs to be taught a lesson so he can get on the right track," or, "You hit your wife because maybe that was the only way you could impress upon her how important this thing is to you—the only way you could be sure she heard you."

Often we address an addict son in terms of the sacrifice he is making. We might say, "You're defending your family like any good, loyal son would," or, "I guess people don't realize how much you care about your family—how much you think about them every day," or, "I

---

*Among the clinicians involved in the program, the two authors and, perhaps, Samuel M. Scott, have been the most likely to employ the technique of noble ascriptions. Later, it was learned that a somewhat similar approach had been adopted by the Milan group,[135] who termed it "positive connotation." Soper and L'Abate[141] subsequently coined the more generic term, "positive interpretation."

know your father doesn't like to worry, but when you get into trouble it does give him a way to show his concern and to occupy his thoughts until a job comes through for him."

Sometimes it is most effective to use an ascription that encompasses subsystems or the whole family, thus placing the problem in a larger, or "meta," context. For instance, if it is revealed and emphasized by a family that the father has a drinking problem, the therapist might state directly to the addict (and indirectly to the father and the rest of the family), "By taking drugs you are letting people know you don't want to be better than your father, or show him up. If you weren't hooked he would be the only one in the family with a problem, and that might not be fair. In a way, you and Dad can be sort of close, because you each use something a lot—you know, 'Like father, like son.' Your being on drugs is a kind of way of telling your dad he isn't such a bad guy and you want to be like him, at least a little bit." Such an ascription could serve, structurally, to connect father and son while not disparaging the commonality that they share, that is, substance abuse.

We also make use of noble ascriptions that speak to the family tradition. One such might be, "This family has had drinkers for generations. Grandad was a heavy drinker; so was Great-uncle Harry and Dad's brother, Jim. Mom's stepfather used to drink a lot, too. This family has had a tradition of rough-and-ready guys who may have drunk too much, but it was part of being a man. And the women in the family always took good care of their men, too. They understood. So now, Joe is using drugs instead of liquor because drugs are more popular these days. He is being loyal and keeping the tradition."

Sometimes the best ascriptions are the most metaphorical. When arriving at an ascription we suggest that the therapist attempt to put himself not only in a nonjudgmental frame of mind, but also in a very positive one, so he can come up with a benevolent rationale. Thinking thoughts of "beauty," "sacrifice," or "wonderfulness" may help, as well as imagining scenes in which these qualities or tones prevail. Such a cognitive "set" or mood will also permit access to one's more creative side, making the emergence of a noble metaphor more likely.

It is perhaps ironic that a family's or a member's response to a noble ascription is so often one of acceptance or agreement. Commonly, family members truly *believe* they are being sacrificial and are relieved that an outsider can recognize it. They see themselves as unappreciated and beset by difficulties at the same time that they are engaging in behaviors that they view as being in the service of their loved ones; they have felt unfairly blamed and may have been reacting either with anger or hopelessness. The therapist's acknowledgment of their noble intentions—an extreme form of joining—can have the effect of "freeing them" (through his consensual validation and approval) and making them more amenable to his subsequent interventions. A greater sense of trust can be established (see Chapter 12).

Obviously, noble ascriptions have a paradoxical flavor to them. However, they are not the same as prescribing the symptom—the kind of tack usually associated with paradoxical interventions. In fact, we do not apply more conventional paradoxical techniques with any regularity when working with addicts' families.* We feel that Haley's[66] general cautions about the use of paradoxical interventions also apply to their use with families of this type. There are several reasons for our position: first, these families are extremely skillful and may foil any but the most experienced therapist in the ways they react to the paradox. Second, there are obvious ethical and legal problems in prescribing that an addict take more drugs. Third, paradoxical injunctions are not advisable during times of crisis,[112, 121, 159, 189] and the majority of these families enter treatment in a crisis and may have additional crises at different points in therapy.

While the ascription of noble intentions is portrayed here only with addicts' families, it is obviously applicable to other symptom groups as well. In fact, both of us frequently employ it with a wide variety of cases in our clinical practices.

## GOALS OF FAMILY TREATMENT

It is best to negotiate the goals for therapy with the family at the very outset of treatment. This is because (1) it provides family members with the sense that treatment will have direction, rather than wandering about aimlessly or having as an endpoint the uncovering of personal pain or feelings; (2) it indicates to them that they may get some return for their efforts, that their energies will not be expended fruitlessly; (3) they can take some satisfaction that the therapist at least seems to know what he is doing, thus possibly instilling in them a sense of hope. All of these features serve to both increase the

---

*Indeed, Chapter 10 presents a case example in which a paradoxical prescription for the couple to fight more often did not have a satisfactory effect.

therapist's leverage and keep the family coming to therapy. A therapy that has no goals, or loses sight of its goals, will be quickly abandoned by addicts' families.

It is also wise to prioritize the goals for therapy. We routinely establish three goals in the following order of priority:

1. Drug usage. The IP will be free of use of both illegal and legal drugs, such as methadone.
2. Productive use of time. The IP will be either gainfully employed (volunteer activities are not acceptable) or involved in some kind of school or training program.
3. Stable and autonomous living situation. If the IP lives with his parents, he will move out and live alone or with a spouse, paramour, or friend.

The above priority ordering is employed partly because it is one most acceptable to families. Usually they appear for treatment because of the IP's drug use. Consequently, they are unlikely to accept a treatment in which, for example, the first priority is that their abusing member move out of the home; they did not come with such a goal in mind and may even consider it superfluous.

In the Addicts and Families Program (AFP) therapists tended to establish at least the first goal and to work on the others more or less in respective order. (It is not always necessary, at the outset, to establish a series of several goals with the family, since a single goal provides adequate justification for therapy to proceed.) Since we were operating within a 10-session limit, we did not always succeed in accomplishing all three goals, depending on the specific situation and "readiness" of a particular family. With some families all were reached, and with others progress was made perhaps only toward elimination or reduction of drug usage.*

Since the use of drugs by the IP is usually the primary issue for therapy with families of addicts, it is best to ask in the first session (or no later than the second), "When is he going to detoxify?" The detoxification can be from a legal drug, such as methadone, or from

*Of course, any given goal can be used as the vehicle for structural change in the family. The discussion here refers more to the content for justifying change rather than the process.

illegal drugs, but it is necessary to get this issue on the docket as early as possible.* Then a process of negotiation can be started as to a date for detoxification and how the family is to prepare for it.

Often questions arise about the feasibility of having the addict become totally drug-free. We have found it critical for the therapist to be committed to this goal and to recognize that as long as the addict is on any drugs, including methadone, he is still labeled as an addict and the basic situation is unchanged (see Chapter 1). It is tempting to think of an addict as similar to a diabetic, implying that he will always need methadone. It is Haley's experience that working from such a model with schizophrenics almost never leads to cure.† Similarly, the therapist working with an addict is hopelessly hamstrung if he sees his job as helping the family to cope with a handicapped person suffering from an inherently chronic, incurable condition.

It needs to be underscored that the goals are negotiated with the family rather than being foisted upon them by the therapist. Thus the agreed-upon goal must be one that makes sense to them. This process begins by first assessing the priorities and competencies of the client and family, then reaching closure on a realistic and achievable goal. Although the therapist recognizes that the family may be ambivalent about a goal, he seeks to have the goal stated publicly in order to urge the family to action and, in a sense, to call their bluff. If, however, a family is extremely resistant at the outset to the idea of having the IP get off drugs (including methadone), the therapist might be better advised to postpone family treatment and obtain an agreement with them to reconvene when they have decided they do not want an addicted member. Otherwise, the purpose of therapy becomes unclear and the chances for retention of the family in therapy and for any real change are very slight.

Once an agreement has been reached about goals for the IP's drug use, family members may raise other issues or problems. As noted in Chapter 4, some other, crisis-laden issue may even underlie the addict's move to initiate treatment (e.g., he might be about to get married). While these problems may be real, they should be regarded

---

*As mentioned in Chapter 2, in the earlier phases of this work we tended to postpone this rather pointed question, sometimes until midtherapy. As we developed and refined our methods we approached the detoxification issue more immediately and directly.

†Jay Haley (personal communication, January 1981).

as red herrings by the therapist—as ways of pulling therapy off track and diverting its thrust. Thus the therapist should question their relevance and require that the members who raise them justify their pertinence to the primary goal. (For example, a discussion of the addict's getting a job would only be considered appropriate if it were seen as important in keeping him off drugs.) The general rule is for the therapist to *keep sessions focused on drug use until stable improvement has been achieved.*

It is crucial that the therapist form an alliance with both parents or parent surrogates in this stage so that they may take an effective stance toward the addict around the chosen goal. The therapist must keep the parents working *together* in the early phases, even siding with them against the addict upon occasion. Sometimes therapists, especially young therapists, are uncomfortable in treating a young adult in this manner. For example, such a therapist might feel uneasy suggesting that the parents negotiate a time when their 27-year-old son should be in the house and off the streets in the evening. What one finds, however, is that the IP is often surprisingly cooperative, even though he may protest the fact that he is being treated as a child. This cooperation can be explained as gratitude in many cases. The addict is secretly grateful for the fact that the parents' relationship is being attended to by the therapist. In general, it is very difficult for the addict to significantly improve his situation and remain that way unless there appears to be some tangible evidence that the therapist is addressing the needs of the parental subsystem.

If freedom from drug taking has been maintained for a month or more, it may be possible to shift emphasis to other treatment goals. Two common ones have been mentioned—gainful employment or schooling and getting the addict out of the home. Underlying both topics are issues of separation—either physical separation or separation through increased competence and the resulting independence of functioning. The therapist should be sensitive to the meaning of such separations for the family and restructure therapeutically in such a way that alternative supports are provided for members who are likely to feel the greatest loss.

Similarly, as progress occurs in all the goals relating to the addict, it becomes possible for the therapist to move flexibly toward dealing with other family issues. As is amply demonstrated in succeeding chapters, such a broadening of goals is important at this stage of therapy, whereas it would have been inappropriate in the initial, acute phase of treatment.

## FOCUSING ON CONCRETE BEHAVIOR

Both Minuchin[100] and Haley[65, 66] emphasize the importance of keeping the therapy focused upon concrete, observable behavior. This emphasis is particularly crucial in working with addicts and their families, since addicts can be especially slippery and difficult to pin down. Similarly, family members often *appear* to be in agreement until an attempt is made to get consensus on specific details, at which point hidden disagreements usually surface.

It is most important to have the parents and the rest of the family focus on "house rules," particularly rules dealing with drug-related behavior. The therapist should also help them to focus on positive, achievable goals, such as specific steps the IP might take in looking for a job.

These rules and positive goals should be negotiated in the session, so that the therapist can observe the behavior during the negotiation process and intervene to increase the likelihood of a successful outcome. Often the agreement will include specific "homework" tasks that stem from session interaction but are performed during the interval between sessions. If resistance in the family is high, the therapist may want to assign tasks that are small and almost unchallengeable (see Chaper 12), such as having the IP look up two jobs or two apartments in the classified section of the newspaper. It is ideal for the parents to participate in these tasks, so that they feel some sense of participation in the IP's eventual success.

One type of specific behavior that has been especially important in our work has been the results of weekly urine tests. They give a tangible indication of progress and do not allow family members (or the therapist) to sidestep this issue. They can also serve as aids in getting the family to take responsibility and put pressure on the IP to remain clean. It usually helps to negotiate the criteria for failure with the family at the outset of treatment. The idea is to get advance agreement that they will believe the urine tests. If the addict protests that someone has switched or will switch urine samples with him, the therapist should get the rest of the family to agree on the number of times they will accept this story before they can finally trust the urinalysis results.

## OBSERVING SEQUENCES AND "ENACTMENT" DURING SESSIONS

Haley[65] has placed particular stress on the importance of symptoms in regulating sequences of behavior in the family. As described in Chapter 1, drug taking and related behaviors often occur in response to parental conflict and have the function of pulling the parents back together. The symptomatic behavior of other family members (parents, siblings, grandparents) also has an important regulatory function in these sequences. For example, a mother's depression may serve as a signal that her son has become too independent, or the father may begin to complain about heart pains when conflict becomes too extreme.

It is best for the therapist to be able to observe these sequences *directly in the session.* Videotape is invaluable in this effort, since subtle signals can trigger almost instantaneous changes. Actual drug taking in sessions is rare, but there are frequent examples of drug-related behavior. This includes various forms of acting out, such as impulsive, angry outbursts, leaving the sessions, or threats of shooting up heroin. Equally important is acting incompetent (i.e., depressed, uncommunicative, helpless) or irrelevant. Frequently, we have also noted behavior by the IP that serves to remind the family that he is a drug addict, such as nodding and scratching.

When these behaviors occur in a session, it is important to formulate hypotheses as to the function they serve in the sequence. The therapist might want to ask himself, (1) "What was happening prior to the symptom?" (watching especially for indications of parental conflict, or pressure on a parent to change); or (2) "What new pattern of behavior is produced?" Often in such instances the parents become united against the addict ("detouring attacking") or attention is diverted into a familiar and unproductive fight between the addict and one parent.

Information about events outside the session can be helpful in confirming and elaborating the hypothesized sequence. It is essential to collect factual data about the events both *prior to* and *following* drug episodes, since it is unusual for families to be aware of their own sequences. Once a sequence has been tentatively identified, the therapist can move in the session to block its usual run. For example, he can elicit parental conflict and then prevent the addict from interrupting and diverting the parents' attention. Finally, as Hoffman[68] notes, all aspects of the repetitive sequence may not have to be shifted, but only enough of them to cause the symptom to disappear.

It needs to be emphasized that this therapy is concerned with the repetitive interactional patterns that *maintain* the drug taking. *The thrust of treatment is to alter these sequences.* Although it is interesting to speculate about the etiology of drug abuse, it is our experience that historical data are generally of very little utility in actually bringing about change.

## RESTRUCTURING

The most basic restructuring move in this therapy—and one emphasized repeatedly in this volume—is to get the parents or parent surrogates to work together vis-à-vis the addict. If this is not done, the basic triadic conflictual pattern between the IP and parents will persist and treatment will probably fail.

In addition to obtaining parental consensus on goals, there are other restructuring moves that can be implemented, often concomitantly. A number of these are demonstrated in the succeeding chapters. Usually they are used as intermediate moves en route to getting the parents to work together more directly. For instance, Haley[66] (see also Chapter 7) and the Milan group[136] often have parents alternate in taking responsibility for the problem person; for example, each parent takes charge for a given period such as a week, or they rotate between odd and even days during the same week. We have not applied this method with any regularity in our work with addicts' families, but it is an option worthy of further exploration.

In cases where, for example, a mother and son are overinvolved, a common strategy is to get the father to take charge of the son (see Chapters 7 and 10). This requires that father and son relate differently in some way, and such an experience must usually be engineered *within a session* before it can be generalized to the home situation. It may be possible to get them engaged in discussing some common interest, such as work, fishing, and so forth. The mother should be present during this exchange and may need the therapist's subtle support while her husband and son are engaged. For instance, the therapist might sit next to her, keep her from interfering in the father–son interaction, and quietly comfort her with statements such as, "They need this [talking together]," or, "You know, you are right. They don't get enough time to talk together as father and son."

Other tactics may also be used, depending on the specific clinical situation. When it appears that the mother endorses the drug behavior of the IP, with the father consistently more punitive, it may be possible to force the mother to deal with the negative behavior of the abuser, thus breaking the alliance with him. Alternatively, the therapist may meet only with the parents to formulate a strategy to which both parents will adhere.

Another approach is to shift the roles of the parents to, for example, either those of grandparents (rather than overinvolved parents), or of parents to any younger children they might have ("You can let him go because you have these other kids to worry about"). Further, if the parents are retired or near retirement (Chapter 11), the therapist may want to work with them on planning this stage of their lives.

Because of the nature of the AFP research design, most of our work has been with families in which two adults of different sex were involved, either as parents or in quasi-parental roles. In cases where only one parent is available—usually the mother—the process differs somewhat.[100] Here, the therapist may temporarily have to fill a parental role toward the IP, and at other times must assume an almost spouse-like role toward the parent. Often the latter is a way of substituting for the pseudospouse role that has been played by the abuser. The next step is to develop alternative structures and supports for the parent through inclusion of relatives, friends, and so on—in other words, to establish or strengthen the natural support system. In this way the parent will be less dependent on the IP and able to move toward greater disengagement, while the therapist will also be able to gradually disengage. When applicable, another approach is to help the parent get a job or develop more outside activities. Still another, stated above, is to transfer some of the attention from the IP to any younger siblings remaining in the family. Again, joining with the parent is a crucial part of the process, and under no conditions should the therapist become engaged in a direct power struggle with the parent over separation with the IP.

## HANDLING CRISES

In many addicts' families, crises are a way of life. It sometimes seems as if they would be unhappy if they did not have a periodic crisis to activate them. They appear to swing from one crisis to the next as a way of charting and maintaining their lives, just as Tarzan swings through the jungle from one supportive vine to another. It is therefore not surprising that a family crisis can be anticipated as change starts to occur in therapy and the addict stops or curtails his drug taking. This is probably a necessary feature of change (see Chapter 8). *It can be expected to occur 3 or 4 weeks into treatment.** Most commonly, it will revolve around the parents' marital relationship, with them talking about, or taking steps toward, separation or divorce. This puts tremendous pressure on the abuser to become dirty again in order to reunite his family. At such times, the therapist will need to devote considerable time and energy to resolving the crisis in a different way than has occurred in the past. He will have to be accessible and perhaps constantly on call. His goal is to get the parents to hold together in relation to the IP and not let them separate, at least until this storm is weathered. If the transition is handled skillfully, treatment is usually on the way to a successful outcome, for succeeding crises will be easier for the family to cope with; a previously recurrent pattern has been broken and real change has occurred.

The therapist wants to *contain the crisis within the family,* preventing matters from getting out of control and avoiding spillover into other systems. At such times it is best to avoid steps that take the pressure off the family, particularly hospitalization, increasing medications such as methadone, or kicking the IP out of the home precipitously. This is partly because the therapist and family rarely have major input or control in these other contexts, including the context of the peer or drug subculture. Their ability to manage or intervene in these social systems is minimal. Equally important, the family of origin is the strongest and most logical support system for dealing with such crises. The IP is one of their own, they have likely had to deal with his crises in the past, and they are usually more motivated to be involved this time. Therefore, it behooves the therapist to mobilize the family around the crisis and put them to work to resolve it.

An additional benefit of generating a crisis is that it brings about a situation in which individuals and systems are more amenable to change.[66] Times of crisis are pivotal points at which the system can move radically in either a functional or a dysfunctional direction. The

---

*In the AFP, we found such crises to be so predictable that we designed much of our program around them (e.g., by not having a therapist commence therapy with a new case if he were to be away during the third or fourth week).

key factor here is that movement is more possible at such times, allowing the therapist maximal influence.

## GENERATING CRISES

As noted, it is usually not difficult to generate a crisis with an addict's family. Often it can be done through simple structural moves made within sessions (as, for example, in the case presented in Chapter 7). In other cases a crisis may have already been building at the time of intake (see Chapter 4). However, some addicts' families are too staid and entrenched for this to happen readily. The evidence presented in Chapter 8 indicates that a crisis is usually necessary for beneficial change to occur, so the therapist may instead have to intentionally induce a crisis in immovable families of this type.[102] As exemplified in Chapter 9, this may be done by increasing intensity, unbalancing, and essentially pushing a family hard within a session. The resulting increase in emotion, with its attendant interactions, can then be managed by the therapist while he is present. Again, it is not necessary to do this with the majority of addicts' families—since milder restructuring will suffice to induce a crisis in most cases—but only in those in which no movement or change is taking place.

### Home Detoxification

When an addict is detoxified in a hospital, or in some other setting external to the family, his family members usually deny any responsibility if the attempt fails or is not sustained. They foist their addicted member on the treatment system and then abdicate responsibility by stating, in effect, to the detox program, "You undertook it. We had nothing to do with it. If it failed it's your fault, not ours." Thus staff in the treatment program, having accepted this yoke, end up feeling responsible, even if the family actively worked to undercut their efforts either during or after the detoxification.

We feel this situation is severely flawed and is exactly the opposite of what it should be. It is the *family* that has been rearing and maintaining this addict, not the treatment program. We believe the family should be the system that shoulders primary responsibility for turning the situation around. What is needed, then, is a treatment paradigm that helps families to feel more competent to change their patterns and to care for their own. One possible approach is to detoxify the addict in the home.

Home detoxification is a kind of planned crisis induction.* It is also a logical extension of the notion of containing the crisis within the family. In this approach family members essentially take charge of the detoxification process within their own home. Chapter 12 presents case material and some elements of a paradigm for carrying it out. The aim is to have the family help the addict detoxify "cold turkey." Instead of entering a hospital, or engaging in the time-honored method of detoxifying amid friends, the addict undertakes it within his family and home setting. While it is better that the detoxification be from heroin or another illegal opiate rather than methadone (since symptoms with the former are more acute and therefore more crisis-like) it can also be done easily from a dosage of, for example, 20 mg of methadone, or even higher.[73]

In planning a home detoxification, the therapist negotiates with the family when this should occur. Commonly, a particular weekend is chosen. A round-the-clock monitoring or "watch" schedule is established that specifies which members are to spend which time periods with the addict. The therapist should also plan to be available 24 hours himself during the period, and to make home visits when possible.

Planning a home detoxification additionally requires that the therapist anticipate problems ahead of time with the family, such as the addict getting out of the house, a sibling or friend bringing him drugs, parents relaxing their vigilance, and so forth. The therapist asks them, "What can possibly go wrong?" Once all the foreseeable contingencies are discussed, it may be wise for the therapist to finalize the planning by making a sort of paradoxical statement, such as, "Well, we've anticipated a lot of things, but we can't think of everything. It's very possible that someone will come up with a problem that we haven't thought of. This is a tough thing to do, and you can expect that at some point something will happen to make it tougher." With this blanket statement he covers all possible resistance moves by the family. He may also rob such moves of their sting, since they are less unexpected and are also not being condemned by him.

It may also be wise for the therapist to negotiate a contract beforehand to undertake the process a second time, in case the first attempt fails; if the family members know they might have to go through it twice, they are more likely to succeed the first time. On the other hand, since they themselves are now involved in the process, if

*We are indebted to Jay Haley for first suggesting the idea of home detoxification.

the attempt fails they are not going to take subsequent drug use by the addict so lightly. They will be angry with him and may in this way be able to establish appropriate distance from him. Thus the therapist can use either success or failure of the first attempt to his (and their) advantage. Obviously a successful home detoxification has the family doing just what it should do, and getting credit for it as well. Conversely, failure can serve a disengaging function.*

There are medical precautions that must be exercised in undertaking a home detox. The addict should be screened medically to rule out certain conditions that contraindicate a rapid (cold turkey) detoxification, such as untreated coronary artery disease, uncontrolled diabetes, untreated pulmonary tuberculosis, or other severe infection. It is also necessary to have "on-call" medical backup available to therapist and family throughout the detoxification and to be aware of the closest emergency room service. In fact, knowledge that these backup systems are in line may help the family to better weather the crisis.

## DEALING WITH PARENTAL ISSUES

Although most of these families come to treatment because of their drug-abusing member, it is not uncommon for parental problems to eventually emerge in therapy. Two common ones, a parental marriage problem and heavy drinking by a parent, are discussed here.

### The Parents' Marriage

As mentioned earlier, when positive change starts to occur in the IP's use of drugs, or he stops drug taking altogether, problems in the parents' marriage are apt to come to the fore. *It is crucial at this time for the therapist to keep the parents working together and not to separate,* at least until the crisis is over. If the therapist puts stress on the marriage by addressing it directly, he increases the likelihood of their separating. Thus he should defer dealing with such marital problems—glossing over them if need be—while emphasizing teamwork and the family's working together toward a positive outcome.

*In 1980 we embarked upon a 3-year, Health, Education and Welfare-funded, controlled clinical research program on home detoxification (NIDA Grant No. RO1 DA 02124). The principles and results learned from this experience will be published at a later date, upon completion of the study.

The main idea is to continue engaging these people in their roles as *parents,* not as spouses.

The inexperienced therapist is most likely to be enticed into (prematurely) leaping to the "hot" marital issue. He tends to think, "Now we're going where the problem *really* lies." He plunges in and is then surprised when the parents or family stop coming to therapy. He fails to recognize that *what motivated these parents to engage in therapy was the problem in their son or daughter, not their own marital problem.* If they had wanted to deal with their marriage, they would have gone to a marriage counselor, but they did not do this.* Usually one or both of them is tentative or denies the marital problem; for example, in the case described in Chapter 7, the father notes a marital problem and the mother sidesteps it, at least initially. Consequently, all the therapist has to go on at this point—his primary source of leverage—is the problem of the IP. It is for this problem, and perhaps no other, that the parents will convene. Conversely, dealing too soon with their marriage usually leads to an aborted therapy— either one or both of them will terminate prematurely—and the entire treatment effort will rapidly deteriorate.

On the other hand, once the IP is stabilized and has been free of drugs for a time, it may be possible to deal with problems within the parents' marriage. Again, this applies only *after* there has been symptomatic improvement. At such a point, several things have to have happened to make a difference: (1) from a theoretical standpoint, the system must have changed in some way; (2) the parents may now possess a sense of accomplishment or even pride in having made progress; (3) they probably feel stronger in general, and perhaps more hopeful or willing to tackle their difficult marital issues; (4) usually they have a sense of being joined with the therapist and are more trusting of him, both because of the way he has supported them and because he has helped them to succeed. This last factor is critical, for, as Haley[66] notes, it is necessary for the parents to be able to lean on the therapist, rather than the IP, as they undergo the stress of dealing with their marriage.

When the focus of therapy shifts to the parental relationship, it is crucial to keep the abuser and other family members from getting involved in the parents' problems. Often the IP will attempt to reenter their relationship after he has been clean for a while, and the

*Certainly in most localities therapists and counselors who deal with marital problems are in abundance. It is rarely a case of insufficient or unavailable services.

therapist must take steps to exclude him and his siblings from the parental battles. This can be done both by blocking the intrusions of offspring during sessions and by meeting separately (or concomitantly) with the parents. The best method is for the parents themselves to resist such intrusions, so the therapist may want to structure his interventions to facilitate their efforts toward this end. If treatment can be orchestrated so that the parents vocally tell their offspring—especially the IP—to stay out of their marital discussion, an acceptable outcome can probably be expected.

## Parental Drinking

As noted earlier, in the majority of families treated within the AFP, at least one parent had a drinking problem. In such a situation, many therapists are inclined to try to deal with this problem first, or at the same time that they deal with the IP's drug abuse, under the assumption that therapeutic progress is otherwise not possible. However, it is our experience that this assumption is wrong, for several reasons. First, it must be reiterated that the parents did not come to therapy for a drinking problem in one (or both) of them; they came to help their son or daughter. To ignore this notion is to misjudge their motives and trade a clear source of therapeutic leverage for one that probably does not exist. The second reason to initially avoid focusing on parental drinking is a structural one. The therapist wants to strengthen the parents as a subsystem and to weaken intergenerational coalitions. If he starts by confronting a parent about his drinking problem, he puts that parent in a one-down and weakened position, relative both to the other parent and to the children. Often the whole family will join the therapist in this attack and the entire enterprise will develop into a kicking game against the drinker. The drinking parent is then likely to become furious, withdraw from treatment, and be henceforth unavailable. He probably thinks to himself, "I went to the session to help my son and all I get is a bunch of crap from my spouse, kids, and that therapist. Who needs it!" By allowing this to happen, the therapist has thus succeeded in turning the therapy exactly counter to its goals.

    In contrast, we recommend that the therapist devote considerable effort to joining the drinking parent—treating him with respect, noting his positive accomplishments, acknowledging his concern for the IP, soliciting his opinion, and even challenging him when he says his opinion has little value—perhaps kidding him with little remarks such as, "Don't give me that. You've been working for 27 years. You know what goes on in the outside world a lot more than anyone else in the family. I want to hear what you think about this matter." By building the drinker up to a level of parity with his spouse, and above that of his children, the therapist sets the stage for the two parents to work together and negotiate a plan for the IP. Again, he works with them in their roles as parents. Of course, he is also indirectly working on their relationship as spouses within the total system, but this is not his expressed goal.

Even when the drinking problem seems unavoidable, such as when it interferes directly in the family's plan for the IP, the therapist can deal with it in such a way that the drinker is not disparaged. For example, if a task is established for the drinker and the IP to spend an hour or so during the week engaged together in a particular activity, it may be possible to negotiate a contract with the parent to postpone his drinking for a brief period before, and also during, the activity, with the agreement that he resume drinking afterward if he feels the necessity. Or, as in Chapter 12, a contract can be drawn up in which the drinker agrees to take no alcohol during the weekend when the son undergoes home detoxification, or at least to abstain both several hours before and during his time on watch duty.

Despite the prevalence of drinking problems among parents in the AFP population, we rarely dealt with them directly, especially in the early and middle phases of therapy. The outcome data presented in Chapter 17 indicate that there may have been some merit to our position.

## SPECIAL ISSUES

### Medication and Management

In dealing with drug abuse it is helpful for the therapist to have at least a basic knowledge of drug pharmacology. This will aid him during the detoxification process and reduce the tendency toward overcaution that sometimes occurs when a therapist is ignorant of drug effects. Many family therapists are naive in this area, and if they are going to treat addiction, we recommend that they get at least brief and appropriate training or tutoring and have a consultant on hand to advise them on specific drug issues. In the AFP we provided unschooled therapists with a "crash" course when they joined the program, plus ongoing consultation from Drug Dependence Treatment Center (DDTC) personnel.

It is crucial in dealing with these cases that the family therapist have major—preferably primary—input into decisions about medications such as methadone. All changes in medication should go through him. We do not think this treatment has much chance of success without this provision.

There is a feature of the medication exercise of which the therapist must remain aware. If he chooses to negotiate increases and decreases in methadone dosage with the client and family, he is in a sense "buying into" or being inducted by the family system. He is acknowledging that the addict is powerless in the face of drugs and therefore an inherently handicapped person—a perception that the family usually shares. By discussing gradual weaning from the opioid, he confirms the family's view that the addict is helpless, fragile, and must be treated with extreme care. On the other hand, if he asserts that he is primarily concerned with the addict's detoxifying and getting off drugs, he is conveying the message that this person can be competent and can function adequately without drugs; he is challenging the family's perception. We strongly advocate that therapists adopt this second position in dealing with families of addicts.

### Control of the Case

As emphasized in Chapter 7, if the therapist is trying to shift responsibility to the family for dealing with the addict's problems, he must first have control of the case himself. This not only includes issues around medications (mentioned above), but also refers to overall case management, including the treatment plan and decisions about hospitalization. Being the primary treater also helps to avoid the kind of triangulation among treatment personnel that addicts can so readily instigate. We are essentially referring here to the structure of the whole therapeutic system and the administrative support that it provides to therapists. We estimate that roughly 50% of the effectiveness with these cases is dependent on the efficiency and cohesion of the therapeutic system; if this system is in disarray, or if it handicaps the therapist in some way, even the most superb family therapy is unlikely to be successful.

One way that we dealt with case control in the AFP was to have therapists wear two hats—that of family therapist and of drug counselor. This (administrative) move had a number of beneficial effects. It aided family recruitment, increased cost-efficiency, made crises more manageable, and clearly improved treatment effectiveness (see Chapters 5 and 16). It is our experience that without an arrangement of this sort, that is, one that gives the family therapist case control, treatment will flounder and probably fail.

## Involving Parents in Decisions

Related to the aforementioned, it should be clear that we prefer that all decisions about the addict's treatment involve his parents. This is partly for structural purposes (to get them working together) and partly because we feel the responsibility—and the caring or concern—are rightly theirs. In addition, if treatment succeeds they (instead of the therapist) will deservedly get credit for it, and will be less likely to have the addict subsequently fail as a way of unseating the therapist.[160]

In cases with a young person who takes drugs the question of responsibility often arises. Who is responsible for his drug use? Often, there is a good deal of squirming in response to this question. Conventional drug-treatment programs get around it by either taking responsibility themselves or thrusting it on the IP. However, when seen in a context where addiction serves a clear family function, the conventional view has shortcomings. It should be remembered that the addicted individual was raised by, and in most cases is still being maintained by, his family of origin. It is thus with the family that responsibility rests, and the therapist should help the family either to accept it or to effectively disengage from the addict so that he must accept it on his own.

## Length, Frequency, and Termination of Therapy

In the AFP we were required by research design to work within a 10 (weekly) session model, with some allowance for exceptions if a family was undergoing a crisis at the end of this period. We consider this model unduly constraining and do not advocate use of such a rigid paradigm. Instead, we recommend that a contract be negotiated with the family at the outset for, say, 8 to 12 sessions. This might be extended to 20 sessions with recontracting, but rarely more unless the family wants to make a new contract for other problems. Even within an 8-session program, however, it is best to space final sessions further apart (e.g., 2 to 6 weeks). An "inoculative" follow-up session should be scheduled 2 to 4 months after termination, with perhaps another 6 to 8 months after that, in order to insure the continuation of positive change and monitor continuity of care. Such a system also seems to make families less hesitant to take the initiative in re-engaging in treatment, since they know they are not committing themselves to interminable therapy if they do contact the therapist.*

Concerning termination, the establishment of a contract for a specific number of sessions helps to avoid its coming as a surprise or appearing to be too abrupt. Of course, the therapist needs to be sensitive to termination issues, and can avoid problems related to this phase, if, during treatment, he helps the family to establish appropriate natural support systems that will remain in place beyond therapy. Generally, termination difficulties will not arise if adequate change has occurred and been maintained long enough for the family to feel a sense of real accomplishment. In this way the therapist can prevent them from becoming fearful and generating crises or other problems in order to keep him involved.

In sum, a brief or time-limited, active, problem-focused therapy makes the most sense. As noted in the excerpt from Haley earlier in this chapter, rather than continual, long-term therapy over years, the treatment should follow a pattern of intense involvement and rapid disengagement, with a provision to reconvene briefly if and when appropriate at some point in the future.

### Caseload

In Chapters 14 and 15 the point is made that working with addicts' families can be both demanding and draining—especially in a brief therapy context. Consequently, while a therapist may be able to maintain many such cases for extended follow-up sessions (i.e., beyond the initial block of sessions), we do not recommend that he carry more than three or four *active* addict cases at a time, particularly while learning these techniques.

## POTENTIAL TRAPS AND PITFALLS

Many of the potential traps and pitfalls in this treatment, such as getting diverted by side issues or dealing prematurely with the parents'

---

*This model of session-spacing is extracted from an earlier publication by Stanton.[149, p. 97] marriage, have been delineated. At the risk of repetition, several of them are emphasized and embellished here.

## Avoiding Power Struggles

At all times the therapist should avoid power struggles with the family, for he will always lose in the end and treatment will falter. One way of preventing this is by going through the appropriate hierarchy—usually the parents—when moving toward change. For instance, in Chapter 10 the therapist first gets mother's tacit approval (father is not present) before challenging the addict about his continued use of illegal drugs; the therapist makes sure that mother will not oppose him on this. In Chapter 11, the therapist takes a different tack and waits the parents out; rather than goading them into taking a stance against the addict, or confronting the addict himself while the parents are still tentative, he gives the addict enough rope to hang himself—through a series of dirty urines—and lets the parents finally rise up in protest against their son's conning behavior.

Before the family becomes involved in treatment, the therapist may have to exert some effort in joining the addict on a one-to-one basis (see Chapters 3 and 4). At such times it is not usually fruitful to strongly challenge the addict about the goals of therapy or get locked in some other kind of rigid stance with him, partly because this will usually make him less willing to include his family in therapy. However, once the family is engaged, the therapist should be much more hesitant to see the addict individually, especially before progress has been made toward becoming drug-free. It is our experience that parents are usually more in favor of the addict's stopping his use of drugs and methadone than is the addict himself. Since the therapist wants them on his side and wants to shift responsibility to them, the move toward stopping drug taking will be much more potent if they (and he) unite against the addict on this issue. On the other hand, if he sees the addict individually he will not have this major source of leverage available and can be more easily drawn into a one-to-one struggle over medications, goals, and so forth. This is a divide-and-conquer move by the addict, and the therapist must remain alert and wary in order to anticipate and neutralize it.

It may help the therapist avoid the pressure to see the addict individually if he remembers that the addict's behavior is protective of the family and is not just an attempt to manipulate him. Many of the addict's actions seem to be based on the assumption that the therapist will criticize and upset other family members without accomplishing anything worthwhile. However, if the therapist is empathic to the family members, and joins well, he can obviate the family's need to be protected by the addict. In this way he nullifies many of the addict's attempts to triangulate (such as screening and distorting communications between therapist and parents, making himself overly central, etc.). He engages each member directly, making it more difficult for the addict to serve as a go-between or as defender of the status quo.

## Avoiding Increased Resistance

We have emphasized repeatedly that there must be no blame of the parents in this therapy, and that resistance can often be neutralized through noble ascriptions and, as in Chapter 12, by eliciting and gradually increasing parents' competencies. Blaming parents usually results in swift and premature termination of therapy.

A major strategy for avoiding resistance is to stick with the presenting problem. When side issues are raised by family members— as they often are—the therapist can avoid getting lost by reorienting the therapy and returning to the primary symptom. In fact, there may be points in therapy when the therapist is deluged by a flood of competing agendas from equally vocal family members. At such times the symptom may provide the only lifeline preventing him and the therapy from getting swept away.

When secondary or superfluous side issues are raised, *it is important for the therapist to raise the question, "How does this relate to his drug problem?" before the family does.* If he gets enticed into a side issue and a family member beats him to this question, he will look foolish and may lose ground in his effort to bring about change. His credibility may be questioned, resulting in erosion of their respect and slippage in his base of leverage. It should be remembered that if they entered therapy to deal with the drug problem, they will be much less cooperative with a therapist who waffles or is easily distracted from this goal.

"Spreading the problem" is another pitfall the therapist must avoid. This technique was particularly prevalent in family therapy's early days, when therapists tended to emphasize, for example, that an IP's siblings had problems, too. However, Haley[65] has cautioned against such an intervention because it usually succeeds in making the parents feel worse. They might think, "We went into therapy with one problem and we came out with *three*!" Consequently, they may end up by increasing their attack upon the IP because he has caused them to be put in a situation in which they are accused of being even more "awful" for fostering a second, or even a third, problem child. Further, spreading the problem to include a parent (e.g., for drinking too much), in addition to the IP, is also fruitless, as has been discussed earlier.

Another practice that frequently engenders resistance is when a therapist works toward developing "insight" in family members. The methods normally used to invoke insight often appear demeaning to family members, as if the therapist is trying to undress them emotionally or get inside their psyches. Thus they respond with irritation and defensiveness. Addicts' families are usually much less concerned with intellectual insight than they are in seeing the presenting problem alleviated. They cannot readily explain "why" they do things—especially the kind of "whys" that many therapists prefer. Consequently, they see this tack as a subtle form of blaming or putting them down in which the therapist, with his advanced education and "knowledge," comes across as a smarty-pants who makes them feel inadequate and guilty. Since change can come about through directly altering the family structure and sequences—much of which occurs outside the members' awareness—we do not consider insight to be a worthwhile goal. In fact, the first author (Stanton) has noted elsewhere [153, 159] that intellectual insight, if it occurs at all in therapy, not infrequently lags about 3 months behind actual change, and thus is obviously not necessary for transformation in such cases.

## DEALING WITH MULTIPLE SYSTEMS

From the foregoing—and certainly from the material to follow—it may be apparent that therapy with addicts' families often involves many systems in addition to the family system. The nature of addiction, with its attendant trappings (e.g., the drug subculture, criminality, etc.), plus the current state of the drug-abuse field, frequently culminate in a cacophony of systems resounding to the addict's situation and impacting upon it in conflicting ways. A listing of these other systems would have to include the legal system (courts, probation officers), the primary treatment system or drug program, medical or medication

systems (including unethical practitioners), backup inpatient programs (e.g., for detoxification), the welfare system, vocational and
educational programs, parental job situations, the peer group, and
intimate, extrafamilial relationships, such as when a male addict is
involved with one or more girlfriends or wives. For example, in the
case presented in Chapter 9, the therapist had to contend not only
with the family and a girlfriend, but also with an ongoing, repetitive
pattern of admissions and discharges from an inpatient detoxification
program.

The involvement of multiple systems makes this treatment more
complex than that encountered in the typical therapy situation. Further,
it is not uncommon to have to deal concomitantly with a number of
these systems under the pressure of an immediate crisis in the
family—the family problem "spills over" and engages other systems.
As a result, treatment truly becomes a therapy of *interpersonal
systems* in which the family may be the primary, but not the only,
component. This situation dictates that the therapist adopt a "meta"
view of the addict and family within their context. He must widen his
lens in order to identify the *systems of import*[158] at play and observe
their interrelating patterns. Only then will he have the information
necessary for deciding how and when to intervene, and who or what
should be included or excluded from his operations. Examples of
some of these "macro-moves" are provided at various points throughout the remainder of this volume.

### Networking

In order to counteract the cumulative negative effect of this plethora
of interacting systems, it may sometimes be advisable to mobilize
additional, constructive resources. Family "network" therapy[143] seems
to offer such potential. This approach may be particularly feasible
when the family system is in crisis and therapeutic leverage is optimal.
We have used it on a small scale in cases where we have been able to
identify resource people outside the nuclear family who could be
mobilized to help in achieving therapeutic goals. However, the more
standard network approach is to involve large numbers of people,
including relatives, friends, and neighbors. Speck and Attneave[143]
give a case example of networking with a drug abuser; approximately
50 people were involved. Callan *et al.*[21] report routine use of networks
within the context of a therapeutic community for drug abusers.

While this therapeutic modality requires a great deal of skill and energy on the part of therapists, we feel that its full potential has not yet been realized.

## Multifamily Methods

Another approach is to produce a kind of artificial network as part of the treatment program. Although less common than therapy with individual families, the practice of seeing parents or members of three or more families together has been instituted by a number of drug programs, particularly those within residential settings.[152] Usually this has taken the form either of parents' groups or of multiple family therapy (MFT). Both these multifamily methods share a common element, the establishment of a support group composed of other families with similar problems. In general, the multifamily approach has the advantage of requiring less therapist time per family. Also, the use of a support group, per se, has several added advantages: (1) it helps to reduce the massive defensiveness so characteristic of drug abusers' families; (2) similarly, it can serve as an icebreaker, introducing families to the experience of therapy, which can set the stage for more intensive family involvement in therapy at a later date; (3) it allows the pressure on therapists for producing change to be spread to a larger group of adjunct "therapists"; and (4) it permits families that may have been socially isolated to draw upon the strengths, objectivity, and role-modeling behaviors of a larger group of peers—a sort of extended family.

The research on outcomes with multifamily approaches is somewhat equivocal. There is some empirical evidence in support of the efficacy of various multifamily methods with drug abusers.[110, 152] The problem, in terms of decision making, is that the existent research has only compared multifamily methods with more conventional treatment modalities; we are aware of no studies that systematically contrast multifamily and individual family therapies as to their effectiveness with drug abusers.

The multifamily approach may also have certain disadvantages, including: (1) the therapist working in a multifamily group has less control of each of his cases, so his ability to induce crises, and to contain crises within a given family, is considerably reduced; this mitigation in therapeutic control would make application of several of the principles set forth elsewhere in this volume much more difficult; (2) the therapist is probably less motivated to get a given family to attend sessions, since his treatment is not as focused on particular families and can continue without full attendence; (3) one might question the advisability of leaning too heavily on an "unnatural" support group composed only of families with problems, especially if, as often happens in MFT, the families continue their mutual relationships outside the sessions. While these families may find solace in their shared difficulties and "failures," it seems more important that each family establish relationships with "normal" families and groups. Otherwise, there is the danger that the multifamily group will unwittingly support a family identity that is founded upon drug abuse. Further, the therapist, by fostering a minisociety of "families with problems," is implicitly conveying to such families that they will never completely succeed in normal society and should be content with the secondary status of families with a "handicapped" member; such a message would seem less likely to foster positive change than to serve to maintain its recipients at a marginal level of functioning.

In sum, we do not consider it advisable that multifamily approaches—at least in their present form—supplant individual family therapy with drug abusers. When multifamily methods are to be used, we suggest that (1) they be applied in conjunction with individual family treatment, following the example of Kaufman and Kaufmann,[79] and (2) their predominant use be in the initial stages of therapy, with early and rapid transition to more natural support groups and more intensive methods; one way to effect this transition would be to utilize MFT during a period of brief inpatient treatment and to move to individual family treatment around the time of discharge to outpatient status. Finally, it may be apparent that many of the principles set forth in this book can be applied by therapists conducting multifamily treatment, and indeed Kaufman and Kaufmann[79] have introduced structural techniques in their work with multifamily groups.


## THERAPIST FACTORS

There are a number of therapist qualities, some of which are discussed further in Chapters 14 and 15, that appear to contribute to the success of this treatment. The ability to be active is important and is a cornerstone of structural therapy in general. Passive, reflective styles usually do not work well. The therapist must be able to be supportive, concerned, accessible, and enthusiastic. A lack of rigidity is also needed, as drug addicts' families are very skillful and will "trip up" an inflexible therapist. Finally, the more a therapist is able to tap into his own creative and intuitive potential, the more likely he will be able to devise interventions that are both appropriate to the situation and effective.

In addition, the therapist needs to be skilled in identifying family and intersystem cycles and sequences. He has to be able to observe what is happening in a family, or within a set of systems, and document it. He also needs to know when to enter the cycle, based in part on the steps within it during which he has the most leverage. For example (as implied earlier), it might not be auspicious for him to try to break a cycle in which, at the moment, the addict is hospitalized to detoxify from heroin—espeically if the therapist has no control over the detoxification process. More prudently, he should wait until the addict returns home and the family system has a more direct influence.

Therapeutic acumen of the above sort is not easy to develop. It requires sharply honed observational skills and the ability to selectively ignore the content of family verbalizations. Attention is best directed toward the *consequences* of particular acts. Even experienced therapists can sometimes become misled by red herring behaviors and overlook the essential elements in a cycle. At the very least, however, this approach requires a different perspective of the addiction process and the people and systems involved in it, plus focus on the sequential, predictable, stable, and functional aspects of interactional behavior.

As mentioned in Chapters 9, 14, and 16, it is helpful for the therapist to have a support system of other therapists and/or supervisors. Sometimes this can be group or peer supervision, perhaps in the form of a team that observes each other's session live. Or, it might meet regularly or periodically to view tapes or discuss clinical and case management issues, as did the group described in Chapter 16. Not only can the group collaborate in designing interventions, but it can also help to increase each member's strength and leverage with his own cases. For instance, a therapist who is attempting to induce a crisis within a session is usually under considerable counterpressure from the family to relent or back off. Having one or more colleagues watching through a one-way mirror draws on the greater pool of all their ideas, serves to spread the pressure among them, and helps the therapist to hold more firmly to his position (see Chapter 9). We would advocate that therapists working with addicts' families take the steps necessary to form such a support group whenever possible.

## OVERVIEW OF SECTION II

The remaining chapters in this section present some of the clinical material with which our therapy model has been applied. The model provides them with a unifying or common thread.

The four case studies (Chapter 7, 9, 10, and 11) were selected for a number of reasons: (1) they all showed some level of success; (2) they represent a cross-section of several different kinds of cases (in regard to life cycle issues, ethnicity, etc.) treated by therapists with varied credentials and styles; (3) they are useful in making different points about the therapy; (4) the therapists involved were interested in preparing them for publication; (5) for each case we had complete, or near complete, videotape sets of 10 sessions, allowing the material presented to be as complete as necessary*; and (6) we had at least 3 years of posttreatment follow-up information on each.

Chapter 7 presents a case that quite clearly depicts most of the features of the therapy model previously covered. In addition, this family was chosen because it is so explicit. Not only do the family members show the process and patterns so frequently seen in other addicts' families, but they *verbalize* them as well (such as when the mother states in no uncertain terms that she does not want her son to marry or to leave home). Other families may give indications of similar sympathies, but they may not verbalize them so unhesitatingly.

Chapter 8 discusses the importance of crises in bringing about change. Rather than presenting a single case, the authors survey crises across 39 cases and the relationship between resolution of these crises and treatment outcome.

Chapter 9 gives an example of crisis induction in a case where the father (rather than the mother) is the parent most indulgent of the addict. The therapist forces the issue of the son's imminent death as a way of initiating change.

Chapter 10 shows the intricacies of therapy with the family of a drug pusher. Lengthy excerpts are presented from the entire course of therapy.

---

*All four, plus the case described in Chapter 12, also happened to be in the Paid Family Therapy group, meaning that they were reimbursed for attending sessions. Since attendance at all sessions was characteristic of this group, Paid families were also more likely to meet this criterion of having 10 complete tapes.

Chapter 11 examines therapy with a family in which the parents have reached retirement. A number of conceptual points and general techniques are also covered.

Chapter 12 presents the elements in a process—with accompanying clinical material—for detoxifying the addict, in this case in the family home. The home detoxification paradigm is experimental—we have applied it with only a few cases—and permits a peek at the future direction of our work. This chapter also presents some excellent material on the necessary conditions and procedures for the use of tasks in family therapy.

Chapter 13 covers treatment strategies and techniques with families in which the drug abuser is an adolescent. A number of differences between these cases and families with a young adult drug abuser are discussed. The therapy approach differs in some ways from the model set forth in the present chapter, being more structural and less strategic in its thrust and operations.

Chapter 14 tunes us into a discussion among three of the clinical supervisors about some of the issues and problems in this kind of work. It deals with some aspects of the therapy that have not received coverage earlier in the volume.

Chapter 15 is a sister chapter to the present one. It was felt that it would be premature to present this material before exposing readers to the clinical matter in Chapters 7 through 14, from which the material was derived. Chapter 15 also deals with some matters of controversy, discusses and contrasts case examples, and extends the therapy model to other populations.

# 7

# HEROIN MY BABY: 
## *A CLINICAL MODEL*

JAY HALEY

ONE WAY TO BEGIN therapy with the family of a problem young person is to have the parents reach agreements by discussing the problem young person with each other. The emphasis is on the parents jointly becoming executives in the family. Their communication about the offspring can resolve the division between them as they jointly head the family hierarchy. Another way to begin is to have the parents take turns being in charge. Conflict between them is avoided if each is in charge of the problem young person for a set period of time. When one is in charge, the other is simply to stay out of it. Such an approach makes it more difficult for the young person to be caught between them, or to turn them against each other. The hierarchy is assumed to have one person at the head, but not a particular person, since the parents can take turns.

Another way to begin therapy is for the therapist to decide which parent is more involved with the problem young person and which is more peripheral, and then to put the peripheral parent in charge of the problem person (the first stage). The more involved parent will object and even attack, bringing out the marital issues (the second stage). This approach is commonly used with children's problems and with many families of young adults. The various stages involved have been described elsewhere.[65] This approach works best with families that seem to lack subtlety in interpersonal skills, such as the families of drug addicts.

In the following case, the intervention placed the father in charge of the son at the first stage of therapy, thereby beginning to

The material in this chapter consists of excerpts from *Leaving Home: The Therapy of Disturbed Young People*, by Jay Haley. New York: McGraw-Hill Book Co., 1980. Copyright © 1980 by Jay Haley. Reprinted with permission from McGraw-Hill Book Co. Comments by the editors of the present volume are in footnotes.

disengage mother and son. The 25-year-old problem son had been a heroin and amphetamine addict for 5 years.*

Present at the session were the addict, his parents, and two younger brothers, ages 14 and 19. The therapist was Sam Kirschner, PhD, and this therapy is based upon the film script of a training film, *Heroin My Baby*, which we edited together.† The family had met with the therapist and a research associate 1 week earlier.‡ At this first therapy interview, Kirschner assumed that he had a contract with the family for therapy. He did not make an opening statement about the agenda of the interview and the goal of the therapy because he had done that in the research interview. He did not think he needed to repeat it. As the family sat down the father mentioned that the family was a sad group, and the therapist explored that. The result was confusion, which required the therapist ultimately to reorient the interview and essentially start over.

*KIRSCHNER:* So—what's doing?

*FATHER:* We got a sad group here.

*KIRSCHNER:* A sad group, huh?

*FATHER:* A very sad group.

*MOTHER:* Yeah, because, uh—I'm not coming back anymore.

*KIRSCHNER:* (*startled*) You're not coming back anymore?

*FATHER:* I didn't say it because of that. I'm just saying it's a sad group.

*SON:* We all have things to do tonight.

*MOTHER:* I don't have anything to do.

*SON:* I did.

*KIRSCHNER:* (*to father*) What's the sadness about?

*FATHER:* In plain words, it's a screwed-up family. In plain words, a real screwed-up family.

*KIRSCHNER:* (*to mother*) And you're not coming back anymore.

---

*Editors' note. The young man had been hospitalized six times for treatment of his addiction and had been detoxified a number of times. The longest time he had been off drugs in those 5 years was 2 months. During the previous 3 years he had been enrolled off and on in the Drug Dependence Treatment Center (DDTC) outpatient methadone program. He had recently reentered the program and was on a dosage of 40 mg.

†*Editors' note.* The clinical supervisor during the first eight sessions of this case was Thomas Todd.

‡*Editors' note.* The Family Evaluation Session (see Appendix C).

*MOTHER:* No, I don't think it's necessary. First of all, I'm moving. He [second son] is going on his own. He leads a life of his own. He [third son] comes with me. He [problem son] can do whatever he wants. He'll be twenty-six years old, and if he ain't gonna start now—that's it. He's already made a mistake since we left here.

*KIRSCHNER:* He's taken dope, you mean?

*SON:* Yeah, once. 'Cause I made more money than the boss of the shop. And he let me go. (*laughs*)

*MOTHER:* I mean it's not—it's not necessary for these—these two [the other sons] to tolerate this.

*SON:* Right.

*MOTHER:* I mean, I mean I'm . . .

*SON:* (*overlapping*) *I'm* not bothering them, *you're* bothering them. Explain to the doctor that. I'm not bothering these boys at all.

*MOTHER:* Well, where do you think this is all coming from?

*SON:* Me. It's been, for five years, you know.

*The son is willing to take the blame for the problem, but he also likes to protest that he is doing his best.*

*SON:* I try. You know how hard it is?

*MOTHER:* You do not try hard enough.

*SON:* Why don't you *think* about trying? Think about how hard it is.

*MOTHER:* You don't even try. Sleep in bed all day.

*SON:* Bullshit, man. Why don't you think about what I'm going through and how hard it is to go through it?

*MOTHER:* I can't imagine, I just can't imagine.

*SON:* That's right, you goddamn can't imagine, can you?

*MOTHER:* No, I can't imagine that I would do such a thing to my parents. I can't imagine it.

*SON:* Oh, I'm doing it to you. You think I'm doing it to you?

*MOTHER:* How long have you been in school?

*SON:* Two weeks.

*MOTHER:* And you didn't go to school yesterday either.

*SON:* I went to school.

*MOTHER:* And you didn't go today.

*SON:* It was snowing out.

*KIRSCHNER:* Somebody fill me in on what has happened since I last saw you. (*to father*) Why don't you fill me in.

*FATHER:* That's it. I just gave it to you all in a few words. This is a screwed-up family.

*SON:* (*interrupting*) I had a job, I lost my job, and I did dope.

*FATHER:* (*continuing*) She should go with him, or he should go with me. She should go her way. I should go my way. This kid [second son] I think he's the most—I pray to God he stays with it.

*KIRSCHNER:* You two want to separate, is that what's happening?

*FATHER:* Well, I—I don't know. I think it's the best thing for us.

*SON:* You think so. You're full of shit.

*FATHER:* I mean it.

*SON:* You're separating 'cause—'cause of me.

*FATHER:* No.

*SON*: Oh yeah?

*The first thing the therapist must do is take charge of the interview. He cannot let everyone speak freely, or the family will go on in the same helpless way and the therapy will fail. At this stage the therapist must organize who is to speak and, as much as possible, what is to be said. To correct the hierarchy, he must put down the son and quiet him.*

*It is assumed that the parents communicate through the son, staying together because of him. When the son begins to leave home and the parents face each other without him, they threaten to separate. At that point the son takes drugs and fails in life so that he remains tied to them. From this view, the son has improved by registering in the methadone program and starting school. The parents threaten separation, and the young man takes drugs and misses school.\**

*KIRSCHNER:* George, shut up.

*SON:* That's the whole thing, man.

*KIRSCHNER:* George, shut up.

*FATHER:* No, it isn't because of you.

*SON:* I'm not shutting up. When—when I want to say something, I'm gonna say it.

---

\**Editors' note.* This process is dealt with at length in the conceptual model presented in Chapter 1.

*KIRSCHNER:* You—everybody in this room has a chance to talk. I'm talking to your father now, man.

*FATHER:* (*to son*) Why are you so incoherent?

*SON:* Because you're just doing this, 'cause you're saying—you—you . . .

*FATHER:* No.

*SON:* You should go your way, she should go hers—because I'm a dope addict . . .

*MOTHER:* Well, how have we been getting along?

*SON:* (*continuing*) . . . trying to make it, you know . . .

*FATHER:* Listen . . .

*SON:* (*continuing*) . . . and you know how hard it is to make it? It's like trying to pull an elephant.

*The therapist has the goal of moving the young man out from between the parents in their marriage. A first step is to move the young man out from between the parents in the room and to place himself there, so he asks the son to change seats with him. The son is reluctant.*

*SON:* I'm twenty-five years old and I can sit where I want.

*KIRSCHNER:* I'm asking you, I'd like you to sit *here.*

*SON:* All right, relax. (*They change seats.*)

*KIRSCHNER:* Thank you.

*SON:* Sit and be happy.

*KIRSCHNER:* OK.

*SON:* They think I shoot dope 'cause I hate them. I want them to suffer.

*KIRSCHNER:* Right.

*SON:* They're all mixed up. They're very mixed up.

*KIRSCHNER:* OK. Let—let me find out—let me find out what—what the fight is all about here. What's been happening in the last, uh . . .

*FATHER:* It's been a constant—constant turmoil between her and him [son and mother].

*SON:* Me?

*FATHER:* Between her and him.

*MOTHER:* Not really.

*FATHER:* She can't cope, and he can't cope.

*SON:* Do you realize that I'm a drug addict?

*That brief sequence illustrates the triangle in the family. As the father says the mother cannot cope, thereby criticizing her and implying a disagreement between them, the son draws them away from each other by making himself the problem. That sequence occurs in many forms in the life of the family. A typical form is one where the son starts an argument with the father at the moment a conflict develops between the parents, so the issue between the parents does not get out of hand and also does not get resolved.*

*KIRSCHNER:* Hold it, we'll get to you. Hold on.

*FATHER:* (*to son*) We're not talking about drug addicts. You made the mistake . . .

*SON:* I made a big mistake, man.

*FATHER:* We made—you made the mistake that time. I mean, it was stupid for you to do it, very stupid.

*SON:* And I'm still using dope.

*FATHER:* Your reason was—first, you wanted an excuse, and you got the cheapest excuse that you could have gotten.

*SON:* I didn't want an excuse.

*FATHER:* Well, you got an excuse.

*SON:* I had fun.

*FATHER:* OK.

*SON:* That was my—I didn't believe—I didn't say . . .

*FATHER:* There you go, you're gonna keep having fun all your life.

*SON:* I didn't say I'm gonna—because I want my mother and father to break up.

*FATHER:* You have nothing to do with this.

*SON:* Or that I want them to drop dead—and die of a heart attack.

*FATHER:* You have nothing to do with this.

*KIRSCHNER:* George, your father is telling you that you have nothing to do with them breaking up.

*SON:* No? Oh, then how come it was mentioned in the beginning?

*FATHER:* You know, our life isn't much . . .

*SON:* (*interrupting*) She's making them crazy [the other two sons] 'cause she yells because of me.

*FATHER:* No.

*SON:* I got her a nervous wreck.

*FATHER:* She yells because of everything.

*KIRSCHNER:* Hold on.

*FATHER:* There's no reason why she shouldn't, 'cause you don't do a goddamn thing.

*KIRSCHNER:* Hold on.

*FATHER:* You understand?

*KIRSCHNER:* Hold on. Uh—I'd like to talk to the two of you alone. George, could you take your two brothers out into the waiting room?

*The therapist now takes charge by essentially starting the interview over. He sees the parents alone and establishes a contract and an agenda with them.\**

*FATHER:* If he's gonna keep looking for excuses like this, little excuses. Now like this incident here, now he'll go out and shoot. Now this is wrong I know it, it's a hundred percent wrong. We are not helping him.

*KIRSCHNER:* That's what we got to try doing.

*FATHER:* The boy is trying to help himself, but we need as much help as him, maybe more. Now this is not your affair. You know what I mean. I mean you've got problems with him.

*When the father says that the problems of the husband and wife are not the therapist's affair, that is a decision point, and how the therapist responds determines the therapeutic approach. He could ask what kind of help the father needs. He could offer to help them with whatever problems they have. He could define the therapy as for the whole family, not just for the son. In the approach presented here, it would be an error to offer to help the husband and wife with their problems. The goal of the therapy is to establish a correct hierarchy, with the parents in charge of the irresponsible son. Any emphasis on their problems would divide the parents at this time of crisis. Divided leadership will fail. The therapist must therefore agree that the problem is the son and keep the focus on the addiction. He*

---

*\*Editors' note.* In addition to trying to gain control of the session, the therapist is starting to reestablish an appropriate family hierarchy. He separates children and parents by placing them in different rooms, thus affirming the boundary between generations. He also reestablishes the hierarchy among the children by asking the oldest boy, George (who was actually behaving more immaturely than his brothers), to take charge of his brothers and escort them to the waiting room.

*can offer help for them at some future time, but he should agree that their problems are not his focus at this time.* *

KIRSCHNER: Right, and that's what we're here for.

FATHER: Right.

KIRSCHNER: OK. Now that's what I'm trying to say. You— the three of us have got to work together so we can help him to help himself, that's all. Now, are you willing? The point is that the three of us as adults have got to straighten him out, and we can do it if we work together. I have worked with more difficult problems with success, and I'm telling you that if the three of us work together we will lick this problem. Then, whatever else comes up between the two of you is another issue.

*The therapist has now stated his agenda. He gets an agreement with the parents that they will continue to work with him to try to cure the son's addiction problem. When he brings the boys back in, he has begun to establish the parents as joint authorities over their son rather than a husband and wife in conflict and struggling helplessly with the problem. He is accomplishing the first interview task: clarifying the agenda of the therapy and correcting a malfunctioning hierarchy.*

*The therapist then brings the three sons back into the interview room. Upon his return, the addict still tries to make an issue of his parents' threat to separate.*

KIRSCHNER: (*to son*) Well, I told you what I have to say in the hall, that any kind of stuff that's going on between your folks has little to do with you.

SON: Right.

KIRSCHNER: All right?

SON: Right. I got that down pat. They don't like each other.

MOTHER: That's not true.

SON: Well, I don't know what's true. You know? What is true?

---

* *Editors' note.* It should be recognized that marital counselors and therapists are plentiful in Philadelphia, but the parents have not sought one for their marital problem. This, alone, should dictate caution in moving toward marital therapy. In this particular case the father identifies a marital problem, but the mother says nothing. They are willing to engage in treatment for their son, but not necessarily to work on their own relationship. In most addicts' families, shifting to the parents' marital problem at this stage will result in one or both of them terminating therapy (see Chapter 6).

*KIRSCHNER:* Let's say this. When they don't get along with each other, it's not necessarily because of you. Is that a fair statement?

*FATHER:* Definitely.

*KIRSCHNER:* OK, that's a fair statement.

*SON:* Oh, no, it's only *ninety* percent me, how's that?

*MOTHER:* No, you're wrong.

*SON: Fifty?*

*MOTHER:* You're wrong.

*SON:* Oh, bullshit, you don't know what it *is*, man. Be realistic with me at least. Have I caused you . . .

*FATHER:* Oh, yeah.

*SON:* . . . heartbreak?

*FATHER:* Oh, yeah, well certainly you have.

*SON:* Well, your boy never got arrested, you—the fast, quick, little jackass, queer, jerk-off never got arrested, but he was a *junkie*, turned into a *junkie*, can you understand? How could you understand it, my own father. Understand all that. (*weeping*) Do you know what hell I'm going through? *Hate* each other, I don't give a shit, I'm trying to do *my* thing. Trying to do it, and it's *hard*, man.

*KIRSCHNER:* OK, tell—tell—why don't you explain to your parents what you're going through?

*SON:* They don't want to hear shit.

*KIRSCHNER:* They're listening now.

*SON:* They want to see me high, every time, check my arms.

*KIRSCHNER:* They're listening.

*SON:* They want to do what *they* want to do.

*KIRSCHNER:* They're listening, they're listening now. Tell your folks what you're going through.

*It could be considered an error for the therapist to encourage the young man to express his feelings if he does so with the idea that the expression of feelings is curative. Any addict has been through group therapy experiences that include the expression of emotions and so the addict will do it well, but it is irrelevant to therapy. It makes a session more exciting but things can be said that may make it difficult to organize the family to change. This therapist encourages the addict to express his despair because it will help bridge the gulf between addict and parents. He argues that most addicts simply do not believe that parents can understand the struggle with addiction.*

*KIRSCHNER:* Tell your folks what you're going through.

*SON:* Hell, man, hell!

*KIRSCHNER:* OK. What's going on?

*SON:* Just—you know, I'll be straight, and as soon as the word "dope"—everything just stops. I don't think of nobody, you—her—nobody. Just Miss Heroin.

*KIRSCHNER:* You were straight—you were straight . . .

*SON:* Miss—when I'm high—

*KIRSCHNER:* Hey, you were straight for how long?

*SON:* Two months.

*KIRSCHNER:* OK.

*SON:* And for free I got it, not even from Tommy or Marion. They get high, but they know how to control it. I'm a *glutton.*

(*later in the interview*)

*KIRSCHNER:* As soon as you get a job, you mean. So the plan is for you to get a job, make some money, and then move out, is that the idea?

*SON:* I don't want to move out.

*KIRSCHNER:* You don't want to move out?

*SON:* 'Cause I think he [the father] needs help too. They both need help, like I need help.

*KIRSCHNER:* That's a different problem. We've already talked about that when you were gone.

*SON:* No, he could drop dead right now. You know, I think of that. More than I think of my own problems. That's how I escape myself, thinking of how I can help my father and mother—from being nervous. But yet I'm crazy. That's crazy, that I'm high and I'm thinking, "How am I helping them?"

*The son expresses the situation nicely. When he's high on drugs, he's thinking of how he is helping the parents. The therapist does just what he should at this point: rather than discussing whether the father needs help (something the son understands better than the therapist), he offers to take on the father's problems himself. This must be done to free the son. The expert who is paid to do the job must help the father, while the son is freed to lead his own life.*

*KIRSCHNER:* Hey, George, could you do me a favor? Do me one favor. Will you turn that job over to me? I'll worry about your father's health.

*SON:* (*weeping*) Yeah, but he made me. He didn't make you, man.

*KIRSCHNER:* That's all right, so what?

*SON:* Do I make any sense coming there with that sentence?

*KIRSCHNER:* I hear you.

*SON: He* made me.

*KIRSCHNER:* So. So what do you have to . . . ?

*SON:* I care.

*KIRSCHNER:* I know you care. OK. I . . .

*SON:* More than anybody else cares.

*KIRSCHNER:* I want to make an agreement with you. If you care about your father's health, right, which I know you do, turn it over to me. And you worry about your own business.*

*SON:* As soon as they move, everything will be cool. Like a happy home. I come in, I want to go and stay with a chick, she has three kids. If I'm having fun, I want to stay. I'm twenty-five. (*to mother*) I feel like I have to report in to the Army, but I want to call you, 'cause I know you're worried, you don't sleep, you're nervous. You understand, Ma, why I call my Ma. "Mommy, I'm at so-and-so's house, and I had a good time last night, and I'm all right." What does that sound like to a twenty-six-year-old girl? That I'm—it sounds like I'm checking in with my sergeant.

*The therapist must take charge and organize action if change is to take place. The goal of the therapy is to draw a generation line where the parents hold together in relation to the son without either one shifting and joining the son against the other. A first step in achieving this end is to ask the parent who seems more peripheral to take charge of the son. The therapist directs the father to be in charge of the son, and he asks the mother to communicate with the son through the father. The father is thus put in the middle of the intense relationship between the son and the mother. Even though this move is defined as for the mother's benefit, she will probably respond by activating her previous involvement with the son. The therapist must block that off. If the therapist can hold the father in the position*

---

*Editors' note.* This might be considered an "isomorphic" change in the family structure (i.e., it takes a similar form). The therapist substitutes himself for the son (earlier he had even traded places with George, seating himself between the parents). Therefore, the parents still have a "helper" between them, but one who may be able to help them in a different way. A move such as this may be appropriate when a therapist senses that complete removal of the third person at this time would be too drastic or upsetting for the parents. It is, of course, a temporary stage in the therapy and is continued only until the therapist senses a readiness by the family for him to extricate himself.

*between mother and son, it is the first step in the ultimate joining of mother and father.*

*KIRSCHNER:* I would like to try something. OK, since George is so upset, I would like to try something.

*SON:* I ain't upset, I'm having fun now. I really feel like a nut.

*KIRSCHNER:* I would, I would like, uh . . . *(long pause)* Yes, this is what I'd like to try—for one week. Just for a week as an experiment, OK, in the house. *(to mother)* If you have any complaints, or you want to check up on George, or whatever you want to do, you know—tell your husband to do it.

*SON:* Everybody's checking up on me, Sam.

*KIRSCHNER:* Hold on. Hold on.

*MOTHER:* Well, that's no problem, because whatever I ask him, he tells me.

*FATHER:* You gave us permission to tell . . .

*SON:* I tell . . .

*KIRSCHNER:* *(overlapping)* No, no, no, no.

*SON:* You know, the last time I got high . . .

*KIRSCHNER:* *(to mother)* But I don't want you to do it.

*SON:* *(continuing)* . . . and how I jumped on—tell him, tell him I'm getting high. I want to tell you, 'cause you don't understand.

*KIRSCHNER:* *(continuing to talk to mother while son talks to father)* I want to give you a rest. Seriously. I want to give you a rest. I mean that. You got a lot of things on your mind, you got a lot . . .

*MOTHER:* He offers that, he tells me. He [the father] says to me, "Please be quiet. When something is wrong, tell *me*, let *me* talk to him." But I just can't seem to keep quiet.

*KIRSCHNER:* OK. Hold on . . .

*MOTHER:* I feel like I'm the only one that's gonna make him better, and I feel like I'm making him worse.

*KIRSCHNER:* Hold on. OK. OK, so let's try it different . . .

*SON:* *(overlapping)* You got to do it, I know that, Mom, you know how much it hurts me when I do dope, huh?

*KIRSCHNER:* George, hold on, we're trying something.

*MOTHER:* I don't feel like him [father], him [second son], or him [third son] is capable of helping him.

*KIRSCHNER:* Well, right now what you're trying is evidently not working. OK? Let's look at the facts—it's not working. You're concerned, but the way you're going about it, it's not working. That's all. You've got a lot of things on your mind, maybe that's why it's not working. You've got a lot of things on your mind now anyway, OK?

*When parents perpetuate a problem with their child, the therapist must change what they are doing. Sometimes he must object to the way they are doing something. If this is done by implying that something is wrong with the parents' character, a great deal of therapeutic time can be wasted by the parents proving their innocence or proving the therapist wrong. If the therapist objects to the opera-tions of the parents in a matter-of-fact way, they will accept his objection. In this comment to the mother, the therapist managed to correct her without being offensive.*

MOTHER: Mm-hmm.

KIRSCHNER: So I'd like to have you worry about your own things, and if you have something that you're concerned about with George, tell your husband and let him tell George. OK? Is that fair enough?

MOTHER: Yeah.

SON: He's been telling me in a pretty good way, too.

KIRSCHNER: OK, hold on.

SON: And I been telling him. We been getting along, haven't we been getting along better, Dad, than ever?

KIRSCHNER: Hold on. Hold on, George. (*to father*) Are you willing to do that?

FATHER: (*puzzled*) Say that again.

KIRSCHNER: If your wife has some kind of thing that she's concerned about with George, that she wants to ask some kind of question, some information, or whatever, would you be willing to do it instead of her?

FATHER: Certainly.

*The father clearly agrees, and in his next statement begins to take charge of the son.*

KIRSCHNER: You're willing.

SON: (*to mother*) When are you moving to the South Side?

MOTHER: We looked at a house there.

FATHER: (*to son*) Did you get your uh . . . did you get your medicine Monday?

SON: Nah, 'cause I was—hell, I can take my medicine, that I'm on now. You know that methadone makes me talk, makes me go nuts. As you say, I'm dopey.

*FATHER:* Did you go to the clinic?

*SON:* Methadone lasts for eighty hours, Dad. I can stay—I can go for four days without getting sick.

*MOTHER:* Well, how come you go every day, then?

*SON:* Why? 'Cause you have to, that's the law. It's the law.

*MOTHER:* Well, then why . . .

*FATHER:* But you didn't go . . .

*KIRSCHNER: (to mother)* Hold on, there you go, you're asking him again. You were asking him again.

*SON:* No, I didn't—'cause I was . . . I just didn't go. I was with a girl. And I was—right, I should have been somewhere.

*FATHER:* You're not being honest with them, because you have to take . . .

*SON:* I lied to you.

*FATHER:* Will you let me talk a minute? They have to take the urine test, right? You didn't take it Monday? Are you having trouble urinating?

*The directive that mother communicate to son only through father seems simple, yet it is a major intervention, and the outcome of the therapy will depend on the therapist's skill in enforcing it. In the interview room the therapist becomes a communication traffic cop, encouraging father and son to talk together and preventing mother from communicating with son about his problems. The therapist must persistently prevent the inertia of the system from causing a relapse to a mother–son intensity with father on the periphery. One can expect that all three family members will take some action to return to the previous system. That action can include threats to leave therapy.*

*SON:* No man. They didn't take it, they know I did heroin. I told Henry. I said, "I did heroin." I do so much that I did forget. But usually I don't forget, I shoot up . . .

*FATHER: (interrupting)* When did you do it? Sunday?

*SON: (continuing)* It hurts me more, when I get high. It makes sense? I can't figure it out either, Mom.

*FATHER: (interrupting)* When did you do it? This Sunday?

*SON:* No, Saturday.

*FATHER:* You did it this past Saturday?

*MOTHER:* Again.

*KIRSCHNER: (restraining mother from talking)* Hold on.

*FATHER:* Why?

*SON:* Why? Why and again? I don't know. It just was there. Nobody understands.

*FATHER:* (*to therapist*) You figure it out.

(*later in the interview*)

*SON:* I ain't coming back, Sam. I'm telling you.

*SON NO. 3:* Well, I'm coming back.

*SON:* I'm asking Henry [his drug counselor] for medicine. You can come back, but I'm not.

*The therapist responds simply and correctly to the young man's threat by making it personal.*

*KIRSCHNER:* I want you to come back. I want you to come back. I want you to come back at least one more week, to see how this works for one week.

*SON:* 'Cause, as soon as—you know, I'm gonna make a loan and get away from them. After I'm away . . .

*MOTHER:* You couldn't make a loan from nobody.

*SON:* No? You want to bet?

*MOTHER:* The only way you're gonna make it is to sell heroin to your friends.

*SON:* Oh, there's ways, Mom, I'll hustle and bustle.

*KIRSCHNER:* (*interrupting*) Hey, George. (*whistles*) Hey, George, one more week. I want to see how this, how this works out.

*SON:* I don't want to come, Sam. You talk to them.

*KIRSCHNER:* I'll talk to you privately then.

*SON:* Yeah—uh, I'll do that.

*KIRSCHNER:* OK, fine. I'll tell you what . . .

*SON:* Nobody understands me, I'm a nut. You know, I'm retarded. I'm a nut, I have a disease . . .

*SON NO. 3:* You *want* to be.

*SON:* Oh, yeah, I want to, sure.

*SON NO. 3:* (*crying*) Then what do you keep on saying it for, huh? How come? It's real funny, ain't it!

*SON:* Oh, see now—I knew you were gonna cry.

*SON NO. 3:* Ah *jerk* off, man, *get* off!

*SON:* See, he's right.

*SON NO. 3:* I'm right. (*runs from the room, crying*)

*SON:* He's right. (*standing up*) You're right, come on in and sit down.

*KIRSCHNER:* He's not going anywhere.

*SON:* I don't care where he goes. I don't care.

*FATHER:* You don't care for nothing.

*SON:* I don't care about nothing, I want . . .

*FATHER:* (*overlapping*) He just don't care.

*SON:* I've tortured these people so much, I don't *want* to care no more. That's why I want to leave.

*FATHER:* (*standing up, as son does*) Sam, we're just holding up your time.

*KIRSCHNER:* You're not holding up my time. (*to son as he goes out the door*) Where are you going now?

*SON:* I'm gonna thumb it home. I don't need a ride.

*A therapist always has a problem when someone gets upset and leaves the interview room. When it is the problem young person, he must decide whether to bring him back and, if so, who should go and get him. Sometimes when a young person leaves, the therapist should merely continue with the parents. He should take the young person's departure as an indication that the parents need to talk with the therapist. In this case, the therapist had already talked with the parents alone, and so this did not seem the way to respond. Typically it is best to send a parent after the problem young person. This defines the hierarchical issue as one within the family. Whoever the therapist is encouraging to take charge should be asked to go after the young person. In this case, it is unclear whether the father, if asked, would have been able to bring the young man back or whether he was there so tentatively himself that he would not himself have left. The therapist acts in what appears to have been the correct way: he goes and gets the young man himself. The problem son and the other two sons reenter to continue the interview. This determination to keep the young man involved could have influenced father to do as he did later, when he pursued his son.*

*KIRSCHNER:* (*sitting down*) We got some other shit to talk about here. OK. (*to father*) You got a cigarette?

*FATHER:* Yeah.

*KIRSCHNER:* (*to son*) OK, so you're upset, and that's why I don't want you to move out of the house.

*SON:* No.

*FATHER:* Did you go to the clinic Monday?

*SON:* What?

*FATHER:* Did you go to the clinic?

*SON:* No, I didn't go nowhere. I don't want to go nowhere.

*KIRSCHNER:* You been to the clinic this week?

*SON:* Huh? Since I got high that one time—oh, yeah, I was there tonight. Henry don't even—I'm gonna talk to him and ask him one more time if he'll bear with me—'cause all I'm doing is jive-assing. If I keep—I'm trying, but it seems like I'm not trying. I'm—I'm like double-talking right now. I am really trying, but it's *impossible* sometimes.

*KIRSCHNER:* I hear you.

*SON:* You understand?

*KIRSCHNER:* I understand.

*SON:* Nobody believes it, that how—all of a sudden, somebody says (*whispering*), "I got some heavy shit." Everything stops! (*sliding off his coat*) My coat falls off, all my clothes, I'm nude, and that's all there is: "Baby, I'm gonna be nice." That's all there is, that's what this does to you.

*MOTHER:* (*to therapist*) Is this a *mental* illness?

*KIRSCHNER:* (*to mother, overlapping*) You understand that?

*MOTHER:* That's not a mental illness?

*SON:* That *is* a mental illness.

*MOTHER:* No, I don't understand.

*SON:* It's a sickness, it's a disease.

*MOTHER:* I don't understand.

*KIRSCHNER:* Hold on. You're saying your mother and father don't understand how hard it is.

*SON:* They don't.

*KIRSCHNER:* Do you understand how hard that is for him to resist that?

*MOTHER:* No.

*SON:* They don't. I love them, but . . .

*MOTHER:* (*interrupting*) Not when a boy says that he loves me, and he loves his father, and he wants . . .

*SON:* (*interrupting, standing, and shouting*) But I forget all *about* you when I see my *baby*, "Heroin."

*MOTHER:* Well, then, you might as well pack your clothes and get out with your baby!

*By the end of this first interview, the therapeutic plan has been set. The therapist has a contract with the family and a plan to follow.*

*He will have father deal with son, and mother deal with father about the son's problems. Predictably this will lead to marital tension and threats of separation. When that happens, the son will relapse to save the parents. The therapist must help the parents to consolidate both their relationship with him and their relationship with each other. The focus should be on the problem that the family wishes to solve: the addiction.*

*At the second interview, the therapist interviews the parents alone.*

KIRSCHNER: The next four weeks are gonna be tough.
MOTHER: For Georgie?
KIRSCHNER: And I wanted to prepare you in advance for that—to know what you're coming up against. It's gonna be a very tough period. And—depending upon what we decide today, in terms of how I can—of how you can use me in the best way, in terms of ensuring that this guy stays off drugs for the next—I would say the next four weeks is going to be critical. You know, how he's gonna react to the detox, and so on.

*During the second week, the young man was detoxified and taken off a massive dose of methadone. As reported in the following interview, the parents had an argument in which the mother threw dishes around the house. This was followed by the son shooting heroin and the father getting into a physical fight with him. The expected sequence therefore took place within just a week: the young man improved; the parents had a fight; the young man relapsed. What was new was that the father got actively involved in stopping the young man from taking heroin.*

*Therapist, parents, and son are present in the interview.*

KIRSCHNER: You're relaxed.
MOTHER: Yeah.
KIRSCHNER: How come you're relaxed?
MOTHER: When everything's fine, I'm fine.
KIRSCHNER: So you had a stormy evening the other evening.
MOTHER: Mm-hmm.
SON: Wasn't too stormy.
KIRSCHNER: (*to father*) You know, I can see that you're making a real effort to get this guy to, uh—to be what he *could* be.

*FATHER:* It's either do or die for him.

*KIRSCHNER:* And you're gonna stick it out, right? You're gonna really . . .

*FATHER:* If he don't do something this time . . . I'm not coming . . .

*KIRSCHNER:* (*to mother*) You must be proud of him, huh?

*MOTHER:* Mm-hmm.

*FATHER:* I don't know why.

*KIRSCHNER:* Were you proud of him?

*SON:* What were you proud of?

*MOTHER:* Well, I didn't stop it.

*SON:* You didn't stop what?

*MOTHER:* I mean, I knew neither one was really gonna hurt each other.

*KIRSCHNER:* (*cutting off George, who is talking*) Hold on, George.

*MOTHER:* He would never hurt his father.

*KIRSCHNER:* Right.

*MOTHER:* And he could have.

*KIRSCHNER:* I know he could have.

*MOTHER:* He could have. He could have killed him.

*FATHER:* And I've been crippled since Monday or Tuesday. (*Everyone laughs.*)

*SON:* No, it ain't that. It's just that he followed me down the street, kept following me down the street, saying, "Come on back, you bastard. Come on back. Are you scared? No? You want to get killed again?"

*FATHER:* I said, "I want to *talk* to you."

*Just as the therapist pursued the son and brought him back after the first interview, so does the father pursue the son in this situation.*

*SON:* Talk to you, yes, and to take another shot. (*demonstrating a blow*) Try another right? That made my head go like this. (*laughs*) Twice. You're getting over the hill, Pete. You taught me how to throw them lefts, Pete. You dropped—you dropped your right so easy that it comes right across the chin. Does it hurt here?

*KIRSCHNER:* But how about, how about the fact that your father is making a real effort to keep you in line, and make sure that you're doing the best thing for yourself.

*SON:* I didn't really—I appreciate it, but I didn't do nothing the other night. I was just standing there. I walked in and all of a sudden lamps were thrown and everything.

*FATHER:* You know what it is. You know how happy we were—last time we spoke about him, we were so happy, he was doing good. And we were sweating out that there, uh—"atressin," whatever they call it.* And then just like that he just gives up everything. So there was a little, uh—medical mistake.

*KIRSCHNER:* Mm-hmm.

*It is important that a therapist reach agreement with his fellow professionals so that nothing medical is done without his permission. If custody or drugs are used without his permission, the therapist will fail. In this case, this medical arrangement was not made at the beginning of therapy. During the second week, the young man was detoxified and placed on a drug that would cause him to reject heroin. This experiment was done without considering the therapy, and it went badly. The young man shot up on heroin again, perhaps in relation to this drug treatment, perhaps in relation to his family.†*

*The therapist should not condemn his fellow professionals but should find something positive in their actions, as the therapist does here when he returns to the subject.*

*FATHER:* So it seemed like that little medical mistake gave him an excuse.

*KIRSCHNER:* Mm-hmm.

*FATHER:* Now I'm almost positive he must have shot after he got out of the hospital. Did you?

SON: Once.

*FATHER:* Once. There you go. He needed that excuse.

*(later in the interview)*

*KIRSCHNER:* Didn't I tell you it was gonna be a tough week?

*MOTHER:* Yeah, you said that, but I figured, you know, a week . . .

---

*Editors' note.* The son was admitted to an inpatient unit and placed on a naltrexone regimen.

†*Editors' note.* The case was nearly lost at this point. The son was admitted to the hospital without Kirschner's knowledge and he had to act swiftly to regain entry into the therapeutic process (e.g., by visiting the son in the hospital, talking to the parents by telephone, coordinating with the drug counselor, etc.).

*FATHER:* When we come here, he had been discharged from the hospital, and that's what disappointed me. He put all that in there, all that effort, and then he just . . .

*MOTHER:* The third time [referring to the detox]. But he looks great, doesn't he?

*KIRSCHNER:* A little tired, but good. Real good, yeah.

*MOTHER:* He looks good, and he says to me that . . .

*KIRSCHNER:* (*interrupting and turning to father*) Wait a minute. Hold on. You said that was a waste?

*SON:* That was not a waste.

*MOTHER:* It is a waste because he doesn't want to do nothing.

*FATHER:* Being in that hospital.

*SON:* I don't want to be on naltrexone.

*KIRSCHNER:* He detoxified, so it's not a waste.

*MOTHER:* Well, I mean, we thought, you know . . .

*SON:* I was on forty milligrams. To come down in six days, you know what it did? You know what it is—forty milligrams? If you and him [meaning father] split it, you'd die.

*MOTHER:* Well, that's what I'm saying . . .

*KIRSCHNER:* So first of all, it wasn't a waste, 'cause he detoxed. That's the first thing. So his system was clean, and that's important.

*FATHER:* And now his system is dirty again.

*SON:* No, it ain't. It's been since last week, last Friday.

*The therapist attempts to shift the focus to the parents' marriage, wishing to bring about the second stage of the therapy.*

*KIRSCHNER:* Now what—now let's get back to work. So, in other words, he was wedged between the two of you, and aggravating the two of you, in addition to anything else that was going on. OK?

*MOTHER:* It makes everything else worse.

*KIRSCHNER:* OK, it makes everything else worse.

*MOTHER:* Right, it makes everything else bigger.

*KIRSCHNER:* OK. Now the question is—the question is, how much longer are you going to let George do that to the two of you? Now you're moving into a new house, and I see that as a fresh beginning.

*It is always good to refer to a fresh start in therapy as a turning point. Later in the interview the therapist tries another approach to the parents' marital problems.*

*KIRSCHNER: (to mother)* Now if your husband is taking over the job of helping his son straighten out, you know, in conjunction with me, is that gonna satisfy you? What more needs to be done in terms of you? I'm concerned because you've got a lot on your mind now. You're moving, and you're doing a lot of things, you got your job, you got a lot of responsibility there—I'm still concerned about you being overworried.

*FATHER:* She can't put him out, she can't stand the thought of him being on the street, and being like a derelict, or starting to steal, or—so that's her problem. She has to be strong. If he isn't gonna help himself—I don't intend to have an invalid in my house. I mean, if he didn't have arms or legs, I mean that's different.

*MOTHER:* And you know what I thought? I'd leave him [the father] and take him [the son].

*KIRSCHNER:* Mm-hmm.

*FATHER:* And you know what I thought? I was gonna do that. I was gonna let—I was gonna leave her and have her take him.

*The therapist has a particularly difficult problem here. Mother has stated the basic issue clearly: she is tempted to ignore the generation line and go live with her son. The father merely agrees. Instead of striving to draw a generational boundary between themselves and their son, the parents accept an absolutely confused hierarchy in a classical Oedipal triangle. The therapist's problem is that if he discusses this situation either as a practical matter or as a philosophical one, he is accepting the premise that this resolution is a tenable one. The therapist chooses an alternative that dismisses the mother's proposal.*

*KIRSCHNER:* You know what I think? That's the shittiest idea I have ever heard.

*MOTHER:* I know it is. *(All laugh.)*

*FATHER:* That—that's the way I feel.

*KIRSCHNER:* What can your husband do for you that will ease the worry about your son?

*MOTHER:* He can't do it. He [the son] has to do it. He—it's what he . . .

*KIRSCHNER:* No, no, we're gonna work—I'm working with Georgie separately, and we're gonna meet together. But what can your husband do for you to make you less worried? Besides he's gonna help Georgie and talk to him and stuff, and check him out, and that kind of stuff. What can he do for you? What can your husband do for you?

*MOTHER:* He can't do nothing for me, because I feel that I'm the only one that can do it.

*FATHER:* (*to mother*) I don't know, I'm stuck there. I don't get what you mean.

*MOTHER:* I feel that I can do a better job than you.

*KIRSCHNER:* Mm-hmm.

*FATHER:* Job with Georgie?

*MOTHER:* I feel like I can.

*SON:* Give in too easy.

*KIRSCHNER:* There we have it, you're saying that you're the one who can do the job, so you don't really want to give over charge to your husband. You're afraid that he's gonna blow it and kick Georgie out of the house, and then you're gonna get upset and leave with Georgie.

*MOTHER:* Well, it's—it's what I think I would do.

*KIRSCHNER:* Right, yeah, right.

*MOTHER:* But I don't know how I could ever manage it.

*KIRSCHNER:* Right, but I'm saying that's how your mind is running, right? That's the way your imagination goes.

*MOTHER:* Mm-hmm.

*KIRSCHNER:* And I'm telling you, and George—George senior has already said it, that because he's a man, he understands his son's problems, and what he needs to do in his life, better than you can, even though you're her—you're his mother.

*Later in the interview, the therapist summarizes what he thinks the husband should be saying but has not said.*

*KIRSCHNER:* Then what you're saying, what you're saying then, is you would like to get your son straightened out so you can get closer to your wife, is that what you're saying?

*The therapist assumes that he and the parents want the same results. He defines the parental job as interfering with conjugal pleasures. Mentioning this interference does not make the parents willing to shift from the parental issue to the conjugal issue. As the therapist states the goal of the parents becoming closer as husband and wife, there are significant pauses and other indications that they prefer to deal with each other through the problem son.*

*FATHER:* If he was straightened out, I'd raise him again from the time he was a child, in this new house.

*KIRSCHNER:* If he was straightened out, then you would get closer to your wife, is that what you're saying?

*FATHER: (after a pause)* Well, naturally. When there's—when there's contentment, peace and contentment in the house, uh—then definitely everything would be straightened out.

*KIRSCHNER: (to mother)* And that's what you want?

*MOTHER: (after a pause)* Yeah, I'd want that with him. But it ain't gonna be if he's [the son] not there—if—if he's not all right. 'Cause I just don't feel right, nothing else matters to me.

*KIRSCHNER:* I know. I know. OK, so that's—that's where we want to go. We want to get him straightened out, and the two of you closer.

*FATHER: (after a pause)* Definitely.

*KIRSCHNER: (to father)* And they are—and as you pointed out, they're wound up with each other. You know, the two of them—like they depend on each other.

*It is better for the therapist to receive the parents' hesitations as indications to him that he has work to do to bring them together. These messages do not merely report how the parents feel, they are guides to the therapist and should be received that way. The therapist pursues this issue by projecting them into the future.*

*KIRSCHNER:* OK, let's say he gets a job, OK, and he starts working for about a month. Things are going well. Then what do you want? I want you to tell George. What do you want George to do then?

*FATHER:* Save his money.

*KIRSCHNER:* Tell him, tell him.

*FATHER:* Save your money. Get what you want, the things you say that you want, which would be great—wonderful. You give your mother a little money for the food. And that's it.

*KIRSCHNER:* You want him to stay at home?

*FATHER: (continuing)* You got your room.

*KIRSCHNER:* You want him to stay at home?

*FATHER:* Yeah, as long as he's . . .

*SON:* I'd like to, Sam, to tell you the truth.

*FATHER:* He can be with us the rest of his life. I mean, we want to see him married, have children, and all.

*SON:* I mean they don't have nobody, you see.

*KIRSCHNER: (noting wife shaking her head)* Your wife—your wife disagrees.

*FATHER:* Oh, she just . . .

*MOTHER:* I don't want him married.

*FATHER:* She doesn't want him married. She wants him the rest of her life.

*SON:* She don't have nobody.

*FATHER: (to therapist)* You—you misunderstood. She wants him the rest of his life. I do too, as long as he's straight.

*SON: (agreeing)* Straight.

*KIRSCHNER:* You want him to live with you for the rest of your life?

*The therapist's values, which represent the wider culture, are contrary to those of the parents. To disengage the addict, the therapist asserts his values in a way that can lead to constructive change.\**

*SON:* Sure.

*MOTHER:* Why not?

*SON:* As long as I'm straight, Sam, I told you that.

*KIRSCHNER:* How about him getting married and having a family, so you can have grandchildren?

*SON:* They don't even care.

*MOTHER:* If it happens, I guess—I mean, what am I gonna do about it? . . . But I prefer that he stay.

*FATHER:* Suppose if I become senile, I start becoming senile, I'll be coming to that age.

*MOTHER:* Especially to have children—I don't want any of my children to have children.

*KIRSCHNER:* Why *not*?

*MOTHER:* I just don't.

*KIRSCHNER:* Let me understand. You want to have him and have to take care of him the rest of your life?

*FATHER:* I'm not gonna take care of him.

*SON:* Naturally, naturally I want to . . .

*KIRSCHNER:* You'll have to feed him, and do all that stuff.

---

\**Editors' note.* The therapist's position is strengthened in this by the values held within the parents' own Italian-American subculture. It is unlikely that their friends, relatives, and neighbors would find acceptable the idea about to be expressed by the mother of intentionally having no grandchildren.

*MOTHER:* I got to feed myself and my husband, so what's one more?

*FATHER:* When he's ready to go.

*SON:* The only way.

*MOTHER:* Yeah, it's up to him. I don't—I'm not insisting.

*KIRSCHNER:* Wait, what—what you're saying though, is you would prefer to have him live with you for the rest of your life.

*FATHER:* No, she prefers him not to get married.

*KIRSCHNER:* Hold on, let's find out.

*MOTHER:* No, if he decides that he's—wants to go on his own, and you know everything's fine, that's good. I mean he could have a place of his own. He's got things he would want to do, and uh—that he wouldn't be able to do at my house.

*KIRSCHNER:* Would that be all right with you, if he moved out?

*MOTHER:* Yeah, if he wanted to, oh yeah.

*KIRSCHNER: (to father)* How about you?

*FATHER:* Certainly.

*SON:* Is that a goal?

*FATHER:* That's a real, that's—that's his goal. That's our goal, that he straightens out, that's our goal.

*The therapist, by persistence, is persuading the parents that they will have to give up their son and deal with each other, even though, as the son says, they feel that they don't have anyone else. The persistence through the hour ultimately pays off, as will be shown. At this point the therapist physically separates the son from the parents.*

*KIRSCHNER:* Sit next to me. (*He pulls over the chair and they sit and watch the parents talk.*)

*SON:* This is ridiculous.

*KIRSCHNER:* Hold on, we're gonna watch this now. Hold on. Hold on.

*SON:* I see it all the time, Sam.

*KIRSCHNER:* Hold on.

*SON:* I don't have to stare and watch.

*KIRSCHNER:* OK. I want you out of it. Could the two of you as parents please discuss what you have in mind for your son and come to an agreement on it? About whether or not—specifically, what your idea as a goal for the future for Georgie is. I want you to tell—tell her, don't tell me.

204 STRATEGIES AND TECHNIQUES OF TREATMENT

*FATHER:* The only disagreement we have is she don't want him to get married. But she still feels, if he—if he was straight, then he'd go out and find a girl.

*MOTHER:* How can you say you don't want someone to get married when they don't even have a girl. There is no girl present, there was never any, anything of this, or close to this. How could I really know how I feel?

*SON:* How do you know I wasn't close to this?

*KIRSCHNER:* Hold on.

*MOTHER:* I know who it was close with, the one who *started* all this shit!

*KIRSCHNER:* You—you're talking to your son again, instead of to your husband.

(*later in the interview*)

*KIRSCHNER:* You want him in a good environment in his own apartment.

*FATHER:* Right.

*KIRSCHNER:* Once he's ready. Is that what you want?

*MOTHER:* That's all right with me.

*KIRSCHNER:* That's OK.

*MOTHER:* Mm-hmm.

*KIRSCHNER:* And you're going to work toward that.

*MOTHER:* (*after a pause*) Toward what?

*KIRSCHNER:* Toward making sure that he's prepared, that he doesn't leave prematurely, that when he leaves—your husband has helped him prepare, you know, the finances, and you know, showing him, going over how much he needs. And then giving him your blessing.

*Although some therapists think of the problem as one of the parents holding on to the child, it is best to keep aware that the child also holds on to the parents. When the parents sound as if they are willing to let the son leave, he responds with a certain reluctance.*\*

---

\**Editors' note.* This example demonstrates the limitations of a linear view of causality. A linear interpretation might lay blame for the problem either at the feet of the parents, or of the son. In contrast, nonlinear or recursive thinking[11] incorporates the contributions of all members—they and their actions are all inseparable parts of the family system, with each making his own contribution to the problem sequence (see Chapters 1 and 6).

*SON:* As much as they don't need me, they think they don't need me, they're gonna need me.

*MOTHER:* Why?

*FATHER:* Why?

*SON:* You'll need me.

*MOTHER:* For what?

*FATHER:* For what?

*SON:* You don't know yet.

*MOTHER:* Well, you must have some idea, George. I mean you're getting me scared, like maybe you know I got some kind of, uh, cancer or something, that I'm gonna die.

*FATHER:* You mean, I may drop dead, and your mother may need you?

*MOTHER:* Hey, you know how nice—I'd love to be (*laughs*) on my own, in my own apartment.

*KIRSCHNER:* Can you tell your son you don't need him?

*MOTHER:* I don't.

*KIRSCHNER:* OK, you tell him that. Tell him that.

*MOTHER:* I don't think anybody needs anybody, if you have yourself.

*KIRSCHNER:* Tell George that you don't need him.

*MOTHER:* I told him that. I told him that coming up in the car.

*KIRSCHNER:* Tell him.

*MOTHER:* Right. I don't need you, George.

*KIRSCHNER:* (*overlapping*) Tell him in the straightest possible way that you do not need him, that when he is straight and together, you don't want him around because you don't need him.

*FATHER:* We love him but we don't need him. He needs himself.

*SON:* Now.

*FATHER:* Now? Later.

*MOTHER:* You need yourself all the time.

*FATHER:* We need each other.

*KIRSCHNER:* You want him to live with you and take care of you, is that what you want?

*MOTHER:* Not the rest of his life, no.

*KIRSCHNER:* You don't want that.

*MOTHER:* Not when we're two old people, how's he gonna benefit from two old people?

*This third interview was a turning point in the therapy. Early in the interview, the mother said this about sons who lived with their mothers.*

MOTHER: There's so many families where sons are still with them, and they're happy. These boys come and go as they please. Sometimes they don't come home for weekends. . . . I know a fellow who works with my other son, his aunt works in my place. This boy is about twenty-eight or thirty years old, and he lives with his mother and father. I guess 'cause they're old. He has older sisters who are married. There's no problem there.

*Toward the end of the interview, after the therapist's persistent efforts, the mother said:*

MOTHER: (*to son*) Maybe you ought to talk to Edgar and see how miserable he is, being with his mother. That he wishes he could put his mother away. That's really how Edgar honestly feels. Not that he don't love her, it's just that he has no mind of his own. None at all. He would *love* to be married. And Edgar *could* have been married. And so could Robert. Robert don't even want to stay in that house where his mother was.

FATHER: Edgar had a miserable life in his house.

MOTHER: He's so unhappy, Edgar, it's pathetic. All that laughing and joking, it's all a front. Just *talk* to Edgar, and *see* how he feels.*

*The interviews continue to focus on a job, school, and disengagement from the parents. The parents are required to talk more to each other—first about the son and then about other aspects of their lives. Three weeks later, in the sixth interview, the progress continues.*

KIRSCHNER: Your son had tremendous cravings for heroin. If he's not taking heroin, it means that big changes are taking place. That's what it means. And it means that what you're doing at home, and what we're doing here, is helping him to get on his feet.

---

*\*Editors' note.* A less obvious factor in the parents'—especially mother's—reversal here has to do with their physical placement in the room. The couple was situated toward a corner and close together. When their son was removed, they appeared to move even closer together. We would view their increased proximity as indicative of, and contributory to, their stronger stance. It is not clear that the change in their attitude toward the son's leaving would have occurred as readily or as forcefully if they had not had each other to lean on—for example, if they had each been seated in different corners.

*FATHER:* That's what I say too.

*MOTHER:* (*to son*) Well, I tell you, I don't want you to be with this boy.

*SON:* I go with who I want to go with.

*MOTHER:* But then this upsets me, 'cause I don't like this boy. And you know that . . .

*KIRSCHNER:* But *you* don't have to go out with him.

*MOTHER:* No, but I—he's gonna entice him again, I know it. He has ways, you can't imagine how . . .

*FATHER:* When he entices him again, that's *his* problem.

*MOTHER:* He really is an evil person.

*KIRSCHNER:* Listen to what your husband is saying. Tell your wife again.

*FATHER:* That's his problem. That's all. When he don't come home one night, that's his problem.

*SON:* Right.

*KIRSCHNER:* What do you mean?

*FATHER:* What I mean, I don't like him staying out overnight. If he's gonna live with us, and he's under treatment, I don't want him staying out overnight.

*KIRSCHNER:* All right. So let's make . . .

*FATHER:* That's all.

*KIRSCHNER:* So make a rule about it.

*MOTHER:* I told him that.

*SON:* You're not making no rules for no twenty-six [his age] . . .

*MOTHER:* Well we got rules over here. Me and your father have to come here, we have things we have to do to help you.

*KIRSCHNER:* (*to son, who is looking in a mirror and combing his hair*) Hey, George, could you stop grooming yourself for just a moment, for that heavy date that you got?

*SON:* I ain't got no date. I'm here to talk about myself.

*KIRSCHNER:* Your folks—your folks are saying that they don't want you to stay out all night.

*SON:* Yeah, so? That's one reason why I'll be getting my place sooner than I think. You know, they don't need me. You don't need me to do this work that I'm doing. You don't—you don't need me. You're just telling me you don't need me.

*KIRSCHNER:* How did you hear it that way?

*SON:* That's the way I heard it.

*KIRSCHNER:* How do you figure?

*SON:* 'Cause if I—if I do the work for them, I'm gonna go out.

*KIRSCHNER:* They're not saying that you can't go out, they're saying that they get, uh . . .

*SON:* Overnight.

*KIRSCHNER:* Yeah, that's what they're uptight about.*

*As the parents and the son face the issue of separation, it becomes more real to them. There is no relapse and the improvement continues. Four weeks later the young man is working and making plans to go to school and to move to his own apartment. One can predict that the parents will develop conflicts with each other as this time of separation from the son approaches. They talk of separating from each other or of substituting someone else for the son.*

*SON:* I've had enough of that frigging area, it makes me sick. I'm moving up to the East, get me a nice little place somewhere up there. And I'll just go to work from there.

*FATHER:* OK.

*SON:* Then you'll know where I'm at. There'll be a phone booth in the apartment building, or whatever I'm in, and you call me if you need any help or something.

*KIRSCHNER:* Right. So the first step then is for you to get a job.

*FATHER:* The second step is, she has to—she has to change her mind about not coming here anymore.

*KIRSCHNER:* OK, George . . .

*MOTHER:* I'm not coming the next couple of weeks. You go.

*KIRSCHNER: (to son)* George, could you excuse us for a few minutes? I'd appreciate it. Here, you can take your college bulletin. I'll meet with you alone; we can discuss some things—maybe I got pointers, 'cause I worked in a college.

*SON:* All right. *(He leaves.)*

*KIRSCHNER: (to mother)* You don't have to—come all the time. I'll give you a breather. If you think that's the best thing.

---

*Editors' note.* The negotiation of "house rules" that transpired here is the same sort that a therapist might promote with a family in which the problem person is an adolescent (see Chapter 13). While the therapist might be tempted to agree with the son that these rules are inappropriate for a 26-year-old, in this family the son and his parents were still functioning as if he were an adolescent. Therapy had to first progress through this stage before he could be treated as a young adult.

Because I think you've had a very—despite the fact that you and George agitate each other—I think you've had a big influence on his getting better. Believe it or not.

*MOTHER:* Well I can't take anymore, I got news for you.

*KIRSCHNER:* But what is it that you can't take anymore?

*MOTHER:* Anything. I'm tired. All I want to do is be left alone.

*KIRSCHNER:* How come you never went dancing in New Jersey to that place with your husband?

*MOTHER:* Where?

*KIRSCHNER:* What was that place you were telling us about?

*FATHER:* I don't know.

*KIRSCHNER:* You just want to be left alone, huh?

*MOTHER:* Hmmm.

*KIRSCHNER:* You and your husband are at your wits' end.

*MOTHER:* You just finding that out?

*KIRSCHNER:* No, I'm not finding it out. (*pause*) I told George [the husband] something on the phone when I spoke to him the other day. That one of the problems that your son has is that he's constantly afraid that the two of you are going to break up.

*MOTHER:* Well, maybe that will bring him right out of it. That's what I've been thinking about.

*KIRSCHNER:* No. This is his greatest fear.

*MOTHER:* Why?

*KIRSCHNER:* 'Cause he feels he's responsible for it. And that is his greatest fear, that the guilt . . .

*MOTHER:* Well, he apparently would be responsible.

*KIRSCHNER:* I don't think so. Why would he be responsible?

*MOTHER:* You don't? Well I don't know, but any time that this boy has been in the hospital, or he ain't been home, we've gotten along fine.

*KIRSCHNER:* You get along better when he's not there?

*MOTHER:* Yep.

*KIRSCHNER:* Is that true? George, is that true?

*FATHER:* (*after a pause*) I'm a little confused.

*MOTHER:* *Only* when he's in the hospital, not when he's out anywhere else. 'Cause I'm still nervous worrying about where he is.

*KIRSCHNER:* Oh, oh, yeah, when he's in the hospital, yeah. Well what about the rest of the time?

*This is a typical reaction in the families of disturbed young people. When the problem person is in the hospital, the family triangle and the parental marriage are stable. Treatment by custody and restraint stabilizes the family by perpetuating the problem.*

*MOTHER:* Well, that's different.

*KIRSCHNER:* So anyway, so that's why, his greatest fear is that, you know, when he's—he's not in the house, you know, and making sure that the two of you are living together. In some crazy way, you know, that's his greatest fear, that he's gonna be responsible for it—for you two breaking up. This is a tremendous fear that he lives with, you can't imagine how powerful this is.

*FATHER:* I don't know what she's gonna accomplish by even thinking of us breaking up.

*KIRSCHNER:* Well, find out. (*suggesting father ask her*)

*MOTHER:* It don't have nothing to do with you, it's *me*. I'm thinking about *me*. You have a fine time, you don't worry about nothing. You come and go as you please, do what you want. I just want an out. I'm going to my brother; I don't know where you think I'm going. I hope you don't think I'm running off with somebody.

*FATHER:* Oh, I wish you would. You need somebody.

*MOTHER:* Yeah, you wish I would.

*FATHER:* I swear to God in heaven.

*MOTHER:* There ain't anybody.

*FATHER:* I wish you would find somebody.

*MOTHER:* They're all the same.

*FATHER:* 'Cause you deserve a better life than you've had, believe me. You definitely do. My word of honor, you really deserve somebody.

*MOTHER:* (*to therapist*) We feel sorry for one another.

*FATHER:* I don't feel sorry for you, I think it's stupid.

*KIRSCHNER:* (*after a pause*) Tell her why it's stupid. I don't think she's—she made it clear. Why is it stupid for her to leave?

*FATHER:* I think it would be the greatest thing in the world if she would find somebody—have a love affair also.

*KIRSCHNER:* You want her to have a love affair?

*MOTHER:* Yeah, I could have a love affair with all this piled up inside of me, right?

*FATHER:* Well, that's what you want.

*MOTHER:* I need some *other* jerk.

*FATHER:* Well, it would take some of it out of your body and your mind.

*MOTHER:* Would it? That's for you, not me.

*KIRSCHNER:* I don't believe it. You're telling your wife to go have a love affair, and she's saying no. (*laughs*) This is a strange discussion.

*MOTHER:* Well, that's the easiest thing to do.

*KIRSCHNER:* What's the easiest thing?

*MOTHER:* To go out and find somebody. It's easy for a girl.

*KIRSCHNER:* But you haven't done it though.

*MOTHER:* Well, I don't care to do it. And he knows—if I find anybody, he'll be the first one to know about it. Because I would leave. I wouldn't make a fool out of him or out of myself.

*KIRSCHNER:* But you haven't done it.

*MOTHER:* No, I'm not interested.

*One should never underestimate how involved a peripheral father actually is and how intense his reaction can be to the son's leaving. It is important that a father–son discussion take place, to lay old issues to rest and to allow the son to begin a new relationship with his father as he disengages. The therapist sees the father and son alone as part of the 11th interview.*

*FATHER:* I am so frigging fed up!

*KIRSCHNER:* Right.

*FATHER:* He's giving me hell. Who is he to give me hell?

*KIRSCHNER:* You're right.

*SON:* I'm giving nobody hell.

*KIRSCHNER:* Right, he's your son.

*FATHER:* You think you don't give me hell?

*SON:* Who is the one that told me, "I'm a jackass, and you'll be a jackass the rest of your life"?

*FATHER:* That's the only saying you've been saying all night!

*SON:* And that's all I dream about.

*FATHER:* That's all you—my goodness, that's all you've been dreaming about?

*SON:* Yes.

*FATHER:* What a terrible statement that is: "I'm a jackass, and he'll be a jackass the rest of his life too." In other words, I've been a stupid ass—I'll admit it.

*KIRSCHNER:* All right, so how do you think that makes your son feel?

*FATHER:* He says it.

*KIRSCHNER:* It makes him feel bad, right?

*FATHER:* Like a jackass, he's a jackass like me.

*KIRSCHNER:* No, it makes him feel bad that his father talks about himself that way. More than what you're saying about him, it makes him feel bad about you.

*FATHER:* You're twenty-five; I'm fifty—twenty-five years older than you.

*SON:* Right.

*FATHER:* What the hell have I got, but a few more laughs? You've got everything ahead of you.

*SON:* A few more laughs? You've got more than a few more laughs.

*KIRSCHNER:* He says you've got more than a few laughs.

*FATHER:* Bullshit.

*The therapist skillfully lightens the tragic air of the interview.*

*KIRSCHNER:* Ah, come on. You got a few good golf games.

*FATHER:* Yeah, I got a few good golf games.

*KIRSCHNER:* What do you shoot in golf, anyway?

*FATHER:* A woman beat me this Sunday. Twenty-one handicap, and I'm an eighteen, and she beat the shit out of me.

*KIRSCHNER:* You were off that day. Now look, I agree with you, you know, it's not good for anybody for him being there [at home]. I agree with that. And I think you're doing the right thing. But we have to plan it in such a way, you know, that he gets out financially okay.

*SON:* Tomorrow I can be out of there—packed up.

*KIRSCHNER:* No, I don't want it done that way, though. You see, when you do it that way . . .

*SON:* When you get out—when you feel you're going to get out, get out as fast as possible so there ain't no more complications.

*KIRSCHNER:* No, there's not—there's no more complications if you leave in two weeks. What's the complication?

*SON:* I'm not leaving in two weeks. He needs me two weeks more like he needs, uh—the black plague.

*KIRSCHNER:* (*to father*) George, do you think you could stand your son another two weeks? If we know that he's leaving, and he's got a room, and you see that he's got his money situation straightened out? Do you think you can live with him for two weeks? You know what I'm saying. I mean I want it to be done right.

*FATHER:* I definitely know what you're saying.

Therapy terminated with this interview, having lasted only a few months of weekly interviews. The son moved out at the end of therapy. After a short time the parents separated. The son moved back home again, and the parents reunited.

In a 2-year follow-up, the parents were still together. The young man had recently moved out of their home. He had a responsible job at a managerial level and was doing well. He no longer took heroin and had not done so during the 2-year period.

Also at around this 2-year point the parents had difficulty with the second son, again pertaining to drugs (primarily occasional use of hallucinogens) and leaving home. They saw a family therapist for two or three sessions and apparently resolved the problem. It is worth noting that the difficulties with this son were neither as severe nor as chronic as with the first son (i.e., he did not develop a 5-year opiate habit).

In a follow-up 4 years later, the oldest son was still off heroin and was working; after living locally in his own apartment, he had moved to another state. The parents were still together.*

*\*Editors' note.* A more detailed report of the long-term posttherapy results with this case are reported in "Case History of a Male Addict and His Family," by M. D. Stanton and G. Zug, prepared for the Services Research Branch, National Institute on Drug Abuse, 1980.

# 8

# CRISIS RESOLUTION
# AND THE ADDICTION CYCLE

DAVID T. MOWATT/DAVID B. HEARD/FREDERICK STEIER/
M. DUNCAN STANTON/THOMAS C. TODD

THE ATMOSPHERE of perpetual crisis and even life-and-death drama in which the heroin addict and his family live is evident in the following excerpt from an initial session:

The addict arrived drunk, having been fired from his job, and having wrecked his truck on the way to see the therapist for their initial meeting. When the therapist suggested that he contact his father, the addict responded by stating, "He wouldn't come down no way; my father has no interest in me whatsoever. I OD'd one time and my father went out and took out a $50,000 insurance policy on me and after 4 months he got mad because I didn't die, and wanted me to start paying for the insurance policy."

In Chapter 1, a conceptualization is presented of drug addiction as part of a complicated, homeostatic system of interlocking feedback mechanisms that allows the family to maintain pseudostability. The dramatic events that characterize these families, such as drug overdose, criminal activities, and episodic involvement in treatment programs, are seen as symptomatic of a larger process—the inability of the addict and his family of origin to separate. In these families it is possible to detect a recurring pattern of the crisis process and how the family "solves" such crises: family tension triggers the addict's drug-related behavior; other family members (e.g., parents) then focus attention upon the addict, thereby diverting their energies from the

Appreciation is extended to Maria Rychlicki, MAC, and Susan Carle for assistance in preparation of the data presented in the latter part of this chapter.

original source of stress. Thus the initial conflictual issue is "resolved," at least for the time being, through denial accompanied by a shift to another problem.

The course of successful treatment can be described as a shift within the parent–addict triad from an initial structure in which the addict is viewed as responsible for the system's instability, to an eventual position of shared responsibility. In this second structure the parents maintain a clear hierarchical status, permitting the addict to leave the system without drugs and without carrying the burden of future family problems. When treatment is successful in allowing the addict to stop "making problems" for his family, the family is faced with an interpersonal crisis. The therapist's ability to guide the family through this crisis—and prevent it from spilling over into extra-familial systems—will determine the extent to which a new structure within the triad can be maintained, allowing for a lasting change.

It is our experience, and the position taken in this book, that this crisis is predictable in families of drug addicts and that successful treatment is largely dependent on the therapist's ability to anticipate the events and phases through which the family passes, as well as to remain in control of them. The present chapter describes (1) the rationale for a crisis-oriented family therapy with drug addicts, (2) the nature of the crisis and its relation to the addiction cycle, and (3) the relation between crisis resolution and outcome in 37 families treated within the Addicts and Families Program (AFP).

## CRISIS-ORIENTED THERAPY

Over 20 years ago, Don Jackson, in his now-classic article "The Question of Family Homeostasis,"[71] noted that improvement of the identified patient was concomitant with changes in behavior among other family intimates. He cited examples of this, such as the treatment of a depressed woman whose improvement was followed by her husband's complaint that she was worsening. Continued improvement in the wife was accompanied by the husband's loss of employment and suicide. Jackson observed that "healthy" intimates of patients attempted to sabotage the patients' improvement to prevent their own downfall. Successful treatment of an individual in isolation of his intimates frequently evoked a crisis among these intimates to the magnitude of death.[71,72] An important clinical consideration, suggested by Jackson, is that the crisis experienced by the intimates may be worse than the problem presented by the identified patient (IP). Such phenomena underlie the rationale for conjoint family therapy, although there is little evidence that simply working with the whole family, per se, insures that the IP can get better without his intimates getting worse.[56]

Langsley and associates[88, 114] attempted to keep acutely disturbed patients out of psychiatric hospitals by providing crisis therapy for the entire family. Pittman *et al.*[114] describe the underlying assumption of this project: that the symptomatic member is a pressure point in a family in which crisis resolution has been faulty. Helping families to resolve crises more successfully was at least as helpful as hospitalization and had a preventive effect in avoiding subsequent hospitalization.[89] By containing the problem within the family, the family's dysfunctional mechanisms for crisis resolution could emerge and be corrected, thus permitting the symptomatic member to improve.

Two of the authors (Mowatt and Heard) participated in a somewhat similar project housed at the Philadelphia Child Guidance Clinic, under the direction of Jay Haley.* This program provided family therapy as an alternative to psychiatric hospitalization for severely disturbed young adults, focusing on the immediate problem as a family crisis and on contracting with the family around a goal of preventing future hospitalizations.

The treatment approach applied in the Schizophrenia Project has been described elsewhere by Haley[66] and is synopsized in Chapter 6 of this book. Basically, the parental dyad was strengthened by the therapist, who helped the parents to adopt a united course of action toward the patient. When this led to symptomatic improvement, parental conflict or some other interpersonal crisis would usually emerge. If the therapist was successful in helping the family through this crisis and avoiding a relapse and rehospitalization, therapy was extremely helpful. Haley[66] reports that 10 of the 14 cases (71%) had not been rehospitalized at the point of follow-up, 2 to 4 years after treatment.

---

*It was known as the "Schizophrenia Project" and the participants are listed in the Preface of this book.

## THE ADDICTION CYCLE AND FAMILY CRISES

As emphasized in Chapter 1, the behavior of the addict is part of a cyclical process of crisis and resolution involving the family of origin. This behavior, including enrollment in treatment programs, being hospitalized, and relapsing, typically serves to detour interpersonal conflicts that the family has been unable to resolve. One of our major therapeutic assumptions (see Chapter 6) is that effective therapy involves keeping the problem within the family so that an interpersonal crisis can emerge, which the therapist can then help the family to resolve. In order to test this assumption, we attempted to ascertain whether successful therapeutic outcome was related to the emergence and resolution of major interpersonal crises.

## *THE NATURE AND RESOLUTION OF THE CRISIS*

Thirty-nine families involved in the AFP were studied for the occurrence of major crises during the course of therapy.* Therapists in the project filled out questionnaires asking them (1) if there was a major crisis during the course of therapy; (2) to describe the nature of this crisis and other crises; (3) if this crisis was successfully resolved; (4) if the therapist considered the treatment of the addict and his family a success.† The crisis could have (1) been intensifying at the time of intake (Chapter 5); (2) resulted from standard restructuring moves within therapy (Chapters 6 and 7); or (3) been intentionally induced by the therapist (Chapter 9).

In 36 of the 39 families a major crisis involving the addict emerged during therapy. The addict's behavior varied from threatening to leave therapy, to the use of illegal drugs, to criminal activity, and, in one case, to a threat of violence within the family therapy session itself. Of the three families without crises, two dropped out of treatment before a crisis emerged, while a third—which remained longer in therapy—simply experienced no crisis. In the group of 36

---

*Information on the remaining seven families was inadequate for this analysis.

†These data (item 4) were not used in analyses because they were almost perfectly correlated with item 3 (i.e., in 36 of 39 cases the answers to 3 and 4 were identical), and because better outcome data were available.

families where there was a clear crisis (usually involving the addict), the therapist worked with family members in an attempt to resolve the crisis manifested by the addict in a way that kept him drug-free; the goal was to interrupt the usual drug cycle in which the addict acted out to "save" the family from other problems.* Commonly, this took the form of urging the parents to pull together against the addict, and, at the same time, encouraging the addict's autonomy from his family. For example, in one family where the addict had been arrested for stealing merchandise, the therapist got the parents to refuse to pay the damages, while also working with the addict around returning to work. In another family (described in Chapter 12) in which the addict had taken illegal drugs, the therapist was in constant contact with the family over a complete weekend as they worked at detoxifying the addict in the family's home.

In these 36 cases with crises the therapist was asked to indicate whether or not the crisis was successfully resolved. Resolution was indicated in 26 cases. In the remaining 10 cases crises occurred but were not resolved (7 cases) or there were multiple crises but only some were resolved (3 cases).

## Family Types without Crisis Resolution

A major hypothesis of this chapter is that much of the crisis-like behavior revolving around the addict is a detour for larger issues in the family, usually involving the parents. Therefore, treatment is more likely to be successful if these larger issues are either overtly or covertly resolved. Conversely, cases in which these issues are *not* resolved tend to follow one of three courses: (1) no crisis occurs and the family aborts treatment (3 of the 13 cases in which no crisis either occurred or was resolved); (2) the addict throws up a smokescreen of crises that prevents the therapist from dealing with the family (4 of these same 13 cases); (3) crises occur in the family early in treatment

---

*We realize that this is a linear, cause-and-effect description of a process of complex interdependency. It is simultaneously true that the addict takes drugs in response to the actions of his parents and other family members *and* that the family organizes itself around the behavior of the addict. However, it can be quite useful therapeutically to offer a one-sided punctuation of this cycle, as a way to engage the parents in treatment or to interrupt behavior that maintains the addiction. It is crucial, however, that the therapist not lose sight of this deliberate oversimplification, and that he constantly remember that the behavior is, again, part of a circular process of mutual interdependence.

that prevent the successful resolution of the addictive crisis—for example, it is impossible to get parents unified enough to establish and adhere to rules for the addict (6 of the 13 cases).

## Family Types with Crisis Resolution

We looked further at the aforementioned 26 families in which the therapist reported successful resolution of the major crisis—a crisis that almost always involved the drug-related behavior of the addict (the addiction cycle). Our assumption was that the continued improvement of the addict would be followed by the emergence of other family problems, usually between the parents. The therapist would then attempt to help the family deal with these additional problems in a way that did not involve the addict. For example, in one case the mother's drinking problem emerged and the father threatened to leave the family. The therapist encouraged the parents to stay together, since a separation at this point might be interpreted by the addict as being his responsibility, encouraging a relapse. At the same time, the addict was told that the therapist was better equipped to handle the problem than the addict, and that the most helpful thing for him to do would be to continue work on his own career interests. The addict's continued improvement seemed assured when the therapist convinced the father to take the mother to Alcoholics Anonymous and become involved in her care.

The successful blocking of the addiction cycle resulted in the emergence of interpersonal problems in the family in all 26 cases; in 17 of them, these later problems assumed crisis proportions. The relationship between the addiction cycle and the masked family problem tended to assume one of four forms:

>    1. In some families, it was possible both to (a) get the family to change its behavior toward the addict and deal successfully with crises around his behavior, and (b) produce major shifts in the parents' behavior without an explicit crisis developing between the two of them. This pattern emerged in 9 of the 26 cases. Examples, such as in Chapters 10 and 11, included the therapist supporting the father to be more effective and the mother less involved, and having the parents accept this shift without other problems developing (such as threats of divorce, the mother becoming depressed, the father drinking, etc.). We

hypothesized that the outcome of this group would be most positive.

2. Another group of cases expected to be successful were those in which the addictive crisis was resolved, and other family problems emerged that also proved to be resolvable. Nine of the 26 cases were of this type. For example, in one case the addict became hysterical as other family problems emerged, threatening suicide, provoking a crisis at his job, and/or using illegal drugs. After the parents pulled together to avert such behavior, and the son was successfully detoxed from methadone, both the mother and the father began to display similar crisis-like behavior. The mother disclosed to the therapist that she was developing "nervous symptoms" and the father revealed that he had a drinking problem that was becoming worse. In this type of family it is important to normalize these complaints as part of the therapeutic process. For example, the therapist explained that this was common during this stage of the treatment. Both parents had worked so hard to cure their son of heroin that they needed to feel a period of nervous exhaustion, or "a bit low," and would probably begin to experience differences between themselves. This set the stage for the emergence of a major family issue: the maternal grandmother had lived in the home for several years. This had become such a long-term taboo topic that both parents feared that discussion of it would destroy the family. However, the experience of working to cure their son of heroin had strengthened the relationship between the parents. They had shared something with each other and were therefore able to deal with the grandmother as well. The decision to put the grandmother in a nursing home was followed by a period of relative peace between the parents and their son continued to improve.

3. In a third type of family, the addiction cycle masked problems in another family member that were not resolvable within the constraints of a concentrated, brief therapy model. In these families, as the addiction cycle was broken, another member of the family became vulnerable and was handicapped in a real way. This was not "deterioration" in the usual sense, but more a maintenance of the status quo, or perhaps of "first-order" change.[186] We found four cases of this type. In one family, the therapist was able to mobilize the parents to thwart the addict's

efforts to leave treatment and his job as he approached the end of a planned period of detoxification from methadone. Yet as the addiction cycle was broken, both parents literally broke down. The father was hospitalized for a heart attack and the mother threatened to leave home. The family responded to this threat in a way that kept the addict uninvolved, although other family members took his place in rescuing the parental couple: the sister divorced her husband and returned home to live, and another sibling began to use illegal drugs. In a similar family, a brother began to use drugs after 2 years of abstinence, following the IP's detox from methadone. In a third family, the father's drinking problem became worse as his son remained free of drugs. The therapist's efforts toward getting the mother to help her husband through this problem initially required psychiatric hospitalization of the father. Treatment was successful in freeing the addict of his addiction and a 1-year follow-up indicated that he had remained drug-free and had completed an apprenticeship that allowed him to become successfully self-employed; yet, he remained living with his mother and in a follow-up interview it appeared that he and his mother talked about his father much in the same way that the mother and father had previously talked about him.

Families of this type may at first appear quite similar to those of Type 2 (above), in that crises occur in other family members. However, the Type 3 families are considerably more persistent in maintaining a symptomatic member once the addiction cycle has been broken, and the crises that they do generate are usually more intense and difficult to manage than in the second type. Further, although the addict's functioning may appear dramatically improved from where he was at the beginning of treatment, the separation from his family may remain marginal, with other family members taking his place in rescuing the family through self-destructive acts. Cases such as this usually require additional sessions to reach a point of stability and reorganization without major problems.

4. In a fourth type of family (four cases), breaking the addiction cycle provoked a crisis worse than the addiction cycle itself. It would appear that these families are tightly enmeshed and that their structures for resolving conflict are so fragile that when stressed to resolve crises in a different way they explode

violently. For instance, in one family[146] the process of treatment was similar to that of other families in the sample: the addict threatened to leave treatment and quit his job as he approached detoxification, and the parents mobilized to prevent this, thus interrupting the addiction cycle. As the addict continued to improve and move away from his family, the parents threatened separation and two siblings overdosed on drugs—one fatally.* This is another instance where a more flexible and extended treatment paradigm might have resolved or prevented these other events from reaching such catastrophic proportions.

## Additional Considerations

Some might view the above typology of crisis resolution as one of "therapeutic systems" rather than of addicts' families *sans* therapist. The four categories were defined ex post facto, having been derived from various classes of observed family behaviors. However, these behaviors emerged within a context that also included a therapist. It is possible that some families might have shown patterns that were more or less dysfunctional than actually occurred here, given a different therapist, or given the same therapist making different interventions. It is difficult to completely separate therapists' contributions from the family events used for categorization.

On the other hand, we do not consider all 26 families to be interchangeable, that is, that they were assigned to one of the four types primarily due to their therapists' operations. In fact, therapeutic factors are partially controlled, since all the families at least resolved the addiction crisis. In sum, we believe the typology has validity as a

*While this might be considered an example of the kind of "deterioration" discussed by Gurman and Kniskern,[56] many of these families show such a propensity for self-destruction (see Chapters 1 and 17) that it is not clear whether family therapy "provoked" the disasterous events, or whether these events might have occurred anyway, without any kind of family intervention. As noted later, our data indicate, in fact, that family therapy probably *prevented* a number of premature deaths.

On another point, one of us (Stanton) has emphasized previously the thin line between addiction and death and how the pervasive self-destruction in addicts' families is usually a collusive family process.[146, 163] Consequently, we are alert to, and concerned about, the need for continued attention to possible deaths of other family members, such as siblings, in these families. However, even though we regard such processes in terms of a systemic model, serious problems in other members can occur despite this concern.

*family* typology, not one of therapeutic systems, per se. At worst, if there has been slippage between the four types due to therapeutic factors, it is our opinion that no family would have shifted more than one category adjacent to its assignment within the schema.

Related to the above, it might be instructive to examine an extreme example of the kind of reaction that can occur in some families when little or no family-oriented intervention is attempted. This case was not seen in family therapy because it was not eligible for our family-treatment program. We knew about them because we initially tried to engage them in therapy, before their ineligibility was determined. The addict continued in the standard methadone program and as he approached detoxification, he became involved in criminal behavior and initiated violence toward the family, seemingly as a harbinger of the events to follow. His actions marked the beginning of a disasterous chain of events within the family that resulted in five deaths. Three brothers and a nephew died of drug overdoses and the father died in the hospital of a heart attack. This family clearly demonstrates the interlocking nature of addicts' families, giving a picture of the extremes to which the dysfunctional cycle can swing.

## THE ADDICTION CYCLE, CRISIS RESOLUTION, AND OUTCOME

We examined the 39 cases to see whether there was the expected relationship between crisis resolution and outcome. The degree of success was measured by the extent to which the addict abstained from legal or illegal opioid use (the addiction cycle) during the 6 months following the end of treatment. In those families where a major crisis did not occur during therapy, we predicted poor outcome, since the addiction cycle had not been challenged. In families where a crisis was manifested by the addict during treatment, and where this crisis was not resolved, treatment was also expected to be unsuccessful.

More positive outcomes were anticipated in cases where the addictive crisis was successfully handled, setting the stage for other family issues to emerge and be resolved. Based upon the typology described earlier, these emerging family problems could take one of four forms, with the particular form expected to be related to outcome. The expected *order* of the forms, from best to worst outcome, was (1) family issues were resolved without reaching crisis proportions; (2) such crises developed and were clearly resolvable by the therapist, which was expected to allow the addict to continue to improve and move toward more autonomy from his family; (3) in families where interparental issues were not resolved, continued improvement on the part of the addict was less likely; to the extent that the addict did improve, such improvement was likely to be offset by physical illness of a parent or the emergence of significant problems in a sibling; (4) in the fourth type of family, the breakdown of the addiction cycle was followed by a chain reaction of violence and even death.

The type of reaction mentioned above, in item 4, was unusual in our sample, occurring in only 4 of 39 cases. When it occurred, the violent reaction was not necessarily precipitated by the therapy, but seemed to be an example of the level of crisis under which some of these families attempted to survive, never seeking professional help.* Exactly what would constitute a helpful intervention in this type of family is beyond the scope of this chapter, but it seems that the development of methods for identifying them prior to treatment would be a fruitful direction for future research.

The topic of interest here is the relationship of crisis occurrence and resolution to outcome. However the family patterns described are, although important, too refined to detect any correlations in our own sample of 39 cases; for example, some "types" had as few as 3 families. Consequently, it was decided to compare outcome based on one distinction: those families where the therapist considered the addictive crisis to be successfully resolved versus those families in which either no crisis occurred or the occurring crisis was not successfully resolved. A listing of the various categories, and the number of families in each, is presented in Table 2.

Outcome data addressing the primary issue of opioid addiction, in the form of days free of legal opiates (e.g., methadone) and days free of illegal opiates during the first 6 months posttreatment, were available for the IP in 37 of the families; for two families these data were incomplete and thus insufficient for inclusion here (see Chapter 17 for a detailed explanation of the methods for obtaining and calculating outcome data). An outcome was classified as "Good" for a given IP if he was free of that particular class of drugs for more than

---

*In fact, data presented in Chapter 17 would indicate that family therapy may actually have prevented a number of deaths from occurring. The rate of premature deaths is abnormally high among addicts,[32, 163] but the mortality rate among family therapy cases was a fraction of that among those not treated in family therapy.

*Table 2.* Breakdown of Cases as to Types of Crisis and Resolution[a]

| WITH CRISIS RESOLUTION ($n=26$) | | WITHOUT CRISIS RESOLUTION ($n=13$) | |
|---|---|---|---|
| Addict crisis resolved without explicit family crisis | $(n=9)$ | Family crisis | $(n=6)$ |
| Moderate family crisis | $(n=9)$ | Addict crisis only | $(n=4)$ |
| New identified patient | $(n=4)$ | No crisis | $(n=3)^{b}$ |
| Severe family crisis | $(n=4)$ | | |

[a]The seven subgroups are listed, from top to bottom, in order of expected positive outcomes. For example, cases with a resolved crisis in the IP, but no explicit family crisis, would be expected to show the best outcomes. Cases with no crisis are anticipated to do most poorly, relative to the other six subgroups.

[b]Two of these cases withdrew from treatment prematurely, before a crisis emerged.

80% of the days within the 6-month period. We then examined the distribution of cases across these two dimensions—"Good" versus "Not Good" outcome, and crisis resolution versus nonresolution (or no crisis)—separately for both legal opiates and illegal opiates.*

Inspection of these distributions revealed that, for illegal opiates, 18 of 25 families in which crisis resolution was attained had Good outcomes (i.e., 72%), whereas Good outcomes occurred in only 5 of 12 (41.7%) of the families in which either no crisis or no crisis resolution occurred. This difference, using a one-tailed† test for the difference between two proportions, was significant at the .05 level. For use of legal opiates, 17 of the 25 families that resolved the crisis (68%) had Good outcomes, while 5 of 12 (41.7%) of the families without crisis resolution had Good outcomes—a difference significant at the .10 level using the same one-tailed test.

These results tend to support the idea that occurrence and resolution of a crisis within the course of therapy are important variables in helping the addict to both get off and remain off opioids, that is, to break the addiction cycle. Certainly this is a topic that merits further investigation with larger samples, more detailed measures, and continuous sampling throughout treatment.

*It should be noted that the follow-up aspects of this program were funded primarily to track change in the drug use of the IP, hence these individual-oriented data. Once this primary obligation is fulfilled for the complete 4-year follow-up period, we hope to be able to examine outcomes with other family members as well.

†One-tailed tests were used here because of the clear direction of our hypotheses.

## SUMMARY

This chapter emphasizes the utility—even the necessity—for crises both to occur and be resolved in family therapy with drug addicts. The therapeutically induced crisis might be seen as the "royal road" to functional reorganization and change in the family. In these families, the lack of a crisis—or the aborting of therapy prior to the occurrence of a crisis—usually means that no change will occur. Addicts' families appear to take one of seven paths in the face of family intervention (with its impending crisis). The particular path or pattern a family manifests may be predictive both of (1) the success of treatment, and (2) the need for continued therapeutic intervention. The occurrence and resolution of crises would appear to be important variables in therapeutic success.

# 9

# DEATH AS A MOTIVATOR: *USING CRISIS INDUCTION TO BREAK THROUGH THE DENIAL SYSTEM*

DAVID B. HEARD

THIS CHAPTER is a clinical presentation of brief family therapy with a case in which the index patient (IP) had used heroin for 9 years and been chronically addicted for 7 years. It emphasizes ways the therapist can prepare and use crisis induction to bring about change. The rationale for using crisis induction[102] rests upon the observation that family patterns of interaction are often stabilized by one member of the family acting in an extremely dysfunctional, life-threatening manner, such as shooting heroin. The recurring pattern of the addiction cycle has been described in Chapter 1; basically, it is a process in which the addict creates a crisis related to drug usage as a way of distracting family members from more threatening inter-personal conflicts within the family. As noted in Chapter 6, the therapist can get this pattern "unstuck" with some families through basic restructuring moves within sessions, such as blocking dysfunctional interactions between the parents and refusing to allow typical unproductive patterns of focusing on drugs. However, some families are more staid or homeostatic than others, remaining relatively un-moved by standard interventions. In such cases the therapist may have to intensify his interventions in order to get the family beyond their impasse-like stability and allow them to progress. Thus he intentionally induces a crisis, thereby temporarily unbalancing the family system. In this way he "opens the system up," providing the opportunity to make significant changes in the way parents align themselves in the family hierarchy.

## CASE MATERIAL

The IP in this case, Jim, was a 23-year-old male of Italian-American extraction whose father was a repairman and whose mother was a homemaker. Jim had an 11th-grade education and had served 2 years in the Army. Prior to treatment he had been arrested once for burglary, but the charges had been dropped. Although he had not been otherwise apprehended, he occasionally engaged in shoplifting and drug selling to sustain his habit.

Most of the transcriptions in this chapter are taken from the ninth session, in which a crisis was planned and implemented. To assist in understanding the context of this session, excerpts from the initial meeting between the addict and the therapist are first presented. The dialogue below takes place when the two of them are alone, having just met for the first time. Earlier in the day, Jim had been told by personnel at the Veterans Administration Drug Dependence Treatment Center (VA DDTC) that the therapist would be his drug counselor and would be in charge of his methadone.

> *HEARD:* OK, Jim, what's your situation?
> *JIM:* I've been doing dope since I was fourteen years old. That's when I first had a spike in my arm. I used to be a "weekend warrior," as they call it. At the age of fourteen I shot dope on weekends. Just for the hell of it, for kicks, with my buddies. I was a follower.
> *HEARD:* How old are you now?
> *JIM:* I am twenty-three years old next month.
> *HEARD:* Do you live at home?
> *JIM:* I live at home.
> *HEARD:* Who else lives in your house?
> *JIM:* I have a mother who is very ill. I have a father who works two jobs. I have an aunt that lives there. I have a [paternal] grandmother that lives there, and I have two younger sisters. That's all my family.
> *HEARD:* How old are they?
> *JIM:* Seventeen and nineteen. . . . Now this is what I want to rap to you about. I called the Veterans up last night because I was withdrawing. I didn't have enough medication. Dr. Woody straightened me out today on that. My arm is in bad shape. You know what I did? I tried to put my fist through one of the walls . . . because I was very

uptight. I was sick as a dog. So I got in contact with my family doctor and he gave me something to settle me down OK, . . . to hold me over till this morning, all right. . . . Putting that aside, my whole problem is like I heard that this place is for to get family together. Now if I don't get my family together, I'll never see my family again, because at Redtown [Hospital] they say I have suicidal and homicidal intentions. Now I told them the only way there'd be suicide is if I OD'd on a bad bag . . . that would be the only way there would be suicide . . . or else if I went on a suicide mission . . . say I flipped out or went nuts. . . . I would kill people, but I would probably in the process kill cops or anybody who got in my way but I'd be killed doing it. That would be the only way I'd do suicide . . . otherwise I have no intensions to slit my wrist. I have no intentions to eat fifty pills. I have no intentions to do that, but I do have homicidal intentions . . . they already proved that. I've been in a depressed mood right now. This has been going on for over a year. I got out of that mood when I had a girlfriend, . . . a steady girl. She set me up. I got both my jaws busted . . . both sides. Ever since then I've been depressed. I can't get over this depression and it bothers me. My mother don't understand too much about drugs. Right away she calls the doctor and screams and yells, "It ain't his fault," saying, "My son, he's messed up in the head. Put him away." I was at Redtown for two weeks, by the way, and I just got out, a couple of weeks ago.

*HEARD:* What were you there for?

*JIM:* I didn't go for AMA [against medical advice]. I went for detox on valium. I was on methadone, which I am still on. . . . I'm on what is called "wesadone" . . . going to use technical words because that what I'm on. It's not methadone . . . you can't call it methadone, it's wesadone. I want to go on LAAM,* but I can't go on LAAM until me and you get together and I have clean urines and all that bullshit. Now what kind of thing is this? Now I told you a little bit about myself.

*HEARD:* How about wanting to get off of it completely?

*JIM:* Sir, . . . I tried it. I tried it six times in the VA hospital, . . . two times at Redtown. One at Johnson-Burns [Hospital]. . . . Sorry, Doctor.

*HEARD:* You've got a long list of failures.

*JIM:* I am a failure. . . . I'm not ready yet.

---

*Levo-alpha-acetylmethadol (a long-acting derivative of methadone).

*This dialogue between therapist and addict clearly indicated that Jim's problem was not simply a drug problem, but that it involved significant interpersonal difficulties within his family. To quote Jim, "My whole problem is like I heard that this place is for to get family together. Now if I don't get my family together, I'll never see my family again, because at Redtown they say I have suicidal and homicidal intentions." Also evident in this statement was a clue to the therapist that suicidal and homicidal threats and actions might become central issues in working with Jim and his family.*

As this session continued, Jim became more agitated and complained of feeling sick. He gave permission for the therapist to phone his home and both parents were home. The therapist introduced himself and explained to the parents that their son had entered a new drug-treatment program that involved participation of the entire family. The parents were asked if they would come to the clinic immediately. The parents agreed, but said that only they were coming, not the daughters or grandmother.

## FIRST (FAMILY) SESSION

Once the parents arrived, Jim's behavior became more agitated and he raised a new subject not previously discussed. Jim began to make threats toward a visiting great-aunt, saying that he had a sawed-off shotgun and that he was going to go home and "shoot the old bitch." The aunt was on the father's side of the family, a sister to the grandmother. She had come to visit the family approximately a week earlier. There was some mention by the grandmother that perhaps the aunt could remain permanently. Mrs. Galvani (Jim's mother) wanted her husband to speak with the grandmother and aunt and try to explain that there simply wasn't room in the house for the aunt to remain permanently. Mr. Galvani felt that he should "not intrude into this delicate situation," as he explained it. The aunt was sleeping in Jim's room. Jim was sleeping on the couch. As the session continued, Jim became increasingly agitated, threatening to kill the aunt "just as soon as all of this stupid bickering stops." The therapist took the position that he hardly knew Jim and that the parents should decide what was to be done to handle this situation. Within a very short period of time, the parents decided that Jim should go to Redtown (a pseudonym for a nearby hospital with an inpatient program). The session ended with an agreement that the entire family would meet again once Jim returned home from Redtown Hospital. This was Jim's second trip to Redtown in a month.

In this family the hospital was like a pressure valve and the therapist came to view hospitalization as an integral element in the addiction cycle. Mounting family tension would set off threatening behavior by the addict. This would be followed by a refocus of all family attention on him and the family would push for him to be hospitalized, thereby diverting attention from their original conflict. It was quite evident how Jim's behavior played a protective function in the family, especially in relationship to his father: Mr. Galvani did not have to speak with the grandmother and the aunt; nonetheless, the situation was resolved. While Jim was checking in at the hospital, he phoned home to inform the aunt that she was responsible for his going into the hospital and making him go crazy. When he was discharged 6 days later, the aunt was gone. This interaction provided important diagnostic information to the therapist in partially understanding the Galvani family. The interaction suggested that Jim was involved in a protective coalition with his father; also, Mr. Galvani was involved in a protective coalition with his own mother.

Based upon this experience, the therapist knew from the very beginning the important function the hospital played in this family and that in all likelihood he would again be faced with an impending hospitalization once another stressful situation presented itself. An individual-oriented therapist might have overlooked this larger cyclical process, which involved the entire family and the hospital, and instead have focused his attention exclusively upon the individual behavior of the addict. In doing so, he would have missed the opportunity to intervene more effectively—such as in modifying the interprotective alliances among family members—and might unknowingly have become part of the intersystem cycle himself.

## SECOND (FAMILY) SESSION

Up to this point the therapist had no working contract with either the family or the addict. They had not agreed upon the goals of therapy, nor had they agreed upon who was to be involved in the therapy. In the second session these two issues were carefully addressed. The therapist took the position that he only worked with addicts who wanted to get off drugs—all drugs, including methadone. The parents agreed that this was indeed an admirable goal, and the addict likewise agreed. When there was some recurring expression of doubt as to whether such a goal was "realistic," the therapist assured them that it was realistic and that he had successfully worked with other cases equally as difficult as Jim's. As for the second question of who should be involved in the therapy, the therapist took the position that all family members should be involved. The mother objected that she didn't want her daughters involved because she "wanted to keep them away from Jim." Again, this kind of information provided valuable diagnostic cues concerning the mother–daughters coalition within the Galvani family. The therapist insisted that the daughters be involved and mother relented. On the question of the grandmother's participation in the therapy, the father objected vigorously on the grounds that her health was poor.

## THIRD, FOURTH, AND FIFTH (FAMILY) SESSIONS

All family members except the grandmother were present during the next three sessions, spanning a period of 6 weeks. The general theme of these three sessions was how the parents were going to make Jim more responsible as long as he continued to live with the family. The therapist strongly emphasized that Jim's stay with the family was only temporary, that is, that he would be moving out on his own. The parents were directed by the therapist to jointly make some concrete decisions concerning Jim's behavior. For example, the parents agreed that he should minimally have three job interviews a day. The parents decided how many friends Jim could invite to the house at any one time and what hours he might have friends in the home. Limits were set on how much alcohol he could consume at home and what the consequences would be if he broke this agreement. Most importantly, the parents agreed to put him out of the house if his urine tests indicated use of illegal drugs.

It is important to emphasize that what is most important is that these rules be jointly negotiated by the parents. Commonly, parents of addicts find it difficult to agree upon much of anything; therefore, the easiest issues to focus upon are related to making concrete rules about what they, as parents, will accept while their son continues to live with them. Again, the implicit message to the parents is that the addict's presence is temporary, but that he will be obliged to follow their jointly developed rules as long as he remains with them.

Mr. Galvani was consistently the more soft-hearted of the parents. He and Jim had a history of periodically staying out late at night drinking. Mrs. Galvani was dissatisfied with the drinking habits of both husband and son. On some cold evenings during the winter, Mr. Galvani would wait up until the local bars closed (2 A.M.) and then go and chauffeur his son home. These examples were used as a basis for challenging Mr. Galvani's paternalistic overindulgence.* Mother appeared annoyed at her husband's permissiveness, but would never openly criticize him within these sessions. During this period of approximately 6 weeks Jim was very cooperative, almost overly so. He steadily reduced his methadone dosage, searched for work diligently, obeyed the new house rules concerning chores, friends, alcohol, and privacy of his sister's rooms. His urine tests were consistently clean.

## SIXTH (INDIVIDUAL) SESSION

The sixth session was not a planned session. Jim telephoned the therapist and said it was urgent that he speak with him alone. On the phone he complained that he was experiencing withdrawal effects from the methadone and that he was getting irritated by the therapist "stirring up all this shit in my family." An individual meeting was arranged within hours and the addict insisted that he was checking into Redtown Hospital immediately. The therapist offered to assist Jim in obtaining additional methadone if that was what he needed, but Jim refused. He was insistent, even becoming belligerent, when the therapist gave some minimal cue that he opposed the idea of Jim going into the hospital at this time. A plan between addict and therapist had been made 6 weeks previously that Jim would enter the hospital only at the point when the outpatient detoxification was nearly complete. A more traditional drug counselor might conceptualize Jim's "panic reaction" as a response to internal anxiety and the safety that the hospital offers the addict as a way of binding anxiety. From a family systems viewpoint, however, this sudden shift in

---

*Editors' note. This family shows a reversal of the usual family pattern with an addicted son. Instead of the mother being the parent who is overinvolved with the addict, the enmeshment in this case is between father and son.

behavior and attitude on Jim's part signaled to the therapist that something unsettling was likely happening in the family and that Jim was assuming his customary role of focusing attention upon himself. The decision as to what to do at this point was a crucial one in terms both of case management and of planning strategy. The therapist could not stop Jim from signing himself into the hospital because he was a veteran and had the right to enter a VA hospital at will. At the same time, his entering himself into the hospital was part of the cyclical crisis process involved in the addiction cycle. If the therapist did not make an intervention at this point, he would lose an opportunity to make really significant changes in the family. It was thought that the best possible solution was not to oppose Jim's desire to enter the hospital, but to insist that it should not happen until the family could meet to discuss the situation. This decision was made primarily on the basis that it is better to try and have some effect upon the direction that a team of runaway horses moves, rather than to be trampled trying to stop them. A family session was scheduled for the next day.

## SEVENTH (FAMILY) SESSION

The goal of this family session was to strongly emphasize how Jim's impending hospitalization and detoxification should be different from past hospitalizations. The therapist consistently underscored the fact that this detox was special and that it would be the last one, ever. Mrs. Galvani and Jim's sisters demonstrated a directness in challenging Jim that had not been manifested in previous sessions. In the past, hospitalization (with detoxification) occurred without family input; that is, it had been purely a decision between drug counselor and addict. In the current situation, the addict was pressed by family members to fight for his right to detoxify, and various family members took committed positions about the impending hospitalization. Present were both parents, Jim, and his two sisters, Susan and Joan.

HEARD: Where are you going to sit, Jim?

JIM: It doesn't matter to me.

MOTHER: You can sit outside.

HEARD: Sit here then. Did you talk to your mom and dad about our session yesterday?

MOTHER: No, not one word.

*JIM:* No, because it was private.

*HEARD:* Oh, it was private?

*MOTHER:* I didn't even ask. I figured if he wanted to tell me anything he would tell me.

*HEARD:* That's a good attitude. How should we start then? I don't know how to raise the topic.

*MOTHER:* How to raise the topic? What topic?

*JIM:* We were talking about, what was it, going in the hospital over at the VA.

*MOTHER:* Going for what?

*JIM:* For the rest of the detox, instead of waiting for, what is it, another four or five weeks.

*HEARD:* Why don't you tell her some of what we said yesterday?

*JIM:* I said I was tired of going up there every day, six days a week.

*MOTHER:* You mentioned before you wanted to get on that other drug program.

*JIM:* No—our whole thing is that when we first come here—by the end of the sessions I was supposed to be drug-free, right? So I figured I'm tired of going back and forth so I wanted to go in the hospital and get it over with—instead of, you know, going back and forth every day. That's what we were talking about . . .

*MOTHER:* I don't know. Do you think he's ready? I don't think he's ready.

*SUSAN:* Neither do I.

*JOAN:* Neither do I.

*HEARD:* Jim, you have three people in your family here. You'd better talk to them. They have questions.

*JIM:* Well, it's up to me. I think I'm ready so I'm going to do it. That difference of four and two weeks don't make much difference.

*HEARD:* Why do they think that? Why did your mom and your two sisters say they didn't think you're ready?

*JIM:* I don't know. I don't care what they think. I'm just saying what I think.

*HEARD:* I agree. I think that what you think is important, but I'm just curious as to why they think that.

*JIM:* I don't know. Ask them.

*HEARD:* Why is that? Why do you think that . . .

*MOTHER:* I don't think he is ready. I think he is rushing himself.

*JOAN:* He's not ready, man.

*HEARD:* How would you know? What are the signs that you would know that he is ready?

*MOTHER:* Past experience.

*JOAN:* When he changes. He is still the same old Jim.

*SUSAN:* That's it. He's just going to go and detox and start over.

*HEARD:* I have to tell a little bit about what we talked about yesterday. I told Jim yesterday, I was kind of kidding him and I said, "You're an old pro at this, you know. You've done it a half a dozen times, and you're going to do it again." But I said, "What I want to know is what is going to be different after you detox this time?"

*FATHER:* He was great one year. I'd like to see him the way he was that one year. It was beautiful. Everything was OK. Remember?

*HEARD:* It's almost like the family has been programmed to expect he can't do much better than maybe a year. I'm talking about doing it for good. (*Sisters giggle.*) The family thinks that's not possible.

*JOAN:* If I'd seen any change I'd say yes, but I don't see any change.

*JIM:* What kind of change? What kind of change?

*JOAN:* A lot of changes!

*JIM:* What kind of change! To your standards? You don't know what kind of change!

*JOAN:* Your attitude! You still are, you know, up here. If you want me to get into it I will . . .

*JIM:* To me it's a bunch of bullshit!

*HEARD:* What is your sister saying?

*JOAN:* That's why I don't even bother saying nothing when I come here . . .

*HEARD:* You know, I don't think you're helping the situation by keeping quiet.

*MOTHER:* Yeah, but he denies everything!

*JOAN:* Yeah, I can't get nowhere with him.

*MOTHER:* What they say, you deny everything. It's true.

*JOAN:* Try to help him and that's what he does: lies and everything.

*Note that the family members' focus of discussion here was not Jim's drug habit per se, but rather the issue of interpersonal relation-*

*ships among family members. His sisters were provided an oppor-*
*tunity to confront him directly concerning their grievances. The*
*therapist maintained a position similar to that of a stage director;*
*that is, he set the stage for the scenes to follow. If the therapist had*
*not carefully prompted the two sisters, and simultaneously restrained*
*the father from being overprotective, the interaction between family*
*members would quickly have ended.*

*HEARD:* You know I think Jim's talking now about going into the hospital, about detoxing. I want this to be—I want it to be the last time Jim ever detoxes . . . and for that to happen I think people need to kind of lay the cards on the table.

*JIM:* It's up to me. They ain't even helping a bit anyway. It's only up to me. I couldn't care less what they think.

*HEARD:* But they know how you've been.

*JIM:* Well yes, so, that's it.

*HEARD:* And so I'm asking them why they think you can't change.

*JIM:* There's what they think, and I don't really care, that's it; I know when I got to stop, that's up to me.

*HEARD:* Yeah, but they're your family and they know you.

*JIM:* Well, so what. I still have feelings and I just don't give a shit.

*HEARD:* What can you say to your sisters?

*JIM:* What do you mean, what can I say?

*HEARD:* About what they are saying.

*JIM:* They got their own opinion.

*HEARD:* All right, do you think they'll be able to trust you when you come out?

*JIM:* I don't really care.

*HEARD:* You don't care if they trust you?

*JIM:* No, I don't.

*FATHER:* What are you saying? You're not coming around!

*JIM:* If I'm doing good when I come out and they still don't trust me, it's up to them. I don't really care.

*FATHER:* Well it's up to you.

*JIM:* That's the way I feel; I'm not gonna have to prove nothing to nobody no more. That's it.

*HEARD: (to family)* What would Jim have to do for you to believe that this detox is really different?

*JOAN:* He would have to change.

*HEARD:* Yeah, but how? In concrete terms, what would he have to do?

*JIM:* Change to her standards, and I ain't changing to nobody's standards.

*MOTHER:* Have to get a job, and get a good job, too.

*JOAN:* And move out . . .

*JIM:* (*to Joan*) And how come you don't leave the house? You're eighteen. You're working.

*JOAN:* 'Cause I'm a girl.

*JIM:* What's that got to do with it?

*MOTHER:* She don't have to leave.

*JOAN:* When I get married. What do I do? I only sleep and eat, that's all.

*FATHER:* (*to therapist*) Just a minute, let me talk a minute. What I was trying to do is get him a job, a government job.

*HEARD:* I'll tell you something. I think that's a mistake. I think it is—I think that's treating him like he is really helpless, like he's a child . . .

*JIM:* What, trying to get me a job?

*HEARD:* Yes.

*JIM:* Jobs are hard to get.

*MOTHER:* That's what he is waiting for. For one of us to get him a job. He keeps telling me, "Why doesn't someone get me a job?"

*JIM:* The mayor promised me a job. All right. Now he [pointing to father] works in the township. So there's nothing wrong by him asking, because the mayor did promise me a job and never got me a job.

*HEARD:* (*talking to two sisters*) The problem that I've seen over and over again, and the one I hope changes, is that Jim has a way of making your mom and dad treat him much younger than he is. You know, he has a way of making them . . .

*MOTHER:* But he wants to be treated that way.

*HEARD:* I know, I know. That's part of it. The other part of it is that he's done a good job of training the two of you to treat him like a child. As far as I'm concerned, if Jim is to stay off drugs, that's the key thing that's going to have to change; that's the key thing. If he's going to stay off drugs, he's got to act like a twenty-three-year-old man, and you're going to have to treat him like a twenty-three-year-old man . . .

*FATHER:* Well, I think a lot of it is environment too. He comes out and goes right out and meets somebody. Come a couple of pushers or what they call them, around, you don't know, it's the same old thing. He was doing beautiful and . . .

*HEARD:* Some kind of way, you don't think Jim can ever straighten out.

*FATHER:* Well, I don't know. We gave him the chance of his life. We did everything for him . . . can't do any more. What else could we do for him? . . .

*JOAN:* This is the last resort though . . .

*HEARD:* (*talking to sisters*) He's trying to be helpful (*pointing to father*), but he's really not being helpful when he treats Jim like . . .

*JOAN:* Sometimes you can treat a person in a way that spoils them. Then he's no good no more, when he's spoiled.

*HEARD:* I know it's hard for you to hear this, Mr. Galvani. I think that it's absolutely true and I think that unless you change, when Jim detoxes, unless you change and unless you let him be a man, he's going to be back on drugs. Because his being on drugs is one of the ways that he remains a child. As long as he is on drugs everyone can say, "Poor Jim," and have to take care of poor Jim. And as long as he's on drugs you'll keep taking care of him. When he gets off drugs, unless you change, I think he'll be back on drugs. That's the whole purpose of our family meeting. Jim's got to change. There's no doubt about it. But you know, the family's got to change too, in the way they deal with Jim. He goes into the hospital and he "detoxes" again, and this must be time number six . . .

*FATHER:* More than that, isn't it, Louise?

*HEARD:* Time number seven, time number eight, you know it's going to be; there will be another—nine and ten and eleven, unless the family changes . . .

*FATHER:* (*to therapist*) See, the thing about looking for a job . . .

*HEARD:* (*to father*) Don't rescue him now, Mr. Galvani. The rest of the family needs to be heard. They've been living through hell, so don't rescue him.

*This session was dramatically different from any previous sessions in that the mother and daughters openly confronted Jim for the first time during the course of therapy. The father was blocked*

*throughout the session from protecting Jim. Mr. Galvani was notice-*
*ably uneasy during the session and much of the therapist's blocking of*
*him was done nonverbally. These examples validate the earlier hy-*
*pothesis that father and son were involved in a protective alliance.*
*Also, the mother and her daughters were involved in a coalition that*
*grew stronger when the father was prevented from protecting Jim.*
*This interaction had important effects upon Jim. It made him account-*
*able to his mother and sisters, something that seldom happened at*
*home. Also, it induced him to fight vigorously with the family for his*
*right to detoxify.*

The session ended by making concrete plans for Jim to check
into a nearby VA hospital for a planned inpatient detoxification.
Should he not carry through with his plans to detoxify completely,
the groundwork had been established for the session to follow.

## EIGHTH (INDIVIDUAL) SESSION

Three days following the seventh session, Jim entered the hospital.
The therapist visited him on his 4th day in the hospital for an eighth
session. Jim complained extensively about the hospital staff, about
the inadequacy of the facilities, about the food, and about the behavior
of the other addicts on the ward. The staff indicated that Jim had been
uncooperative and felt that he would probably leave the hospital
against medical advice within a day or two.

## NINTH (FAMILY) SESSION

Two days after Heard's visit, on a Saturday, Jim left the hospital after
having been there for a total of 6 days. The therapist had already
made plans to meet with the parents alone on Monday evening, to
underscore the fact that this hospitalization was special and that it
was meant to be the last one, ever, for Jim. The therapist decided to
stick to his plan of meeting with the parents alone because he felt it
would be easier to create a crisis atmosphere if Jim was not present.

This session was intentionally long, lasting almost 3 hours. A
colleague of the therapist, Paul Riley, was observing through the one-
way mirror. The session began with the parents talking rather franti-
cally. In contrast, the therapist assumed a slow pace and his mood
reflected an attitude of pessimism and defeat.

The strategy adopted in this session was to disqualify hospitals, doctors, and drug rehabilitation programs as the panecea for Jim's drug problem and to place responsibility for solutions squarely on the parents' shoulders. The session began with both parents absolving Jim of responsibility, suggesting that the hospital was inadequate for his needs. The therapist intentionally refused to provide the optimistic assurances and encouragement that had so readily been proffered in the past and instead introduced the question of when Jim would next shoot up. Gradually the therapist expounded on his attitude of pessimism and defeat as he projected what family life would be like in the future years. Once the issue of death was introduced into the discussion, the differences between the parents became more crystalized; this issue thus served as the vehicle for a confrontation between the parents.

*FATHER:* So Jimmy came home Saturday, did you hear?

*HEARD:* Yeah, I knew that.

*FATHER:* I didn't know. I got a call at five o'clock Saturday night. Said, "I'm here at the terminal." I says, "What terminal? Aren't you in the hospital?" He says, "No, I'm coming home." I didn't know he was coming home Saturday.

*HEARD:* Well, I didn't either.

*MOTHER:* I think he signed himself out.

*FATHER:* Now wait. He was complaining about. . . . He was with some men there. He was complaining about one person. I don't know . . .

*MOTHER:* He said, "It's an awful place to be."

*FATHER:* He was telling me he wanted to get the heck out of there. I don't know.

*HEARD:* I saw him Thursday, and he was not very happy.

*MOTHER:* No?

*FATHER:* I don't think he was happy in there, probably. Maybe it's somebody who he was with who he didn't know. Maybe that's part of it. I don't know. I figured he would stay in there for the two weeks. Didn't you, Louise? That's what we thought, that he'd be in there for two weeks. *(to therapist)* Did he say something to you? He didn't tell us much, just said it was a very bad place to be and it's dirty . . .

*HEARD:* You know, when I saw him Thursday, I left feeling very bad.

*MOTHER:* Somebody gave him the impression to leave there; even the doctors told him he shouldn't be there. I don't know if he's just telling me a story.

*FATHER:* You don't know what Jim's telling sometimes.

*HEARD:* Well, what did he tell you?

*FATHER:* There was one party was there was throwing stuff on his bed. Things like that and it was aggravating him and this is why he left.

*MOTHER:* He couldn't stand the filth, the dirt. They didn't get washed. It stunk.

*FATHER:* It was dirty. They didn't get washed. Something like that.

*MOTHER:* This is not the first time he's been in those places. You don't know what they are.

*FATHER:* He wanted to go in himself. He admitted that, right? So I mean, I couldn't figure that.

*HEARD:* So where do we go from here?

*MOTHER:* I don't know, because we're not making any headway, to tell the truth. He's home since Saturday and just sitting around.

*FATHER:* He hasn't got a job and I told him to go see the councilman; go in the house and talk to him. He knows who he is, he'll get a job. That's better; I don't go try to get him a job. It wouldn't be right for me getting him a job. I've done it before and this is it. I told him to go down and he'll have to go in there and speak to him and see if he can get it . . .

*HEARD:* How long do you think it'll be before he shoots up on some heroin now?

*MOTHER:* Oh, I don't know. I don't trust him.

*HEARD:* How many weeks do you give him?

*MOTHER:* I don't know. With him you don't know . . .

*HEARD:* (*to father*) I'm wondering, what did you expect when he went into the hospital? You know your wife was pretty pessimistic. She'd been through this so many times.

*FATHER:* I am—I'm very—I'm still pessimistic about it.

*HEARD:* Did you expect something . . . to occur?

*FATHER:* There is something wrong because, well . . .

*MOTHER:* Did you think he'd turn out fine again?

*FATHER:* When we were here the last time, you remember, and all of a sudden he wanted to go in, detox in the hospital, right?

*HEARD:* Why do you think he changed all of a sudden like that and wanted to go in and detox in the hospital?

*FATHER:* I don't know.

*MOTHER:* He does that on the spur of the moment. He will do that, and then you give him a day or two and he just changes his mind. Then he goes the other way. Now the same thing. He calls me up at the hospital and he says, "Well, there's doctors, they want to run tests on me." I says, "Are you going to be acting as a guinea pig?" He says, "No. I'm going to make money on it." Then two days later he calls me, "I'm not going through that deal I told you the other day."

*HEARD:* (*to mother*) You don't have too much faith in hospitals like that. It seems that your husband has more faith in the hospital's ability.

*FATHER:* Yeah.

*MOTHER:* Not what he's gone through. He went through it too many times. I'm the type of person, if you get caught once. . . . All right, the second time you give him a chance, but after the second time, forget it.

*HEARD:* Look, I don't have a lot of faith in hospitals either.

*MOTHER:* I forget it after that. So, I'll get burned twice but after that I . . .

*HEARD:* And you've been burned, how many times?

*MOTHER:* This is eight, nine times.

*HEARD:* Eight or nine times. My goodness. (*to father*) Do you think the hospital is the answer?

*FATHER:* I don't know. Well, the last time he went through the . . . went through the hospital here, time seven, taking the methadone, he went through it and he was detoxed down and he did pretty good, didn't he, considering I mean, I mean let's talk about . . .

*MOTHER:* For a while.

*FATHER:* Well, he wasn't taking any; he was drinking, there's no doubt about that, but he wasn't taking any methadone. But they gave us the number of a place to go in Atlantic City, if he needed it.

*HEARD:* Let me ask you, how old are you?

*FATHER:* Me? I'm fifty-three.

*HEARD:* When do you expect to retire?

*FATHER:* Well, I'm going on my twenty-fourth year and I think your retirement may be twenty-five but you have to be sixty.

*HEARD:* So, you have how many more years before you retire?

*MOTHER:* Maybe seven years.

*HEARD:* Between now and the time you retire, how many times do you think Jim will go into the hospital and come out again?

*FATHER:* I really don't know.

*HEARD:* Just take a guess.

*FATHER:* Oh, you mean go in again? Oh, he'll eventually go in again.

*HEARD:* I know, but how many times?

*FATHER:* Oh, you mean since I've had . . .

*HEARD:* No, I mean between now—between this time that he's checked out and the time you retire—how many times do you think Jim's going to go in and out of the hospital?

*MOTHER:* In the next seven years?

*HEARD:* In the next seven years. What's your guess?

*MOTHER:* It's like every other year to me, or every year maybe.

*HEARD:* Every year? So you think . . .

*MOTHER:* I think he's eventually going to kill himself. I think he's eventually going to just fade on us. That's it.

*HEARD:* Do you think the hospital will ever cure him?

*FATHER:* Well, the hospital can do so much, but they can't do everything for you. I mean, it's up to him to help himself. It looks like he don't want to help himself, but, of course, the environment around you. I don't know who he's traveling with. Could be the same thing.

*MOTHER:* The hospital is no answer for him. I don't think so. He has to be—like I said the very first time—be put away for a very long time.

*FATHER:* He needs a spot where he can't get out and where he has to stay there whether he likes or not. Maybe that would be the only thing, but just like I say . . .

*MOTHER:* They should work these boys, give them hard labor, get their minds off the stuff. They should use a different system altogether. I don't think . . .

*HEARD:* Got to get tough with them, huh?

*MOTHER:* Oh yeah, I think they should be out in the open, get the air, and work hard.

*HEARD:* But do you think it's the hospital who are the people that need to get tough with him?

*MOTHER:* Well, maybe not the hospital. I don't know. There should be some kind of thing that could help these boys out.

*HEARD:* For someone like Jim, I'm very pessimistic about hospitals. I think seven times between now and your retirement is probably a conservative estimate. I mean, Jim goes in and out of hospitals like a lot of people go to movies.

*MOTHER:* Like it's nothing, right.

*HEARD:* I think I'm more inclined to agree with your wife. I think the hospital . . .

*MOTHER:* It's no answer, 'cause I've seen it. I don't know if it's eight or nine times. He comes out. He's all right maybe for a little while and then, back again. So, I can't see where the answer to that is.

*HEARD:* (*to mother*) You seem to have a little more insight into Jim's weakness.

*MOTHER:* Well, I observe him more, maybe because I'm more with him.

*HEARD:* What do you think it's going to take?

*MOTHER:* I don't know if there's any more hope for that boy. I don't think there is. I hate to say it, but I don't think there is.

*HEARD:* If you had to say what his last chance is, what would you say it is?

*MOTHER:* What's his last chance?

*HEARD:* Yeah. I mean the hospital's not going to do it.

*MOTHER:* No, the doctors are not doing him any good. He doesn't want to help himself.

*HEARD:* I can't do it.

*MOTHER:* He can't even do it himself. I think it's gotten to the point that he can't even do it himself now. I think he's just hollering for help, just, "Help me; here I am and do whatever you want."

*HEARD:* Who can do it?

*MOTHER:* I don't know. I don't know who can do it anymore now.

*HEARD:* Do you think the two of you have the strength?

*FATHER:* I don't know.

*MOTHER:* I need a lot of backing up, which is hard to get.

*FATHER:* What do you mean? On what?

*The issue between the parents became clear for the first time: the mother felt that the father was not willing to back her in struggling with Jim. Their split had been made explicit through crisis induction. Because the doctors and hospitals had failed, the therapist was able to continue to emphasize the point that no one else could save their son. The mother had introduced the death issue by saying, "He's eventually going to kill himself." Riley phoned into the therapist and suggested he push harder concerning Jim's dying prematurely, that this should be the direction to move. These two issues—father-mother misalliances and the real possibility of death—would be the focus for the remainder of the session.*

*HEARD:* What stops you from getting tough?

*MOTHER:* I can't do it by myself.

*HEARD:* Whose help do you need?

*MOTHER:* I think my husband should help out.

*HEARD:* You mean he's not willing?

*MOTHER:* Well, he says he wants to, but down deep he doesn't want to.

*HEARD:* You think down deep he's really kind of a softie.

*MOTHER:* Yeah, oh, yeah. He can't do it. Like, you want to but you can't. He does a lot of hollering but it doesn't mean anything . . .

*HEARD:* Much too soft for Jim's own good.

*MOTHER:* And Jimmy knows it.

*HEARD:* Sure he does. I thought in Italian families the mother is supposed to be the one with the soft heart.

*MOTHER:* I'm not really mean. I do a lot hollering too, but then I feel sorry afterward. I want to see this boy straighten out. That's what I'm screaming and hollering about, but if you don't get any backing up—back me up, that's all!

*HEARD:* But your husband doesn't?

*MOTHER:* Like I said, he just can't do it; I don't think he can.

*HEARD:* What does he say when you tell him this?

*MOTHER:* He'll agree with you.

*HEARD:* All right, ask him now.

*MOTHER:* I don't want to make him feel bad by putting it on him.

*HEARD:* We're only talking about your son's life.

*FATHER:* If he is nervous you've got to watch how the heck you talk to him . . .

*MOTHER:* (*to therapist*) He's afraid of talking to him. He's afraid of telling him anything.

*FATHER:* You got to tell him in a nicer way.

*HEARD:* (*to mother*) Stand up for one minute, please, so I can move your chair around. (*Therapist positions parents' chairs facing one another.*)

MOTHER: (*to therapist*) I dictated this. I told him so many times this here story I'm telling you, but it's just that I'm sick and tired of keep repeating and repeating the same thing over and over again.

HEARD: We're only talking about your son's life.

MOTHER: (*to therapist*) I did explain to him.

HEARD: I'm going to walk out, because if I'm here the two of you are going to talk to me. I'm going to be behind the mirror.

MOTHER: He knows what I'm trying; I mean you know what I'm trying to tell you.

HEARD: I think you're one hundred percent right, but I think he doesn't hear you.

MOTHER: He's not going to hear, Doctor. I know he's not because I've been saying this for years.

HEARD: Then try saying it in a way that he can hear you. (*Therapist leaves the room and joins Riley behind mirror.*)

MOTHER: Are you listening?

FATHER: Yes.

MOTHER: I told you what you've got to do with him. You've got to be firm with him and mean it. You just have to tell him, once and for all. You can't just say, this, that, and that, and he knows you don't mean it. He knows it.

FATHER: I told him today to start to . . .

MOTHER: No, the way you tell him, it's just like pussying around.

FATHER: What do you want? How do you want me to tell him?

MOTHER: Mean it!

FATHER: Did he work today? Did he work today? Was I with him and he worked, right?

MOTHER: Yes, but look what you have to do to make him do it. You have to get all aggravated. You have to scream and holler.

FATHER: Not all the time. He's all right after—when he gets started. He can do it alone soon.

MOTHER: He could do it alone. Why can't he do it alone? Why?

FATHER: The stuff was too heavy for him.

MOTHER: He could have started. He could have started and

then if he said, "I can't do it by myself," then you could have helped him. You had to take a day off from work to help him out.

*FATHER:* I had to take a day off anyhow. He did a lot of work today. Now don't say he didn't 'cause he did.

*MOTHER:* You both did!

*The parents continued this discussion for approximately 20 minutes without any resolution. Mother persisted in her insistence that her husband was too soft and forgiving. Father partially agreed, but insisted that his wife did not fully appreciate Jim's fragile nature, and that, besides, he wasn't really that terrible. Meanwhile, Heard and Riley were discussing the goings-on and Riley emphasized that more pressure needed to be applied to the father. Heard agreed, then reentered the room in order to extricate the couple from their quagmire and unbalance the system. He did not want pseudoagreement and a reduction in therapeutic tension. He once again introduced the topic of Jim's death. In doing so, the intensity of the interaction increased sharply. The therapist aligned himself firmly with the mother, insisting that the father had failed to appreciate the seriousness of the situation. He worked from the premise that only by making the split genuinely open, and by preventing premature closure, would they arrive at a different method for problem solving.*

*HEARD:* Let me ask you something. How do you think you'd feel if Jim was no longer with us?

*FATHER:* You mean here? You mean not with us at all? You mean at home?

*HEARD:* Yes. If Jim was just—if he passed away. How do you think you'd feel?

*MOTHER:* I think I would be resting in peace with him.

*HEARD:* Talk about that. Talk about how you'd feel, because Jim's life is on the line every time he sticks that needle in his arm.

*MOTHER:* It is on the line. It is. That's why any time I have fear, I just wait—that something is going to happen to him, and that's going to end everything. Because if we don't do anything now, that's what it's coming to. That's what he's heading for. You know that, don't you? Could be any time. He don't have no life anymore now. He has no life. That's not living; that's not living. None of us, in fact. It's misery all the time. That's why I say, you have to be firm. You have to just tell him and mean it. (*silence*)

*HEARD:* I think your husband underestimates the seriousness of what we're talking about. I'm talking about the life and death of your son.

*MOTHER:* I know. He doesn't have much more to go if he just continues what he's doing now.

*HEARD:* I don't think he hears that.

*FATHER:* (*to therapist*) How the hell can you help. . . . How could you help that?

*HEARD:* Discuss that. The two of you discuss it.

*MOTHER:* I've been repeating!

*FATHER:* Louise, we haven't done a darn thing. Even if you told him to go out he wouldn't go out.

*MOTHER:* You make him go out. Say, "This is it! I want you to get up this morning and go out looking for work and don't come back until you find a job." You tell him. See what happens. You tell him that. Say, "Jim, get up. I want you to go out and don't come back until you get a job, 'cause I can't support you anymore."

*FATHER:* I haven't gave him any money at all. I haven't gave him anything.

*MOTHER:* We gave him his room back. He promised me he was gonna get a job. On account of him we're going back and back in things and you know it. He wants to live there, he has to work. If not, he has to get out. His sisters feel bad about it because Susan is working and she's paying her way through there. Is he better than her? You keep saying he is sick, he's gotta be helped. Yes, he's sick. He's gotta be helped. Not the way you're helping him. You're not helping him.

*FATHER:* Did I call him up in the hospital?

*MOTHER:* Well, you thought he was going to be coming back all cured. I knew he wasn't. It was a mistake, him going in, in the first place. We went through it so many times. I have no more hope for him going in the hospital and expecting somebody else to do what you're supposed to be doing.

*FATHER:* He has to have his methadone. That's about all you can do with him, right now.

*MOTHER:* Is that how you want him to live, on methadone? How long is he going to live on methadone?

*FATHER:* I don't want him to, but how is he going to stop now, when he's hooked on it so fast? Could he stop today, tomorrow? Could he stop tomorrow?

*MOTHER:* It's up to him. He was at the hospital. Why didn't he stay there and get the help he was supposed to get?

*FATHER:* I agree with you. You're right. He should of stood in there. He didn't.

*MOTHER:* Well, why didn't you give him the dickens when he came home? You should have told him, "Why did you come out? Why didn't you stay in there?"

*FATHER:* Well, we did tell him that: "Why didn't you stay in for the rest of the . . ."

*MOTHER:* It was his idea of going in there, not ours.

*FATHER:* He blamed somebody else for it.

*MOTHER:* He's always blaming. He's always blaming and we believe like stupid fools. Sure he's going to stay home. He's going to sit home now and just wait for somebody to get him a job. He's not going to do anything about it.

*This interaction between the parents continued for more than half an hour. It was intense and the father was near tears. Although it was somewhat difficult for the therapist, he decided to push harder on the issue of death. The mother was excused and the therapist met alone with the father for the next hour. The following transcription is the first exchange after mother had left the room.*

*HEARD:* I think maybe you underestimated the seriousness of this.

*FATHER:* I don't underestimate it. I know. I understand this. I understand it very well, Doctor. Now, my wife is a little jumpy at times. When the kid was a lot younger—I'm talking about going back—all these problems could have started from the beginning.

*HEARD:* I'm talking about losing your son. I'm talking about having your son no longer with you.

*FATHER:* Well, what can we do with him now? What can we do with him now?

*HEARD:* I don't think you're hearing your wife. I think she's telling you and I think you don't want to hear it. I think you have a very soft spot in your heart that is much too good for your son's own welfare. I'm afraid that your soft spot in your heart may be responsible for some very terrible tragedy on your son's part.

*FATHER:* There's no doubt about that. That probably will come. There's no doubt about it.

*HEARD:* How do you think you would feel, if Jim's no longer with us?

Death as a Motivator   227

*FATHER:* Well, you know, Doc, I'll tell you frankly, it puts me on the spot. You know why it puts me on the spot? Because when my dad died, the first thing he told me, he said, "Look out for him." And I tried all my best to look out for him, and he ends up with drugs.

*HEARD:* You're too good. You shelter him. You protect him.

*FATHER:* Not all the time. I told everything that goes on. I don't lie to her. I told the truth . . .

*HEARD:* You know, you're treating Jim as if he's sick. You're really supporting his habit.

*FATHER:* He don't get nothing from me. I don't give him anything, as far as money or anything like that.

*HEARD:* He gets a roof over his head, gets food on the table, probably gets clothes. He gets all the necessary things from you, so that his whole life can just be focused on how to go and get that needle and stick it in his arm. He doesn't have to worry about where he's going to sleep, he don't even have to worry about coming home sober. Dad will come find him. Dad will pick him up out of the street.

*FATHER:* He don't call after me no more.

*HEARD:* Dad will pick him up out of the bar. Dad will come at two o'clock in the morning on a cold night and chauffeur him home.

*FATHER:* I haven't done that anymore. I used to pick him up and I don't do it anymore. He comes home. Somebody takes him home, but I don't pick him up, and she knows that.

*HEARD:* I think you have such a big heart, that it's liable to be the downfall of your son. You know your wife knows this, but you don't hear.

*FATHER:* I don't know. I don't know what to say here. I know it's a problem. I know it. I've been to so damn many hospitals. I've been back to Redtown. I've been all over.

*HEARD:* Do you think hospitals are the answer?

*FATHER:* I've been to the [military] hospital too. They haven't a darn thing there, either.

*HEARD:* Can you put him out?

*FATHER:* Oh, we can put him out. Yes.

*HEARD:* I don't believe you.

*FATHER:* We wanted to put him out last time. He won't leave. He refused to leave.

*HEARD:* Then you can't put him out. . . . You say you can do it, but he won't leave. I don't think you can. Even though it may be the thing that saves your son's life. I don't think you can get tough with him.

*FATHER:* You think if we threw him out we'd save his life? I doubt it. I don't think so, because he's so—he's depressed. He's been awful depressed, but if he goes out, it ain't gonna be on account of me, because I'm—I mean if he wants to go out, we'll put him out, but where the hell is he going to stay? Where? There won't be no place for him, because I know it's . . .

*HEARD:* Why should he want to go out? He's got the good life.

*FATHER:* Well, I know it.

*HEARD:* You're too good.

*FATHER:* Well, I don't know what to say.

*HEARD:* You know, your goodness, I'm afraid, is not helpful. Have you thought about what his funeral would be like?

*FATHER:* I don't know. I really don't know yet. He's not getting supported by me.

*HEARD:* But he is.

*FATHER:* I haven't gave him anything.

*HEARD:* You give him a house. You give him shelter. You give him food.

*FATHER:* Well, but that means I have to put him out then. That's the only way to do it.

*HEARD:* I don't think you can. I think you're too soft. I think you're absolutely too soft. Was your father a soft man?

*At this point the discussion changed to an intergenerational issue: what Mr. Galvani's father would advise if he were alive. Jim was the first grandchild in the family and the only male grandchild. In many respects he was very special to his grandfather, who had lived in the same house. Listening for the advice of an important ghost figure added a new dimension in motivating the father to get tough with Jim. Mr. Galvani noted that in many respects Jim's grandfather had been more influential in raising Jim than he had been. The grandfather was described as an influential man who was both strong and soft. At a point near death the grandfather had asked Mr. Galvani to take "special care" of Jim since he was the only male grandchild and heir of the family name. Mr. Galvani related the fact that he had promised his dying father to take "special care" of Jim. To him, "special care" meant protecting Jim from hardships. Once this issue of the deathbed promise became known, the therapist moved to explore with the father what the relationship had been between himself and his own father. Mr. Galvani noted again that his father had been a man with a combination of firmness and support. This admission opened the possibility that perhaps Mr. Galvani had misunderstood what his father had meant when on his deathbed he requested that Mr. Galvani take "special care" of Jim, that is, that perhaps recovering the firmness of Jim's grandfather was a very helpful and necessary step.*

*The closing remarks of the session illustrate two important points. First, Mr. Galvani had been moved by the session. He was suggesting that perhaps his wife was correct and that they needed to become more firm with Jim. He made specific references to jobs, Jim's moving out of the family, and that Jim should perhaps pay board while he remained in the parents' home. The second important point is that despite the fact that the session had been a grueling one for Mr. Galvani, the relationship between him and the therapist remained strong.*

*The therapist terminated the session with an admonition.*

HEARD: Let's stop for now, you know, because I think you need to do some soul searching. I know you are a man who is tremendously concerned about your son, but I'm afraid you show your concern in the wrong way.

FATHER: My wife read something in the paper one time to throw him out of the house. That was a long time ago, but we. . . . She did try to throw him out.

HEARD: If it were up to her she probably would . . .

FATHER: He wouldn't leave. He wouldn't leave for nothing, and I know what he would have done if we would have thrown him out. He would have went in when we're not there, went in and took some TVs out, a couple TVs we have upstairs, or something like that. It's been done before. It's been done before.

HEARD: I'm sure you could find lots of reasons why it wouldn't work. Now, I want you to think about what we talked about tonight. You know, I think it would be a dreadful thing to not have Jim around anymore. I think it would be unbearable for you.

FATHER: Who's to say that he can't get a job now, all of a sudden?

HEARD: Why should he?

FATHER: I know he's went to the employment officer and they had nothing for him.

*HEARD:* I don't think Jim's going to get a job. Why should he? He's got Dad to bring home a paycheck. He's got Dad to put food on the table. He's got Dad to pay the mortgage . . .

*FATHER:* Well, she did tell me this. We were talking about him. He's going to have to pay. He's going to have to do something. He's going to have to pay his board there. I know it's tough on us. It's really tough on us because he's been hitting us pretty hard. I know that. And when we get to a point when I feel like I'm going to throw him out, I will throw him out at the time. Maybe it'll do the best thing in the world. Maybe it won't. Either one way or another. If he gets me mad enough, then I'm probably going to end up doing it, throwing him the heck out. Maybe it'll be the best thing in the world.

*HEARD:* I'd like to meet with you next week. Next Wednesday. It gives you and your wife a chance to talk about this at length. Now, I think it's one of the most important decisions you'll make in your life because I think your son's life, quite literally, is in your hands. I don't say this lightly. This is my job. This is what I do and I work with families. You know, many of them are like yours and there is always someone in families with drug addicts with a heart that's too soft.

*FATHER:* Yes, that's true.

*HEARD:* And they mean well but they're not helping. I think you mean well. It's just that it's not helpful for your son.

As noted earlier, this session lasted a full 3 hours. The expanded time dimension allowed for the intensity of the session to build. The session also gained intensity from the fact that a very limited number of issues were addressed. First, and perhaps most important for this family, the hospital personnel were disqualified as the people who were going to resolve Jim's problem. The hospital was an especially important pressure valve in the family and only after disqualifying the hospital could the therapist be successful in placing the responsibility upon the parent's shoulders. Not all families are as dependent upon the hospital for stress reduction as was the Galvani family. In this case, the shifting of responsibility was accomplished by including the parents from the very beginning in planning the detoxification, and constantly emphasizing that this detox was special—that it would be the last detoxification, ever. Working in this way, the therapist has several options, depending upon the outcome of the detoxification. If the detoxification is successful it can be applauded and viewed as the rite of passage that makes the addict a "normal citizen" with normal responsibilities. If the detoxification is a failure, as with the case of Jim, the hospital personnel can be disqualified as the people who can solve the problem.

The second major issue constantly emphasized throughout the session was that Mr. Galvani's indulgence of his son made it impossible for his wife and daughters to demand that Jim act as a responsible member of the family.* Some of the historical reasons why Mr. Galvani indulged Jim surfaced during this session and it was possible to use the grandfather's ghost figure in challenging Mr. Galvani's indulgence. Pressure was also brought on the father by the mother, as the therapist supported her throughout the session and encouraged her to express her feelings of frustration, anger, and sense of nonsupport from her husband.

The third major issue that arose in the session was the use of death as a motivator. Death is an issue that is seldom distant in the addict's life. Parents appear to outwardly deny and desensitize themselves to the constant proximity of death to a family member. Mr. and Mrs. Galvani admitted the likelihood of their son's dying by the

---

*Editors' note.* By ostensibly laying the blame on the father for Jim's addiction, the therapist's actions might be viewed as contradicting our dictum (Chapters 5 and 6) of not blaming parents. However, there are several important considerations here that must be kept in mind. First, the therapist had been meeting with this family for several months up to this point and had become firmly joined with both father and mother—they respected, liked, and appreciated him. Thus he held a position of leverage and power upon which he could "borrow" in pressuring the father. Second, the therapist usually prefaced his challenges to father with noble ascriptions, noting that he had a "big heart," was "tremendously concerned," meant well, and was "too good" to Jim—having a "soft spot" for his son. By prefacing challenges in this way he both softened the father for the harder material to follow, and conveyed the message that father's *intentions* were not under fire, only his methods. This approach served to make the father more amenable to the therapist's firmer message about culpability (and, in fact, the therapist and the father did conclude the session amicably and respectfully). Third, while the therapist seemed to lay the blame at the father's feet, in his own mind he conceptualized the family in systemic terms, knowing that Jim, his mother, and the other family members were probably contributing to the problem also. (For instance, if the mother felt so strongly about her husband's treatment of Jim, why did she not exert more pressure on him, even making a move to leave him if he did not tighten his control of Jim?) Thus the therapist increased intensity and unbalanced as a way of initiating a change process in the whole system. He risked parental defensiveness only because he had to get the family system moving, while also recognizing (given the "positive" factors described above) that chances were minimal for such defensiveness to well up to the point of neutralizing his primary intervention. Given these (usually necessary) preconditions, it is possible to modify the nonblaming stance and combine it with a seeming message of criticism.

needle. Mrs. Galvani went so far as to say, "I would be resting in peace with him"; and, "It would solve a lot of problems" if Jim were dead. These responses seem to offer support to Stanton's[146] observation that the parents appear to show a preference for having a dead son, rather than "losing" him to friends, spouse, or other outsiders. The fact that the death issue was presented so graphically (asking what Jim's funeral would be like) and emphasized so heavily throughout the session is seen by the author as an important element in explaining why the family system changed. The parents, particularly the father, could no longer ignore it. The therapist would not let them ignore it.* While, as Stanton suggests, there is often an unconscious wish in these families for the addict to die, when this possibility is stressed to them so palpably that they cannot sidestep it, their values come to bear; they may then renounce any wish for his death—hopefully taking action to prevent it (as occurred here and also in Vignette 8, Chapter 5). Further, in this case the father was faced with a conscious dilemma: there was no way he could abide by his own father's injunction to take care of Jim (as the only son and bearer of the family name) and at the same time allow Jim to die prematurely. In being forced to accept the possibility of Jim's demise, he was also forced to try to avert it. If Jim died at an early age, the father would be countermanding his own father's deathbed wish, thereby incurring upon himself the guilt and brand of a disloyal son.

## TERMINATION

In the final therapy session, a week later, Mrs. Galvani reported that she and her husband had worked "very closely together in straightening Jim out." Mr. Galvani gave Jim an ultimatum about the rules for living within the family. Mrs. Galvani reported that she refused to call the dentist for Jim's toothache, telling him that it was "your tooth

---

*Editors' note. The importance of having a supportive colleague, or a team of supportive colleagues, who can observe and help the therapist during crisis induction needs to be emphasized (see also Chapters 6 and 16). The demands on a therapist at this time can be very great—especially in a case such as this one, where the content is emotionally laden and one or more members appear close to breaking down. During such a process the therapist can use a support group to help hold the line and not relax his pressure prematurely. If he begins to let feelings of empathy take over, so that he backs off from the task too soon, the effectiveness of the crisis induction will be compromised. A support group also helps insure that the emotional outburst that often occurs during crisis induction will not get out of hand.

and your ache." Mr. Galvani agreed that Mrs. Galvani had done the proper thing.

Within a period of 30 days following the crisis induction session, Jim announced that he had a girlfriend and was planning to move out of the family home and live with his girlfriend. The relationship with the girlfriend had existed for months, but he had kept it a secret. He also obtained a job on his own within this 30-day period and detoxified himself from methadone without help from the hospital or drug counselor.

## EPILOGUE

Although the therapist would have preferred a few more sessions to negotiate and implement a plan for Jim's moving out of the parents' home, he considered the therapy to be successful. In interviews held with Jim and both parents at the conclusion of treatment, all concurred with the therapist about the success of the therapy and noted that they were very satisfied with it.

Posttreatment follow-up information has been obtained on this case over a 41-month period since termination of family therapy. During the first 18 months following termination, Jim was not using illegal drugs and was not on methadone. He drank moderately (one to six cans of beer a day), a pattern that continued throughout the whole 41 months. He worked full-time in a nursing home through the ninth month, was unemployed for several months, then obtained another full-time job as a truck driver. Eight months after therapy had concluded he got married. He lived with his in-laws for a time, then he, his wife, and child moved out on their own.

In the 18th month Jim started taking prescribed Valium on a daily basis. A month later he enrolled at the DDTC, went on methadone maintenance for 3 weeks, and then detoxified. Two months later he reenrolled, and remained on methadone through the 35th month (with one detox attempt). In the 36th month he switched to long-acting methadone (LAAM) and remained on it at least until the end of the follow-up period. At several points between the 26th and 41st months he supplemented his methadone with various illegal drugs, mostly nonopiates taken over brief (e.g., 2 to 3 day) periods. In the 23rd month he separated from his wife and moved back with his parents. He had continued his full-time job as a truck driver but lost it in the 29th month when his employer learned he was in a drug program; at this point he went on welfare, while occasionally taking odd jobs. He did not become involved with the law during the 41 months.

In sum, the positive effects of therapy with this case appeared to hold up for 18 months. During this period Jim was functioning well in all areas of life—family, occupation, and drugs. While he continued to work for most of 29 months posttreatment, problems later developed in the areas of drugs (methadone maintenance in the 19th month) and the family (23rd month). It seems fair to assume that some kind of family life cycle crisis occurred around the 18th month—perhaps having to do with one of Jim's parents, sisters, or grandparents (our data are not clear on the details). However, this case demonstrates the utility of a more flexible model for number and spacing of sessions, as advocated in Chapter 6. Such a model would allow the family and therapist to reconvene when the family gets "stuck" at some future point. In this instance, it might have permitted later problems to be nipped in the bud, thus extending the period of positive outcome.

# 10

## A FAIR EXCHANGE
## IS NO ROBBERY:
## *A CASE WITH A PUSHER*

THOMAS C. TODD
PAUL RILEY
DAVID B. HEARD
M. DUNCAN STANTON

THIS CHAPTER is a comprehensive case presentation. Since it presents an entire case in some detail, it is necessarily long. In reading it, however, one will perhaps be impressed with the artistic aspect of the therapy. The material underscores the point that a high success rate with these difficult cases is dependent not only upon the utility of the theoretical model being employed, but also upon the therapist's ability to use himself as an effective clinical instrument. This model of treatment is based upon a theory that is rather simple, especially when compared to some of the more elaborate and sophisticated theoretical frameworks developed in the mental health field over the years. The real challenge to a clinician working within an interpersonal systems model is related to the development of strategy, that is, how to move effectively in bringing about change in relationships.

The case is presented sequentially, session by session. Organizing the material in this way permits the reader to follow the therapist's strategy. The lengthy transcriptions allow the reader to see for himself what cues and information the therapist was given and how this information affected the development of his strategy. The authors' comments and analysis are intended, in part, to relate the specific examples used in this case to our general treatment model.

## CASE MATERIAL

The addict, Ed, was a Black male and an only child. At intake he was age 27 and living with his parents. His father was a custodian and his mother a homemaker. He first used marijuana at age 15 and started snorting heroin at age 16. During the last 6 of his 11 years of heroin use, he had been addicted to it. He had been treated once for drug addiction 6 years earlier, having been hospitalized for 7 days. He had spent 3 years in the Army, including 18 months in Vietnam. He had obtained a high school equivalency diploma and had recently applied for entrance to a community college, but he had been unemployed for 2½ years.

Although the therapist did not learn it until the third family session, Ed was a drug pusher. He had also spent time in a penitentiary for armed robbery. While involved in pushing he maintained a certain level of addiction himself, partly so that he could test his wares and maintain "quality control." However, due to increased tension in his home, he had begun to shoot considerably more heroin in recent months.

Prior to the first family session the therapist, Paul Riley, Family Counselor, had one brief meeting with Ed in order to convince him to allow Riley to phone his parents and arrange for them to engage in the therapy. Riley was not only the family therapist but also Ed's drug counselor, which meant that he controlled the methadone dosage that Ed received.

### FIRST SESSION

Very often with families that have an addicted member, the therapist quickly notes that the family hierarchy is in chaos. As emphasized in Chapters 6 and 7, this treatment model assumes that parents should be in charge of children. So long as offspring remain living in the parents' home, it is the parents who should make decisions concerning the rules and regulations of the house. For this to happen in a family with an addicted member, it is often necessary for the therapist to clearly take control of the therapy session and then to gradually assist the parents in asserting themselves to assume the dominant position within the family hierarchy. This struggle for control of the session begins almost instantly as Ed and his parents seat themselves for the initial family session.

*ED:* I called you, telling you that my medication wasn't holding me, right? You said you would check into it, right?

*RILEY:* Is it always customary for you to keep your hat on while you are in a building?

*ED:* Not really, it's just a habit. Sometimes I just don't take it off. If it bothers you, I'll take it off.

*RILEY:* Well, I think that's part of relating when you come into a building. It's a different domain.*

*ED:* Well, you know, it ain't no problem. It's just something, like I usually have it on because usually I be outside. When I'm in the house I take it off. (*Removes hat.*) And like my medication, right. You said that you would talk to the doctor and have it straightened out. Well, as far as like I feel, I haven't seen any change.

*RILEY:* Well, I did talk to Dr. Woody and he did say . . .

*ED:* You see, it seems like my dose is getting smaller. I never did see the difference in the increase, you know, after the last time I talked to you.

*RILEY:* I'll double-check on it.

*ED:* All right. I'd appreciate that because I haven't seen the difference. No difference at all.

*RILEY:* I'll take care of that. I'm wondering if you will take care of what I gave you to take care of.

*ED:* What's that?

*RILEY:* Remember I told you I would like you to go to give two urine tests down at the Center next week?

*ED:* Yeah. I thought I would be on the list.

*RILEY:* Yeah, but I told you I wanted two urine tests. So, in other words, I want to know for myself.

*ED:* I forgot that. You know, when I come in there I look on the list every day. And when I don't see my name for urine, I just go ahead and take the medication.

---

*Note how the addict initiates the discussion by trying to put the therapist on the defensive. Riley neatly sidesteps this (medication) issue and counters with an issue (the hat), which (1) gives him more control, (2) derogates the addict, and, (3) in contrasting the addict's discourteous behavior with the propriety of his parents, simultaneously elevates the parents and connects them to Riley.

*RILEY:* I said that I want you to see that you take two urines.
*ED:* All right.
*RILEY:* And it's going to be on your record. But, if it ain't on your record . . . you still are following me? I said I want two urines.
*ED:* Right.
*RILEY:* We ain't doing no game playing now.
*MOTHER:* That's right. That's right.
*RILEY:* And that's what we got to follow.
*MOTHER:* That's really true.

*The therapist noted Mother's support for his position, slight as it might have been. Ed continued to complain about being physically ill as a result of being on too low a dosage of methadone. The therapist knew that in all likelihood this was true, because for medical safety addicts are generally started on a lower methadone dosage than is required to compensate for their heroin addiction.*

*The topic of conversation moved to whether or not Ed was working. He was not, but he reported that in the past few years he had had five well-paying jobs of various types: in heavy industry, the Post Office, assembly line work, and the like. In contrast to Ed's employment history, the therapist noted that Mr. E (the father) had been employed at his present factory job for the past 22 years; Riley thus supported the father's position, holding him up as a model, and decentralizing Ed somewhat.*

*In a casual way, the therapist then changed the topic of conversation by asking whether Ed had any children. To the therapist's surprise, he learned that Ed had two children and he pursued this topic.*

*RILEY:* You got any children?
*ED:* I got two children.
*RILEY:* You have two children?
*ED:* Yes, I do.
*RILEY:* Where are they at?
*ED:* They're with me.
*RILEY:* They're with you?
*ED:* In the house.
*RILEY:* Where's the mother?
*ED:* She's there too.
*RILEY:* Why didn't she come?
*ED:* Because she has to stay with the children.

*RILEY:* You could have brought them along.

*ED:* Well, the baby is only a little over a month old, you know, and like, uh . . .

*RILEY:* I've got a family. I've had babies, too.

*ED:* Well, this is my decision, you know. I figured it was best if she stayed home.

*RILEY:* She's part of the family, isn't she?

*ED:* Right, she's part of the family, but, you know, right now she should be there taking care of the family while I'm gone, you know. There's certain things she has to do and a schedule for the baby she has to keep. Like this might interfere with that.

*RILEY:* Maybe next time you can have a babysitter and the mother can come along with the others.

*ED:* Well, see, a babysitter. . . . Right now there is no one I would trust other than my mother with my son. You know, that's it. I just wouldn't put it on a babysitter.

*RILEY:* The reason why I would like her to be present—because I'm working with the whole family and that's part of the family. And then that's a piece missing. You know, that's a piece of your life missing. I can't even get the whole picture. I can get yours but I can't get hers. You know, there she is. . . . She can't tell me nothing.

*ED:* Yeah, I can understand that.

*RILEY:* See, I'm just getting your words. I want to see how these things go together. You know, how she can sit down and say, "Well, you feeling bad, stay in bed, don't worry about it." You know, or, "Hey, get yourself together. What's going on?" How can I solve a problem if I don't get all the pieces of the puzzle?

*ED:* I can understand your point, but, you know, this is just how I see the situation right now. You know, it's not possible for her to make it. I guess some kind of arrangement could be made.

*RILEY:* You see, how long have you been trying to solve this situation?

*ED:* What situation?

*RILEY:* This drug behavior. How long have you been trying to get off it?

*ED:* Well, since I've been on this program.

*RILEY:* And even before, you tried to get rid of it, hadn't you?

*ED:* Right.

*RILEY:* OK. So you haven't succeeded on your own.

*ED:* Not really. Or else I wouldn't be here.

*RILEY:* Right. So we're going to try something different. And for me to try anything different, I need everything together. That's how I work. I work with all pieces, you know. You have a thing to do. She has a thing to do. Mother has a thing to do. Father has a thing to do. And I have a thing to do. And that's how we work together. We got to get to the root of it. You know, it sounds like you are the spokesman for the family.

*ED:* No. I just speak what I'm thinking. You know, I don't mean to speak for the family. You know, I just speak for myself.

*RILEY:* (*to mother*) Do you understand what he's saying?

*MOTHER:* Yeah, I understand.

*RILEY:* Did you accept it?

*MOTHER:* Beg your pardon?

*RILEY:* Did you expect the missus to be here too?

*MOTHER:* Sure, she should.

*RILEY:* Man, she's part of the family.

*This was the first major therapeutic change and one of enormous significance. The therapist had been successful in standing toe-to-toe with the addict and in specifying his ground rules for treatment: if he were to be successful, he must have all pieces of the puzzle. In addition, he raised the question directly to the mother, asking whether she expected Ed's spouse to be present.\* In responding affirmatively in support of the therapist's position, the foundation was laid for a weak but significant alliance between Mrs. E (the mother) and the therapist.*

*Riley then redirected the topic of conversation to the issue of Ed's not being employed. Note the way he skillfully applied the newly acquired knowledge that Ed had a spouse and children, using it to support the parents (together) as competent and consequently weakening Ed's position in the hierarchy.*

*RILEY:* (*to Ed*) These [the parents] are good models. How come you didn't pick up neither one of them?

*ED:* Well, I guess I never really tried to follow their type of model that they were setting for me.

*RILEY:* You couldn't follow it?

---

\*Actually, as the therapist learned later, Ed and Linda had never been formally married.

*ED:* I wasn't trying, not that I couldn't. I wasn't trying.

*RILEY:* He wasn't trying . . . well, what about your wife and kids? Now, it just so happens that you're living home with your family and if it wasn't for them, what would happen?

*ED:* What would happen? Well, I would be living somewhere else.

*RILEY:* No, but who's going to pay?

*ED:* Me.

*RILEY:* How are you going to pay without a job?

*ED:* Well, you know just as well as I do, there are other ways of surviving out here without working.

*RILEY:* What, on welfare?

*ED:* No, not welfare. There are other ways.

*RILEY:* OK. How are you going to survive?

*ED:* There are other means for survival. If necessary, if push come to shove, if you want to take care of yourself, you going to do it right or wrong?

*RILEY:* Yeah, but we got family and we can't go—how would you say—take a chance on certain things.

*ED:* Sometimes that comes about. You try to avoid it.

*RILEY:* You try to avoid it, but hey, that big brick wall [prison] is full of people trying to avoid it.

*ED:* Well, I'm aware of that.

*RILEY:* You're aware of that?

*ED:* Very aware of that.

*RILEY:* So nothing is foolproof.

*ED:* That's right.

*RILEY:* And there's always someone got another plan on how to trap you. The Man's got a plan too.

*ED:* That's true. That's a known fact.

*RILEY:* But would you put your wife and children through that kind of strain?

*ED:* No.

*RILEY:* But push come to shove. You know, excuse me, they (*pointing to parents*) may not live forever.

*ED:* Well, see, if I had any intentions of doing this or anything, I wouldn't have come to this program. You know, the point is that I'm sick of the game and I see that I have a family that is growing up in front of me. I'm the man and I'm supposed to take care of them.

*RILEY:* Now, that's why I want her here! That's why I want her here. Hold it. That's why I want her here. I want her to be here when you're telling me that. I want her here!

*ED:* I see what you saying.

*RILEY:* Yeah, you're telling me. I don't know if you tell her this. You understand. So, I want her to be here on the scene. Now, I want to see if she's going to support you or if she's gonna say, "Hey, you told me that before." I don't know where she's at. You understand. I wanna see where she's at. I wanna see if she's gonna say, "Hey, wait a minute, he can make it. I'll support him," or say, "Hey, no, he told me that before." Now sometimes women can get—how you say—uptight when things get kind of touchy, you know. Here she's having the baby; there's a lot of things she don't need.

*From these last statements we get a hint as to what the thera- pist's future strategy would be—with Ed's spouse present. In the closing minutes of the session the therapist returned to the issue of how the mother and father were overburdened. The therapist ad- dressed them as grandparents this time.*

*RILEY:* Grandparents are good, but they get exhausted too.

*MOTHER:* That's right.

*ED:* Well, really you're not supposed to even use them, you know. I don't even like the idea of having my children under the same roof. Well, that's what I mean.

*RILEY:* OK. Well, we're gonna do something about it. We're gonna start working on it.

*MOTHER:* Yes, that's what needs to be done and that's the same thing that I tell him. A grandparent is supposed to be a grandparent is true, but you don't look for a grandparent to do as a parent, unless they just have to, you know. I would like to enjoy them coming and going, whenever I want them. I enjoy them now, because if we didn't, they wouldn't be there. I don't want to see them out. But I want him to realize how to take care of them on his own. Because he's far past the age of playing games. Far, far past it.

*RILEY:* I guess you and the mister had a lot of talks about this.

*MOTHER:* Quite a few, quite a few.

*RILEY:* (*to father*) How did these talks come out? I'm quite sure you had many long times sitting there just discussing what's happening.

*FATHER:* Oh yeah, we still ain't quite eye-to-eye in finding out what he's doing. I can't quite put my finger on what's been going down.

RILEY: So in other words, you two don't have it together?

FATHER: Not really, not really. We try, you know.

*This was the first time the issue of Ed's moving out of the home had been raised and the therapist quickly but briefly committed himself to "doing something about it" in the future. It would have been premature, at this point, to push for Ed to move out. It is generally safer to assume that the glue binding addict to parents is like steel, and that moving the addict out is better postponed to a later stage of therapy. What must first be accomplished is getting the addict off all drugs and getting him to work, school, or a similar age-appropriate activity.*

*Mr. E's statement that "we still ain't quite eye-to-eye" is indicative of what exists between parents with an addicted son. In many such families it is generally difficult for the parents to agree upon much of anything. One way to begin to change this state of constant disagreement is for the therapist to take an expert's position and say that what is absolutely necessary is that the parents need to agree upon some rules for their son. The actual rules themselves are often irrelevant, but the* process of getting the parents to agree within the session *marks the beginning of an important transformation.*

*The therapist then moved to terminate the session.*

RILEY: I want you to fix me with two urines and I would like you to fix me with your madam here next week.

ED: I'll do it.

RILEY: 'Cause then we going to have it together that way. OK? I'm not going to keep you here any longer and thank you for coming. I'd like to see you next week with the missus. And, I hope it's a beautiful day—bring the baby. It's too early to bring the baby out, isn't it?

ED: Yeah, he can come out if it's nice.

RILEY: What is it—a boy or a girl?

ED: A boy.

RILEY: You got a boy and a girl or two boys?

ED: One of each.

RILEY: Oh, you got a rich man's family. Now, you need a rich job.

ED: Yeah, I'm going to be a rich man; I'm trying to work at it.

*MOTHER:* He needs a whole, whole lot.
*FATHER:* Uh-huh.
*ED:* I'll get it.
*RILEY:* You'll get it. When you say get it, which way you going to get it?
*ED:* The right way; I mean work for it.
*RILEY:* Them shortcuts, they get you something.
*ED:* A lot of time. (*laughs*)

*These closing remarks between therapist and addict were surprisingly light in tone, given the fact that the therapist had continually challenged and opposed the addict during the meeting. This may have been partly due to the very positive way the therapist had joined Ed's parents throughout the session. However, we consider the prime factor to be one of relief and security for Ed in knowing that he was with an "expert." During the session Ed and Riley negotiated a lot of issues in an indirect way, and Riley indicated he was up to playing a con game with Ed and winning. Riley had demonstrated his mastery of the situation.*

## SECOND SESSION

The second session was held a week later. Present were Ed, both his parents, Ed's spouse (Linda), and both their children. The plan in this session was to support all family members in challenging the addict's drug taking and long-term irresponsible behavior toward his family.

*RILEY:* The promise you said last week when she wasn't here. Now could you tell her that?
*ED:* I wanted to get rid of my drug habit, to take care of you and our family because the way I was doing, there was no means I could take care of them—not trying to keep up a drug habit and take care of a family. My drug habit, like man, like ran anywhere from thirty-five to sixty dollars a day. You know, you can't take care of a family after that. All things got to come to an end.
*RILEY:* (*to Ed*) Let me hold the baby. You seem like you're uncomfortable. Let me hold him. (*Riley takes baby.*) Yeah, I've had babies. Now, you tell her that. I could hold the baby. Tell her that. Tell her the promises you was telling me.

*ED:* Promises? It wasn't promises, just something I said I was going to do. I was going to leave the drugs alone so I could take care of my family. You know and she knows that she's part of the family which I want to have along with the children.

*RILEY:* Tell her, not the baby.

*ED:* Yeah, well, I want to look both ways 'cause that's my child.

*RILEY:* The child is in good hands. Say, "I got a grandmother and grandfather watching over top of me." So don't worry about the child. There's your wife over there. We're babysitting.

*ED:* (*to Linda*) No, that's really all there is. I feel like she's gonna stick by me because she stuck by me this long. She helped, you know, she wasn't a problem when I was messing around. No, for the mere reason she didn't constantly harass me about what I was doing. And, I still respect her for that even though what I was doing was wrong.

*RILEY:* (*to Linda*) How many times has he told you that?

*LINDA:* Quite a few times.

*RILEY:* How do you feel about it after he told you quite a few times?

*LINDA:* Well, I think that he meant it, but I just wish that he had started this earlier—but like he said, I never pressured him about it.

*RILEY:* Why?

*LINDA:* Because I thought he would do it in his own time if he was sincere in doing it.

*RILEY:* And that's been quite a few years, so how come you just still pass it by?

*LINDA:* I just do, that's all.

*RILEY:* Then you keep passing the same thing by; the same thing keeps happening, doesn't it?

*LINDA:* Uh-huh.

*RILEY:* Uh-huh. Now how old are you?

*LINDA:* Twenty-two.

*RILEY:* What will happen if the same thing be passing when you're twenty-nine? And how old will she be? (*Points to five-year-old daughter.*)

*LINDA:* Eleven.

*RILEY:* Uh-huh. And, this little one, will be?

*LINDA:* About seven.

*RILEY:* About seven. Uh-huh.

*LINDA:* I never really thought about it.

*RILEY:* You never really thought about it? You don't think about the future?

*LINDA:* I think about the future. I never really just sat down and thought about this. I just never realized it myself.

*Using the children and projecting ahead into the future makes the consideration even more concrete. Throughout the course of treatment the therapist would again and again return to the issue of the children's welfare. It would become the primary issue that the therapist used to motivate Linda to challenge Ed's drug usage. The children would also become a primary issue between the grandparents and the addict in future discussions.*

*RILEY:* Do you have a hard time confronting him about issues?

*LINDA:* Sometimes.

*RILEY:* Like what issues do you have a hard time confronting him with?

*LINDA:* I really think it would be a hard time to confront him with anything. I wait until he's not in a mood.

*RILEY:* When he's in a mood, when's that?

*LINDA:* When he's in a mood, we usually argue.

*RILEY:* Especially when there's an issue pressing?

*LINDA:* Uh-huh.

*RILEY:* OK. I got one good issue. Money.

*LINDA:* Well, we don't always argue about money.

*RILEY:* How do you deal with it? Would you deal with it as nice as you deal with the baby? Right now you're lacking, aren't you?

*LINDA:* Yes.

*RILEY:* What would you like to have?

*LINDA:* Some things I need for my children first.

*RILEY:* OK. Like what. Tell him. Don't tell me.

*LINDA:* Well, I'd like for them to have a home.

*RILEY:* To have a home?

*LINDA:* Right. They have a home now with their grandparents, but a home, you know, of our own.

*RILEY:* You know, I'm very ugly. So why don't you look at him [Ed]. You seem like you just keep looking at me. 'Cause I got the baby, huh? All right, here, you take the baby. (*Gives the baby to Linda.*) What do you feed him, puffed rice?

*LINDA:* He eats a little bit of everything.

*RILEY:* OK. Now you can talk to him. You seem like you keep looking at me. (*Riley moves his chair.*)

*LINDA:* I would like to have a home for my children. A comfortable home. I want them to be happy. I want them to be with us. Not with me or just with you. And, all the necessary things that they have to have.

*RILEY:* Have you ever talked about your loneliness?

*LINDA:* No.

*RILEY:* It seems like you don't challenge him. Why wouldn't you challenge him?

*LINDA:* I just don't.

*RILEY:* You don't challenge him, and do you know what, his mother and father don't challenge him. How come?

*MOTHER:* I wouldn't say that I don't challenge him. I listen to him, you know, listen to what he has to say. But it's not a fact that I don't challenge him.

*RILEY:* How about your point—does it get across?

*MOTHER:* It gets across. Eventually. Maybe not right when I first start talking. You see, I don't let up when I talk to him.

*RILEY:* How about you, sir?

*FATHER:* Challenge him about what?

*RILEY:* You pick 'em. Gee, there's a lot to pick from.

*FATHER:* Oh, about what he's done? I've never challenged him about what he's done.

*RILEY:* You never challenged him about what he's doing? Why?

*FATHER:* I figured he's old; he knows what he's going to do to himself.

*RILEY:* But, as I was saying, you have to take the brunt of it.

*FATHER:* I just never have.

*RILEY:* He's twenty-seven years old. And, when he's not working, you support him. You have to have a roof over your head and food to eat, right? So, don't you challenge that sometime when you're out there getting up at five-thirty in the morning and he's still laying in bed sleeping, and when you come home, he just got up and left. Don't you challenge that issue?

*FATHER:* No.

*RILEY:* Why?

*FATHER:* I figured he would wake up one day and find out.

*RILEY:* You figured he'd wake up one day and find out. You sound just like him. Waiting. You both are waiting. And what about you? (*pointing to mother*) You said you challenge him too. But, he's still the same, isn't he? So, in other words, it went in one ear and out the other.

*MOTHER:* Sometimes, he gets a little better. There has been times when he has actually did good, you know. And then he fell back in the same rut.

*RILEY:* What did you both step your foot down on? Together.

*MOTHER:* Concerning him? Him working, his habit with drugs.

*RILEY:* All right. About working. What happens? Is he out looking for a job?

*MOTHER:* He says he goes looking for jobs. He goes to the employment agency.

*RILEY:* Well then, when he goes looking for jobs, when does he get up?

*The topic of conversation had moved to a very concrete discussion of looking for a job and what Ed was doing about it. The family had been reluctant to make any specific demands concerning what time he should get up in the morning and how many jobs he should interview for in a given week. Based upon previous interaction, it appeared that the mother was the one most able to stand up to Ed and offer some minimal challenge, though even that appeared weak.*

*In the following segment the therapist took an even more direct step in challenging the addict. It is important to emphasize that the therapist's role is a temporary one and that a successful outcome is likely only if the therapist is able to mobilize other family members to become more direct in dealing with the addict, rather than continuing to challenge the addict himself.*

*RILEY:* The reason why I brought up the work—I was thinking about, you know, he gave me a list of jobs, good jobs he had. In three years, you have five different jobs. Five good jobs and some of them you just left on account of you just gave it up.

*ED:* No, only one.

*RILEY:* I remember you saying two. I know it was two you said.

*ED:* That was U.S. Steel. The Standard Press job, I was laid off. At the Post Office, laid off. Philco. Yeah, two.

*RILEY:* (*to Linda*) You couldn't bank on nothing, could you?

*ED:* She wasn't on the scene.

*RILEY:* She wasn't on the scene?

*ED:* No.

*RILEY:* When she came on the scene, how about then?

*ED:* Well, I saw Linda as someone I would marry, as my woman; she came on the scene about . . .

*RILEY:* Hey, what did you say!

*ED:* As my woman, someone I would marry.

*RILEY:* Yeah.

*ED:* She came on the scene around seventy-one maybe. As a friend, I knew her before that.

*RILEY:* I'm—the way you said that. Came on the scene.

*ED:* Right.

*RILEY:* And the woman I would marry?

*ED:* Yeah, as the woman I would marry, as the woman I cared about.

*RILEY:* Uh-huh.

*ED:* Before I knew her as a friend.

*RILEY:* But when you both met, you had a plan, didn't you?

*ED:* Eventually, a plan came about.

*RILEY:* (*to Linda*) Did you have a plan?

*LINDA:* No.

*RILEY:* Not at first? When you was pregnant, did you have a plan?

*LINDA:* When I was pregnant? Yeah.

*RILEY:* What was your plan?

*LINDA:* My plan was that I wanted to get married.

*RILEY:* (*to Ed*) Why didn't you tie it up?

*ED:* Well, presently, you can't say that. Well, because it sounds like I'm not taking care of my responsibility as a man toward her. You know, it's not my intentions for it to be that way; it never was, you know, but by me having the drug habit, you know, things worked out that way; it wasn't because I planned it that way. I rarely—I say as far as I'm concerned, I don't like to ask my parents to do anything for me. You know, I live under their roof, you know, and I don't like the idea of living under their roof.

*RILEY:* You see, that's the whole thing. You don't like to but they are the parents and they feel that's their responsibilities. . . . Your mother and father, they need a life of their own . . .

*ED:* Well, see, that I can't speak on. I don't know. You know, I suppose they have a life of their own, to some extent. You see, because

I'm their son, they're not obligated to me to be there. That's a part of life that they want or else they wouldn't be here with me. I'm not speaking on the drugs, I'm speaking on as a family.

*RILEY:* (*to mother*) Do you think you have a life of your own, Mrs. E?

*MOTHER:* Well, there's a part of life of wanting to be a grandmother, a grandparent. But, the other part about him being out on his own, that's another different part. I'd rather see him being out on his own, you know, clear of drugs, with a job, and out on his own; and if he has to marry somebody, I'd prefer he marry the mother of his kids. He knows that because I told him that before.

*Mrs. E's last statement appeared to carry a mixed message. She said that she wanted to see her son off drugs, have a job, and out on his own. As for her feelings about Ed's relationship to a woman, she was somewhat ambivalent. Mother stated, "If he has to marry somebody, I'd prefer he marry the mother of his kids." Linda was not addressed by name, but rather as "the mother of his children." This was important diagnostic information for the therapist, as it gave a clue to the quality of the relationship between Linda and Ed's mother. Earlier in this same segment, Ed had said something very similar, which provoked the therapist's sharpest response to date. Ed had said, "Well, I saw Linda as someone I would marry, as my woman; she came on the scene about. . . ." The therapist responded with a clear, unambiguous challenge: "Hey, what did you say!" Both of the statements of Ed and his mother seemed to be unusual statements to say in the context of a therapy in which Linda and the two children were present.*

*The session ended with an agreement between the therapist and father. The therapist repeated several times that he would take the responsibility of dealing with Ed on matters pertaining to drugs. The father was to assume responsibility for dealing with his son on the job issue. Often it is possible to get parents to agree that they will be responsible to enforce the rules pertaining to drugs. For example, a therapist may be able to obtain an agreement between the parents that they will put their son out of the house if he uses drugs, steals from the home, or abuses alcohol. In this case, the therapist chose not to work this way, due largely to the fact that these parents were not yet prepared to accept such a responsibility. The alternative chosen by Riley is perhaps more difficult and requires greater skill on a thera-*

*pist's part, because it will likely dictate that the therapist directly confront the addict.*

> *RILEY: (to father)* You don't speak much. Why?
> *FATHER:* Well, I guess I always never had too much to say.
> *RILEY:* But you are affected. What's going to help this change? What can you do to help this change?
> *FATHER:* Well, get behind him, like you say, to get it done.
> *RILEY:* Well, I'll be taking care of the drug; now, what about the job?
> *FATHER:* Well, he'll have to look for his job because that's beyond me. I can't find employment for him.

## THIRD SESSION

Session three became a confrontation between therapist and addict. Riley considers it one in which he "stripped the addict of his power." It was a turning point in the course of the therapy, because it clearly established the therapist as the person in charge. It also served the purpose of modeling for the mother (the father was absent). She had an opportunity to see that someone could stand face-to-face with her son, confront him very directly, and come out on top. Linda and the children were also in attendance.

> *RILEY:* I remember last time I left you; I put you on thirty milligrams, right?
> *ED:* Yeah.
> *RILEY:* And you said that wasn't enough, right?
> *ED:* Right.
> *RILEY:* And I raised you ten more?
> *ED:* Right, and that wasn't enough.
> *RILEY:* And you say that's not enough?
> *ED:* I'm sticking with it because, you know, it seems to me like it's becoming a thing of inconvenience to everyone involved, including myself. It appears like I'm getting an image from everybody I'm dealing with that I'm jiving about this. So, like, to tell you the truth, I'm getting tired of going through this all the time, you know: "Wait three days here, see what happens." Then you go on vacation and tell me, "Hold on and see if you can make it for two weeks." What was I supposed to do in that two weeks' time?

*RILEY:* You're supposed to hang in there.

*ED:* Hang in there?

*RILEY:* Right.

*ED:* You don't feel as I feel everyday.

*RILEY:* OK. Since you mention it, you know, since you're saying you feel it, let's talk. I told you to go two times a week to give me your urine, right? OK.

*ED:* I've been there.

RILEY: OK. But, look what you've been doing. On August nineteenth you came, and on August twentieth. On August nineteenth and August twentieth you have quinine in your urine. Both tests. Then you went to the twenty-third and you had quinine, you know; twenty-fourth, quinine; and then September first you not only had quinine, you had morphine. Now I've been raising you, but the part about it, you are using outside the raise. Now, if I've been raising you and you're still taking quinine, you know, I want to know what the raise is doing. You're still—how you say—you're still *using*!

*ED:* I'm going to tell you what I'm using. I've been taking Valiums to hold me to go to sleep at night. That's the maximum I use. Why the quinine is showing up, I don't know. If anything, the Valiums should be showing up. That I am taking.

*RILEY:* Where does the morphine come from?

*ED:* I'm taking Valiums. So, I don't know where the morphine is coming from.

*RILEY:* Well, this is in your urine.

*ED:* That must be somebody else's urine; I'm telling you what I took.

*RILEY:* Look, these are your urines. This is you. (*Riley opens urine record book and places it in the middle of the floor.*)

*ED:* Well, all right, this is me.

*RILEY:* Now there, you can see it right there. (*pointing to the book*)

*ED:* Everything be all mixed up down there [at the Drug Dependence Treatment Center], you know; you can't tell who's getting whose urine down there. I noticed that myself just in the period of time I've been down there. What you do, you go in there, you take a urine, right, you get a slip with your name on it. You personally wrap it around your bottle; they put it in the cabinet there. Anybody can do anything they want to do all day long. Because the man who's in charge of the urine, he's not there twenty-four hours a day; he's not there all the time watching people. You know, I've seen stuff myself going on in there. You know—but it's not my job to supervise that.

*RILEY:* So, in other words, uh . . .

*ED:* In other words, what I'm telling you, if anything should be in there, it should be Valium. Quinine, I don't know where that's coming from. That ain't me.

*RILEY:* That ain't you.

*ED:* It shouldn't be me.

*RILEY:* But, there it is. That must be wrong, right?

*ED:* It could be wrong. You know, that's what I'm saying. I don't see why quinine should be in my system.

*RILEY:* Where's the quinine coming from?

*ED:* That means that I'm shooting dope. You know, it's just as easy for me to sit here and tell you I'm shooting dope as it is for me to tell you I'm taking Valium. You know, what's the difference? One is not better than the other.

*RILEY:* You're not supposed to be taking anything.

*ED:* The fact of the matter is that the medication wasn't holding me.

*RILEY:* I already raised the medication. Now, didn't I raise it? Didn't I raise it? I raised it, each time, each time! I raised it the first time; you said it wasn't good enough. I raised it a second time; you said it wasn't good enough. Now, I raised it a third time; you said it ain't good enough. Now, the part about it, I don't know if you even let it work because each time, from the first time until now, you still been messing around!

*ED:* No!

*RILEY:* Here, it's in the book! Is the book wrong?

*ED:* I don't care what the book says; I know what I do.

*RILEY:* You know what you do. I'll tell you what you're gonna do. We'll take a urine here.

*ED:* That's up to you.

*RILEY:* And I'll have it and we'll see. You're saying that place is wrong—well, I'm going to take one myself.

*ED:* You know, I don't care who takes the urine.

*RILEY:* Then, we could be sure.

*ED:* No, it makes no difference. What's going to come up is going to come up.

*RILEY:* So, in other words, you really don't care. (*Therapist turns toward mother.*)

*ED:* Tell me something, who is this on, me or my mother? You know I'm the one who's going to suffer. Not them.

*RILEY:* We are going to get it together. We didn't come here just to play. We come to try to help you get over it. I'm talking to the whole family.

*ED:* There's no playing. Two children are right there. Those are the two children. You know everyone else in here is an adult. There's no time to play. I'm not playing.

*RILEY:* I didn't come here to play.

*ED:* Do you think I'm playing?

*RILEY:* This is what I'm playing on. Right there, that's it. (*pointing to the book*)

*ED:* I'm gonna take care of business.

*RILEY:* All right. You're gonna take care of business.

*ED:* Sure, you know, I took Valium, but I ain't had no fun on it. You know, that's my admission there. That's my guilt; I did that.

*RILEY:* You know you're not supposed to take Valium?

*ED:* Right.

*RILEY:* But you went on and did it.

*ED:* That's right. Because I'm not going to sit back, feel bad, and don't get nothing out of it. I might as well go back out on the street and shoot dope.

*RILEY:* I couldn't stop you!

*ED:* That's right. Ain't nobody could stop me!

*RILEY:* Who are you killing, you or me?

*ED:* I be killing myself.

*RILEY:* It's you you're abusing, not me. Now, what I'm going to do; I'm gonna raise you ten more, but I don't want to see anything else in your urine. Now, if you have to suffer a little, you gotta suffer a little if you want to try and get over it.

*ED:* You know I don't mind suffering a little.

*RILEY:* That's going to be one thing; you're going to have to suffer some. It ain't going to come overnight. Now, I don't want this cheating.

*ED:* I can understand that. Just like you wanna understand, I want to understand.

*RILEY:* OK. Now I want an understanding that I'm going to raise you but I don't want that quinine or morphine in there. If you can't sleep, maybe you just walk around and suffer awhile.

*ED:* Walk around and suffer awhile. I do that. (*pointing to spouse*) I think that she can bear witness to it more than my mother can. I've been fighting all my life.

*RILEY:* They've been fighting for you.

*A significant aspect of this confrontation was that for the first time it became clearly defined that the drug issue was something that the entire family was involved with. Midway through the above segment the addict said, "Who is this on, me or my mother? You know I'm the one who's going to suffer." The therapist responded by saying that the whole family was involved and that he was addressing all family members. Following this confrontation the family members became much more spontaneous in asserting themselves and saying how Ed's addiction affected them.*

*After approximately 30 minutes of this "stripping the addict of his power," the therapist asked to meet with the addict alone. This was the first such individual meeting and it was a remarkably honest exchange. Riley explains the unusual candidness as a result of the addict having developed respect for the therapist, because the therapist had just publicly whipped him. It was also the first time that the therapist learned that Ed was more than just an addict, that he was a pusher.*

*RILEY:* How did your mother come to know what's happening?

*ED:* You know, a dope fiend doesn't have any respect for hours and time. Well, regardless of what I say, there's a few that's gonna try me anyway. Those few start adding up. It might not happen every day, but maybe somebody might ring the bell two or three o'clock in the morning, right? I'd been out in the street, I might have missed a few, and they done came out looking for me. Some of the people I associated with, my mother didn't know, but others she knew what they were doing and when they started coming more and more frequently to my house, everything started adding up.

*RILEY:* What did Dad do?

*ED:* Well, he was patient for a while. He didn't get wind of it until way later. But when he really found out what I was doing, he really, you know, verbally attacked me. He did everything but physically hit me. He set down what he wanted; he wouldn't have it any other way. It came to a point where if he had to he was going to get me jailed. That was going to be the solution to it 'cause you know it seemed like word of mouth wasn't going to stop anything. What he couldn't understand was that the way it was set up and the way the traffic was going, I just couldn't cut it off like that. You know, I had to wean people off. Gradually, I had to change my whole pattern. You know, I had to go directly outside, you know, which means taking my merchandise outside with me. And that's a bust. I've been out of the penitentiary since seventy-three and I don't intend to go back. Sooner or later, doing that out in the street, wide open, it's more likely for you to be jammed than if somebody be calling you, you meeting them or coming to your house, because they're not going to be coming in a mob anyway. You know, that's the kind of law that I had set up. If a group of individuals wanted to do some business, I'd work something out, come to see me.

*RILEY:* There's only one hang-up in it. It's like, you know, you was making good money. It's like an entertainer, being a star, on top; you follow me? What happens when the entertainer is not on top no more—he lost his voice, he's down low, you know. Some people can't go along with the loss. Like, if the opportunity presents itself again, who knows, you may go back. Why won't you go back?

*ED:* Why, because of the problems that really arose from that. Let me try to explain it to you this way. You read the paper, right? Well, there's a lot of friction about the narcotics control in this city. I live in North Philly. Let's say, hypothetically, that my man is from West Philly. So, I got his merchandise, you know, and I'm selling it in North Philly. But, in North Philly, there's a man who has his merchandise there, but I'm not associated with him. I know him, but because I live there, but I'm not doing his business. There's confusion amongst the ones who are dealing. See, there was some matters that really had to be straightened out 'cause you know, a couple times people stepped up to me with pistols and told me I can't do this. I said I'm gonna do this and we got to make some kind of arrangements to work this out. So, it came to a point where I had a certain location. I gave my bond that I wouldn't do business anywhere else. It took some weight off of me, but it didn't take all the weight off of me because like I'm not up on the top. You know, even though I was able to juggle, I'm not the top man. There was brothers around me that was over me. I was expendable, to tell you the truth. You know, I ain't nobody.

## FOURTH AND FIFTH SESSIONS

The father was absent from both these sessions. Riley met first with the whole family, and then spent most of each session with Ed and

Linda. The three of them discussed the fact that arguments seemed to never end between the couple. In the fifth session, Riley assigned them the somewhat paradoxical task of going home and fighting for at least 5 minutes that night. The directive was that they should not go to sleep before they finished the argument.

## SIXTH SESSION

One of the things that became more obvious as sessions continued was the special relationship that existed between Ed's mother and her 5-year-old granddaughter, Tina. Tina spent most of the day with Mrs. E and in the sessions it was Mrs. E who answered questions and gave directives to her. Although Linda, Tina, and Mrs. E were regularly at home together during the day, there was little evidence to suggest that Mrs. E and Linda had much of a relationship other than issues related to Tina. There was also little evidence to suggest that the mother and father shared much in common other than the concern they had for their son, Ed, and the affection they had for their granddaughter, Tina. In striking contrast, Mr. and Mrs. E appeared to be almost oblivious to the 2-month-old infant. It was clear that the new infant was Linda's baby, because she constantly fixed her eyes upon him no matter who was holding him or how quiet he was.

From the above (and other) observations, a picture of the family's structure and developmental stage began to emerge. Ed appeared to have "bought" freedom from his parents through his daughter, Tina. Before Tina appeared, the parents had focused their attention on Ed—he served to detour their conflict. Soon after Tina was born, Ed and Linda essentially "gave" her to his parents. Mr. and Mrs. E concurred in this contract, thereby relaxing their attention toward Ed. Linda's benefit in the trade-off was that, by releasing her daughter to her in-laws, she was able to gain the home and family of which she had felt deprived; she was in a sense trading motherhood for a continued daughterhood, tenuous as the latter might have been. This, in part, explained her "inability" to discipline Tina, a chore left to her in-laws. The structure was thus composed of an enmeshed triad involving Tina and her grandparents, plus a more overtly conflictual dyad of Ed and Linda. However, the trade-off of Tina was not complete, and Ed was still somewhat enmeshed with his parents also. He managed to attenuate his parents' fear of losing him completely by living in the home and by manifesting only a tenuous spouse-like relationship with Linda (see Chapter 1).

The family life cycle event—with its accompanying family crisis—that eventually brought the case to treatment was the birth of the baby boy 1 month earlier. Mr. and Mrs. E were neither prepared for nor receptive to this new addition. They did not want the added responsibility of another child to raise, but could not resist the urge to assume it, partly because their "daughter" Linda was not competent in their eyes. They were the child-rearing experts in the household, and felt a "natural" tendency to nurture the baby. Linda was not well schooled in child rearing and became involved in a cycle with her in-laws in which she might be remiss in a particular action, they would tell her what to do or criticize her, she would get resentful of their interference and their treatment of her as incompetent, and she would thus hold the baby even closer, and so on. However, they were more overt in criticizing Ed about having the child than they were toward Linda. Further, Ed and (particularly) Linda felt more parental toward the new baby than toward Tina and believed they had done enough in giving Mr. and Mrs. E their first child. The second child was not "for sale" and they fought back, at least in subtle ways. Thus an escalating series of conflictual cycles had developed, leading to more pressure on Ed, who increased his drug intake and not long thereafter appeared for treatment on a level of addiction that exceeded his manageable limits.

In light of these revelations, Riley had begun (in the fourth meeting) to alter his procedure within sessions by first seeing the entire family together for a brief period, and then dividing the family into smaller subsystems and seeing these separately. By the sixth session, he was primarily concerned with Mr. and Mrs. E as a couple and with Ed and Linda as a couple. The 5-year-old, Tina, became important in this process because it was primarily through her that the two couples related. With increasing frequency Riley began to use Tina's welfare as justification for change.

Many years had passed since Mr. and Mrs. E had done anything of a recreational nature together as a couple. In the sixth session Riley began by trying to engage these parents in some common interest or activity. However, it is important to note that he made certain that the plans and hospitality provided to the parents arose jointly both from himself *and* Ed.

*RILEY:* Do you like plays?
*MOTHER:* I like plays.

*FATHER:* I'm not too crazy about them.

*RILEY:* You know what, I was like you. I never did like plays; I thought it was too faggoty to like something like that, you know—until I was working. If you want to see a play that would make you crack up—I went to see one last week—it's a little theater down at Seventeenth and Delancey. If you go and don't enjoy it, I'll pay for it.

*FATHER:* I might check it out.

*RILEY:* You might check it out? (*talking to Ed*) You know, they'll make excuses. They really would make excuses. Now, how are we going to get them out? How can we get them to go to the show?

*ED:* Maybe if I pay their way, they'll go.

*RILEY:* You pay their way, they'll go? OK. Ed and I are gonna pay your way and we're not going to take any excuses. Now, let's see, how we gonna fix that up? Now they'll find something to do or something is in their way or some kind of obligation, like, "I got to get up early in the morning," or something like that, you know. Or, "I don't have my housework done," or, "Food hasn't been cooked," and all like that, right?

*ED:* We'll fix that up. Say, Friday would be good, wouldn't it?

*RILEY:* 'Cause you don't have to work Saturday. Well, Friday should be a fairly good day. I'll tell you what. I'll have it already set up for you. Your tickets will be at the window and all you have to ask for is my name and it's taken care of. Me and Ed will discuss it. Now, if you enjoy it, you're gonna have to pay Ed his five dollars back. You understand? It's a beautiful comedy; it's everyday life and you're really gonna crack up.

*The remainder of the session was spent with Ed and Linda alone. They appeared withdrawn and distant from one another. When the therapist inquired as to whether they had followed his directive to fight at home, they said they had not. The session became focused on an exploration of the differences that existed between the two of them.*

*LINDA:* Sometimes I feel it's best not to say anything. Maybe it's the way I express things, 'cause sometimes I don't say what I originally started out to say.

*RILEY:* Sometimes not to say anything creates that much more problems.

*LINDA:* Oh, please, you should be brothers.

*(later in the interview)*

*ED:* You have to pry all the time, you know; you never come right out and say exactly what you mean.

*RILEY:* Well, first we have to have a subject. Give me one of those little things. Is it pertaining to your feelings?

*LINDA:* Mostly.

*RILEY:* OK. Is it pertaining sometimes to getting you upset or depressed?

*LINDA:* No. Making me happy. I'd just like some happiness.

*RILEY:* Now, concerning your happiness. Come up with what would make you happy.

*LINDA:* Oh, he can give you a list as long as . . .

*ED:* But the point is getting her to understand the necessity of it.

*LINDA:* It's not that I don't understand.

*ED:* You see—like, I see it now. It's more giving than receiving. You know that—like my giving would be outward and hers would be inwardly done, you know.

*RILEY:* Control?

*ED:* Yeah, control, so to speak, whereas I could just come out and relate to "This is this; I'm doing this for this reason." But her, I'm supposed to understand because of our relationship toward each other. I can't see—well, if it's that way, why not say so, rather than letting me deal with the fact that I should know.

*RILEY:* I'm getting the message. The message is that you are the aggressor.

*ED:* Yeah.

*LINDA:* Oh, please.

*ED:* That's what it is. I'm the aggressor. I'm the one that's always trying to force, so to speak, and she's sitting there more or less submitting. It makes it like she's just doing it. It ain't nothing really to it, no emotions in it, no feelings. You know, it's just, well, "I'm supposed to do this, so I'll do it," or "I'm not going to do it." One or the other. She hears me; that's why she's trying to go on to something else. She'll do that, if I'm talking to her; she'll go on to something else.

*RILEY:* How long has this been going on?

*ED:* Ever since I've known her.

*RILEY:* And your feelings are somewhat damaged?

*ED:* And when I express this it becomes a thing whereas I might express it a little too forcefully, but then that's where I'm at. That's how it comes out, you know, more dominant than anything else. It might appear as though I'm trying to be superior because this is what she throws back—that I'm taking total charge; I'm putting myself up on a pedestal—but it's just a point that I have expressed so much in our relationship that I don't see nothing coming my way on her behalf that it makes me emotional. It makes me steamed up, you know; so I might really get built up into expressing that . . .

*(later in the interview)*

*RILEY:* Now, what do you want from him?
*LINDA:* What do I want from him?
*RILEY:* Yeah. He spoke on what he wants from you.
*LINDA:* Number one—and it will always be number one—I want him to be a very good father to our two children. I want him to be a good provider for our two children. And for me, what I really want of him—for myself—I just want him, you know, to really get himself together, find out exactly where he's going.
*RILEY:* Get himself together? Hasn't he got himself together?
*LINDA:* Well, see, he's doing it now, you know, but I don't want him to slip back. He's changed a lot of his old habits and I would prefer if he didn't slip back into them. I guess he would say the same thing about me; there's a lot of my old habits which I need to change.
*RILEY:* OK. So, if he changed his habits—then, are you happy with him?
*LINDA:* With the habits that he's changed.
*RILEY:* Now, why can't you give him what he wants? So he would see that he's *really* touching base. What's wrong with that?
*LINDA:* That's easier said than it is done.
*RILEY:* But what are *you* doing about it?
*LINDA:* Well, I'm trying; I'm working with myself on that. He doesn't even know about that.
*RILEY:* Well, why shouldn't he know? He should be the subject.
*LINDA:* No, not really. It's not easy.

*(later in the interview)*

*RILEY:* Why do you think there are so many call girls and people out there—because they're not satisfied at home. Now, do you want to protect your interests? Or do you just want to even up the score?

*LINDA:* I don't want to make trouble over little things just to even up the score.

*RILEY:* Well, this is what happens if you don't. Now it's your interests and the children's interests—what do you say? "What I'm looking for is I want him to be a good provider. I want this." Now, a fair exchange is no robbery. (*long pause*) Now what do you think about your interests?

*LINDA:* Well, I want to protect my interests. That's clear.

*RILEY:* Well, how you gonna go about protecting your interests?

*LINDA:* Like I said, I was trying to.

*RILEY:* OK. You was trying to. Have you accomplished anything?

*LINDA:* I think I have, but you'll have to ask him that, really. You know, because he's the dissatisfied party.

*RILEY:* (*to Ed*) Are you satisfied?

*LINDA:* I'm not satisfied, but I don't think I'm quite as dissatisfied as he is, I mean.

*RILEY:* Well, you can't speak for him.

*LINDA:* I'm not aggressive; it's never been my nature.

*RILEY:* Why?

*LINDA:* Because that's the way I've always been; I have no explanation why. I've been like that as long as I can remember.

*RILEY:* OK. You've been like that as long as you can remember. Now, you went into one motherhood; your body changed; you changed. So, you made some changes, right? Now, if you said it ain't your nature—people change things from nature.

*LINDA:* You know, from where you're sitting, it's probably easy for you to say that I should. But from where I'm sitting, I know things differently.

*RILEY:* You've been through it; I haven't.

*LINDA:* Let me ask you a question. If I sat here and knocked everything that you said or if everything that you said I tore completely apart and made it look like I didn't even exist—you know—and you saw me next week, would you have anything to say?

*RILEY:* OK. Now, the difference. Now, lots of times some people live together and it's sort of like a sparring match. You follow me? There is no referee to break it up and to deal with it. It's more like a power thing. You follow me? If I can't beat you this way, I'll beat you that way. Now, you're in the conflict all the time. Now, my job is to air these feelings out, to be the referee. So, we'll go over some values which you really feel. Now, from here on you two are able to be open with each other rather than to use a device to harm each other. Now, who knows, he might be using drugs as a scapegoat.

*LINDA:* To harm me?

*RILEY:* I hope he didn't. I know you didn't like it, him using drugs.

*LINDA:* If he was doing that to harm me, he would have harmed me, true; but he harmed himself more.

*RILEY:* Hey, but the fear of him getting knocked off or something happening to him . . .

*LINDA:* That's the everyday fear that I had.

*RILEY:* So, it's like pitting one against the other. But the only thing, you're using different things. And who are you harming, but each other? Now why can't you be enjoying yourself more so than using it as a weapon? And why can't he be enjoying himself more? And to just come out and say, "So and so, I didn't like this and this is the way so and so happened; let's deal with this and let's not have this coming up again and misunderstanding my feelings." You want someone to understand your feelings; they have feelings too.

(*Riley leaves the room to observe through a one-way mirror. The couple does not reach resolution. Riley reenters.*)

*ED:* We never work it out because there's always no response.

*RILEY:* No. There's no response 'cause you don't give her time to respond.

*ED:* Maybe I'm too impatient, you know; I sit and wait but I don't sit and wait too long.

*RILEY:* And you can get very upset waiting. . . . "What's the matter with you?"

*ED:* Right. 'Cause I do.

*RILEY:* So, that turns the whole subject around.

*LINDA:* It changes the whole subject. The position I'm put in then is like I'm looking up to my father; he's telling me, "Yeah, do this and do that." And that really aggravates me. It puts me to a point where, like I said, I'm a very vengeful person; so just to aggravate him even more, because of the way I feel, you know, I won't open my mouth. I might have fifteen million things I might want to say to him, but I won't say a word. I'll sit there and act like he's not even in the room with me.

*Riley asked Ed to give Linda 5 minutes to explain her views. Ed cooperated and the session continued for a time with this structure.*

*RILEY:* Why did you say, "He sounds like my father"?

*LINDA:* Because, you see, that's the way he comes off—he comes off so authoritarian.

*RILEY:* OK. So, he brings back a picture of your father.

*LINDA:* Only in the sense of being so authoritative, domineering.

*Even though it was a difficult session, especially for Linda, it seems that Linda's closing remarks indicated that she felt she had been understood and accepted by the therapist.*

*LINDA:* Have you and Ed ever talked about this before?

*RILEY:* No. Like I said, I've been with families and couples for a long time.

*LINDA:* You know, 'cause it's just the way you are dealing with our situation—it suggests that even though you say you haven't, I'll accept your word for it, you know; I don't want you to think I'm calling you a liar. It seems as though you two have talked about me before.

*RILEY:* No. We ain't talked about you; we talked about drugs. You see, I've been working with many families and handling many problems.

*Riley concluded the session with a task: if Linda or Ed had a subject to bring up or a bone to pick with the other, the other person was to give the first person 5 minutes to talk about or explain it before responding. This was obviously an extension of the exercise that had been undertaken in the session.*

## SEVENTH SESSION

The whole family appeared. The parents had attended the play the week before and the mother reported that she had enjoyed it immensely. The father noted that he had not realized that a play could be such fun. The therapist saw Ed and Linda alone at the end of the session to review their task and the time they had spent discussing things together as a couple.

## EIGHTH SESSION

In this session the therapist continued his strategy of getting the parents to support the couple (Ed and Linda), then getting the couple to deal with each other. He began by asking the parents what they thought about Ed and Linda getting married.

*MOTHER:* I don't know. If they got married? You know, I don't even let that cross my mind.

*RILEY:* Wait a minute, I got to ask them that.

*MOTHER:* 'Cause I have talked about it.

*RILEY:* Them two getting married—what do you think about that?

*FATHER:* I think it would be a very nice thing. If they'd make a go of it.

*MOTHER:* And the next thing to think about is them two there [grandchildren]. And after awhile, this one [Tina] will be asking sixty million questions. You know, it doesn't take too long.

*Having obtain this "blessing" from mother and father, the therapist then excused them and Tina from the session and focused on the couple.\* He used the theme of marriage to continue to explore relationship issues between the couple.*

*RILEY:* What would you look for if you were dating to be married?

*LINDA:* What would I be looking for?

*RILEY:* Yeah. 'Cause it's altogether different now.

*LINDA:* I never really thought about it.

*RILEY:* Don't you think it's time to think about it—because, you know, you would have something, a foundation, you know? That's a part about it—how would you say—it's an altogether whole different ball game, you know. What do you think about it?

---

\*As noted in Chapter 1 and 6, such a blessing, or "freeing up" of the addict by his parent(s) is almost invariably necessary before he can establish a viable heterosexual relationship. Parental permission of this sort is also a crucial requisite for successful marital treatment with addicts.

*ED:* That's the completion of the relationship, as far as I see it. It's one of the steps we should be taking now.

*RILEY:* You mean, your roles have to change?

*ED:* Some of 'em, I think, you know; I don't think all of them should change because I feel like, in a sense, part of the role of a married man—I'm taking that now. So like I really don't see too much else is left really.

*RILEY:* Well that makes her a missus.

*ED:* True, but I relate to her as missus now.

*The therapist encountered some resistance from the spouses, who each claimed that marriage would make no real difference. He countered this by making the marriage more vivid—first, by asking what they would wear, then by asking who they would invite. This led naturally to a discussion of Linda's relationship to her father. Both Ed and Linda talked about their feelings toward him around issues such as his lack of respect for them and his indifference toward her first baby. The therapist accepted their strong negative feelings, but was careful not to accept Linda's rejection of him.*

*RILEY:* He's very important, in a manner of speaking.

*LINDA:* No, he ain't important.

*ED:* Yeah, he is important.

*RILEY:* He *is* important, in a way. From the way that you would like his respect.

*ED:* Yeah, he is important.

*Riley then brought the discussion around to the issue of Ed's leaving home. Although Ed continued to maintain that he was free to come and go, Riley suggested that the parents also worry and hold on, and that Ed might not be as independent as he would like others to believe.*

*RILEY:* Sometimes parents are scared. They think that off-spring won't succeed.

*ED:* It's never no one else can offer enough to your offspring. I think it's false. 'Cause it's not you that's gonna have to accept that, it's the offspring who are going to have to accept it. I think the whole should be that—like, my children need me, you understand. I feel as though it never comes to a point where they need to come back and want to come back; it's there. But there's no thing that they have to or there's no thing that I'm pulling them back.

*RILEY:* I don't know; we can't talk that far.

*ED:* This is how I feel.

*RILEY:* This is how you feel now. What you think you would like.

*ED:* I, like, I'm trying, you know, as they grow, to keep that frame of mind. You know, this is how it's supposed to be, regardless of the situation, you know, because that's how it is with my own upbringing—you know, how I came up, how things are for me. I feel as though if I leave—you know, if there is a necessity that I come back—I think the doors will be open, but also I know that they're not pulling me back there.

*RILEY:* How old are you now?

*ED:* Twenty-seven.

*RILEY:* Twenty-seven. You been living at home all your life?

*ED:* Yeah, you know, give and take the time spurts, I stayed away for a while, you know, the time I was in the service, but like my mother's home was always home whether I spent a period of time somewhere else or not.

*RILEY:* OK. Now, how come—you know—you wasn't able to start seeking for yourself and start your own foundation?

*ED:* Well, I did start foundations of my own; I just didn't stay.

*RILEY:* Why?

*ED:* Why? Either the situation came up whereas where, who, or how I was doing, wasn't suitable . . .

*RILEY:* For who?

*ED:* For me. I needed to regroup so this is where I went to regroup.

*RILEY:* How old were you when you first left?

*ED:* About seventeen, I guess.

*RILEY:* You were seventeen.

*ED:* You know, it was a thing where I lived with my parents; there was no commitment to my being there. I had freedom to go and come as I pleased.

*RILEY:* At seventeen, you left, right? What did you get, an apartment?

*ED:* Right.

*RILEY:* How long did you stay?

*ED:* Well, this is a small period of time, then, because right then I went into the service.

*RILEY:* But how long?

*ED:* This is like a couple of months. This is a thing that wasn't even with the knowledge of my parents. They didn't even know what was going on.

*RILEY:* Oh, in other words, they wasn't sure you left?

*ED:* Right. This is on my own. This spot was mine on the side.

*RILEY:* But really you were still at home.

*ED:* You know, that was the foundation there. This spot was security that I wanted elsewhere.

*RILEY:* So—that even fell out, later on. You said you'd been there a couple of months.

*ED:* Right. Then I went into the service.

*RILEY:* All right. When you went into the service, how long did you stay?

*ED:* Three years.

*RILEY:* OK. Three years. When you came back out of the service, you came back home, right? And then you was working these various jobs? Then did you get another place?

*ED:* Yeah, I had a couple of spots, to tell you the truth.

*RILEY:* Were those spots just to transact business?

*ED:* More or less.

*RILEY:* So, in other words, you still haven't . . .

*ED:* See it wasn't a thing that I was just saying, "Well I'm going." I didn't make that move.

*RILEY:* Why?

*ED:* 'Cause if I would have made that move, I wouldn't be there now.

*RILEY:* OK. Why didn't they say, "Go"?

*ED:* Why didn't they say, "Go"? That I don't know.

*RILEY:* You don't?

*ED:* No. You know, that's something that they know. Because I look at it this way. The period of time I was in the service, I wasn't there—right? When I came out of the service, you know, the choice was mine whether to keep going or come back home, you know. I came back home. It was never a thing of a demand put on me to leave but it was a situation where I knew if I wanted to leave, I could leave. If I no longer wanted to stay under their roof, I could go.

*RILEY:* OK. Now, you and Linda are fixed up together. Did you get a place of your own?

*ED:* No.

*RILEY:* Why?

*ED:* Why? That isn't what I wanted, financial needs, and a hell of a narcotic habit.

*RILEY:* You brought her in your mother's house.

*ED:* That was the security that I had.

*RILEY:* This is—how you say—you care for the woman, right? Now you should give a woman a place that she has of her own.

*ED:* Right. But, regardless of how much you care, when you're not financially able in the situation . . .

*RILEY:* But you were financially able at that spot.

*ED:* No, I wasn't. If I was, I would have done it.

*RILEY:* Do you think he was financially able to do it?

*LINDA:* No, he wasn't.

## NINTH SESSION

This was an individual session with Ed that took place following a brief family meeting (Linda was absent due to illness). The major themes were Linda's family and Ed's (related) concern about her. Riley emphasized the mysteries and secrets in Linda's family and the stress it placed on Linda and on her relationship with Ed.

*ED:* It puts a dent in out relationship, too.

*RILEY:* That's what I was going to get around to.

*ED:* It's a thing of trust; it's like if she don't want to be put in a possibility whereas she is gonna be hurt. That seems to be her main problem—she doesn't want to be hurt. This is what's always related to me, anything to keep from being hurt. She don't want to experience no pain, no emotional pain at all.

*RILEY:* That's why she stays in mostly?

*ED:* I don't think that's why she stays in mostly; I guess she really just doesn't see any comfort around anybody else.

*RILEY:* Doesn't this put a burden on you?

*ED:* Quite. You know, in a sense, something I have to adjust to.

*RILEY:* Have you really adjusted to it?

*ED:* Not completely. I'm still working with it. Because it stops a whole lot of my movement. In a sense, it will change my ways a lot. You know, I could see something wrong, Paul, but I can't say nothing. You know, for the mere reason that it's going to lead to something a little heavier than what I want to get into.

*RILEY:* But, don't you think—how would you say—she would have to feel your feelings and know what you're going through that maybe—how would you say—need to take all her past and put it together and push it away and "Hey let's start."

*ED:* You see, that's the problem, I can't get all of it out of her. I could pry and get a portion here; four or five months from now, I might get another portion.

*RILEY:* So you see your life for the job already.

*ED:* You know it's the thing that I'm trying to get the trust, you know, and the understanding from her.

*RILEY:* Why did you take up psychology?

*ED:* Why? Because I want to know about people.

*RILEY:* Mainly her.

*ED:* Right. And my children.

*RILEY:* Yeah. Particularly children. Children come into that too.

*ED:* And certain things that I see that I wanna know more thoroughly about, other than from my street knowledge—like, why certain things might, in dealing with children, you know, certain ways to react to them, and there's got to be a reason for them. It's like sometimes I see something that somebody else had done, and she's doing it to them, you know, and it moves me. You see, I don't want to attack her about it. Know what I mean? I'm trying to find out; it seems like it's a treatment that she got, or she didn't get—and she's like, trying to make adjustments for.

*RILEY:* Why should the children be the guinea pigs of solving her situation?

*ED:* Well, not be guinea pigs . . .

*RILEY:* Yeah, well, the part about it—they would be—how would you say—like sometimes you say you may see her acting out, and you recall some of the things that she's said and she is doing identical the same thing.

*ED:* Right.

*RILEY:* Is there anything wrong with her head, you know? Or, why does she do this?

*ED:* See, that's why—you know—what I'm trying to do, to get out of her: the reason for it, and I can't get all of those.

*RILEY:* Uh-huh. You've been struggling all along.

*ED:* Yes. Ever since our daughter was born, you know, I've been questioning.

*Riley then continued the discussion about Linda. He made it clear that he was not blaming Linda, or encouraging Ed to do so, but that he thought it important to help Linda wipe the slate clean as far as her past was concerned. The discussion had the further benefit of strengthening Ed's role as a responsible parent.*

*RILEY:* She does need help.

*ED:* She needs strokes, too. You know, I'm trying to be just right to her, but there's a problem trying to get through that shield.

*RILEY:* Well, that's what I was intending to do where I was going to help you get through some of the things which you have been trying to get through and bring it to the surface and wipe it up and get rid of it. So you don't have to deal with that. So she don't have to say, "Hey this is my makeup, I got to follow this."

*ED:* That's something she definitely has to get out of her.

*RILEY:* Yeah, 'cause it's a wonder how she dealt with all these crises, you know, all these things. Here's her whole family, you know; she couldn't even count how many was in her family—wait a minute, six, no, seven—you know, it's like they wasn't there. It's like she wants to wipe them out but she doesn't even know who she's wiping out.

*ED:* Well, I guess she looks at it as the fact that nothing beneficial came out of having a family—you know, as far as her makeup was concerned. She misses that familiness.

*RILEY:* Is she glad she had the children?

*ED:* Yeah. 'Cause she loves the children.

*RILEY:* Maybe sometimes when she sort of gets chastizing them or whatever, it comes out, or something they do, that she acts strange.

*ED:* Well, say, like the reaction of a child. A child can be stubborn at times, you know; they'll want to play, and sometimes you have to disregard what you're doing, you know, take your enjoyment away, to deal with them. You know, 'cause I think that's part of the makeup of being a parent. It's to see to it that the child has the understanding 'cause you should already have your basic amount of understanding by the time you're able to think about start producing a child. It's like sometimes she just don't know how to solve that problem, her own emotions. You know, she'll let our daughter get her emotionally upset when she shouldn't. You know, my daughter is very intelligent; she plays on that. You know, she really doesn't know that she is playing on it, but her natural ability makes her antagonize her a little bit more, you know, a little bit more, when she sees her mother is getting more and more hostile.

*RILEY:* When your wife gets upset, what happens?

*ED:* She becomes very loud, you know; you see a nervousness come out of her. She doesn't really know what to do with herself so she tries to yell, so to speak, to block out everything. Do you know what I mean? Like strong, harsh words will make—a child is not gonna stop, a child continues on if she continues on. Then it's a thing of her against the child, and it shouldn't be like that because she is the mother, you know; it should be that she holds the authority, not the child. It's a thing where almost that my daughter has the authority sometimes. You know, she's letting my daughter make the move and it shouldn't be like that. She's got to make the move for her, because by her being a woman, she has to set an example for her.

*The therapist continued to interweave discussion of Ed and Linda's relationship with a discussion of Ed's relationship with his parents and also what Linda brought to the relationship from her past. As in previous sessions, Riley implied that Ed had some unfinished business with his parents and also that he needed to work out his problems with Linda so that he could move away from his parents. Ed contrasted his home life and background with Linda's.*

*ED:* I wasn't subjected to all that. You know, all of the wrong that I got, I got out on the street on my own. You know, I didn't get it from the house. You know, I just picked that up because I became streetwise. You know, by being there with no brother or sister, you know, I seen that that was my alternative. I didn't have to come out that way, but that's the way I came out. 'Cause I guess I had a little knowledge because my parents instilled knowledge on me. You know, but like I wanted to be out there, you know, to show some type of independence. You know, I didn't want to be stuck with one of my parents.

*RILEY:* And now, you're stuck up in their house?

*ED:* Right. That's about what it is. 'Cause, you know, my activities are limited.

*RILEY:* I'm just thinking—how would you say—if it would be that your parents are going away you would really have a time, in a way of speaking, without Linda's adjusting to what you want and what's good for the kids and how things should be. You thought of that, haven't you?

*ED:* See now, I want to tell you, how it would be like—she would try.

*RILEY:* You going to work.

*ED:* Right.

*RILEY:* And she's home with the kids.

*ED:* Right.

*RILEY:* How would you feel?

*ED:* Well, we've had a little experience like that. When I was working at warehouses, she was staying at the house; then, I'd say for maybe three months, she attempted to put out her best. You know, she would wait up for me when I was on second shift, you know, would warm my dinner for me, you know, things of that nature. Things would be in pretty much order, but, you know, I guess she had all day to do what she wanted to do. But like there were times when you might come home, you're not in the best of moods, after you worked all day, and like you might not want nothing to eat that night. I might not have a whole lot of conversation. And, she takes a negative attitude, very quickly, you know, without thinking things out thoroughly; you know, she would jump the gun. Like she wasn't doing nothing to satisfy me.

*RILEY:* You said she wants everything her way?

*ED:* She would like to be independent, more or less. You know, meaning she really wouldn't like anybody telling her what to do.

*RILEY:* 'Cause she has from her past—they was telling her what to do.

*ED:* Right, same as always, you know. Guiding her, and didn't seem to be guiding her right. And she thinks she knows the direction she wants to go, and if she makes the mistake, she'll be the one what will have to suffer, but it's no longer like that. There's those around her that care now, who suffer also.

*RILEY:* Her father, you know, her father's brother, who raised her with him—it's like you still hunting for whether it will be okay to get some of these things out from him. 'Cause I guess he knows quite a bit, doesn't he?

*ED:* I don't know. 'Cause I don't think he really had time to do anything. You know, it was more or less like he was just there for the image, not for the responsibility. So he really don't know what's going on.

*RILEY:* Is his wife still living?

*ED:* No.

*RILEY:* She died?

*ED:* She died. Maybe in seventy-something. It might have been maybe a year before that, if I'm not mistaken, because I don't recall directly if she was living when I met her [Linda] or not. She might have been. If she was, she died in seventy.

*RILEY:* It seems like all the females in that family, something mysterious happens to them, you know, and I was just saying, "Hey, you know, I want to know if she's thinking that her time may be up, too."

*ED:* I don't think so.

*RILEY:* 'Cause so many mysterious things have happened to them like, what provoked their spouse or whoever it may be to—how you say—to do them bodily harm? Like you say her mother was poisoned, then her older sister got killed, and then the other one got strangled. This was done by someone else. Now, what does the female do to provoke that? You understand? Is this female you have the same, that provokes you to do the same thing?

*ED:* Yeah, I could see what you're saying, 'cause like at times I guess she can provoke you into really doing something to her. She has that way about her. You know, like you want to take her head off, you know, but the point is, it's way past that.

*RILEY:* But where does it come from? In other words . . .

*ED:* Right. Is it heredity?

*RILEY:* And is it—how would you say—part of her destiny? It was with the rest of them, and that may be thrown upon you in such a way that you may continue the same cycle that has been going on.

*ED:* Well, I'm gonna tell you like this. I hope not.

*RILEY:* You hope not.

*ED:* In the period of our relationship, right; I think it was about four times I had to go upside her head. You know, the last time, I told myself that I would never touch her again. And, I haven't since then. No matter what she do, I just bypass it. If it means that I got to leave, I do that.

*RILEY:* Well, how does she upset you?

*ED:* Uh, her whole general attitude. Twice, if I'm not mistaken, it was dealing with my daughter, you know; it was something she didn't do, you know. She was angry with me, and she took it out on my daughter. You know, she used my daughter as a crutch. All of the anger she had at me came out on her. And I put up with it all day and half the night until I got tired of it, you know.

*RILEY:* So, it was by her using her daughter that can make you uncontrollable, in a way of speaking. All these little things—how would you say—that come into play, you know, how her actions and her behavior toward you can build up to such a mountain, you understand.

*ED:* And it has, you know, but I try to adjust to it, to a point where I don't let it happen. You know, and so far I've been successful.

*RILEY:* But I want to get rid of that, because if we keep building, if little things keep building, I don't care, you can say, "Hey I try to get rid of and put it aside," but you keep putting it aside, it—sort of like—it goes. God knows when the explosion is gonna come.

*Riley ended the session by suggesting that the three of them continue this effort to put Linda's past to rest.*

*RILEY:* I guess the best thing we can do for it is all three of us to get together and see what we can do that way and to go—how would you say—to go into her past.

*ED:* Maybe she'll do it. I don't know.

*RILEY:* Well, she started to do it.

*ED:* There's no telling, Paul, she might freeze up on me again. You know, that's been my experience with it.

*RILEY:* Well, together I think she may open up and then we can start digging so we can *end* some of this, because the girl—how you say—may be scared half to death and not know who she is, and what is her history, and what is the family's history. You know?

This session was an example of extremely skillful restructuring on the part of the therapist. Riley used the addict's propensity to be helpful by essentially making Ed a cotherapist for his wife. Riley had channeled Ed's involvement with Linda into helping her overcome her problems, rather than attacking her in an unproductive way. He provided Ed with a rationale for responding to Linda nonviolently. Further, by elevating Ed and making Linda the "patient," Ed was no longer the problem person in the family. Instead, he had become a concerned, helpful husband. This session punctuated a shift in the direction of the therapy.

*TENTH SESSION*

Prior to the 10th session, Ed's urine test indicated that he had taken a narcotic in addition to methadone. This was an unexpected occurrence, as he had stabilized on methadone and had embarked on a smooth and gradual decrease in dosage. The therapist saw the whole family (except the father, who had "had a hard day") and confronted them with the evidence. While Riley did not deny that this was a step backward, he handled the issue differently than in the third session. This time he emphasized that he already had evidence that Ed could handle the drug issue and was capable of staying off of heroin. This created a clear expectation that Ed could and would do this.

> *RILEY: (to Ed)* How are you doing?
>
> *ED:* So-so.
>
> *RILEY:* You know, I have "so-so" feelings too. Last week, your urine was dirty. I have feelings and I wonder why you come up dirty. You know, you were doing so good, all the way down [during the "detox"], and I'll give you credit for all the good you've done. Tell me why you stopped?
>
> *ED:* I didn't stop. I ain't got no explanation for that.
>
> *RILEY:* You don't have no explanation?
>
> *ED:* None whatsoever. I ain't got nothing to say about that.
>
> *RILEY: (to mother)* How do you feel about it?
>
> *MOTHER:* I really don't know what to say, since he had done so good so far. I was trusting that he'd continue.
>
> *RILEY:* How do you feel about it?
>
> *MOTHER:* What?
>
> *RILEY:* The good he done.
>
> *MOTHER:* I feel good about the good he's done, but I feel bad about this turning up.
>
> *RILEY:* OK. Well, how about giving him the good?
>
> *MOTHER:* How about giving him the good?
>
> *RILEY:* Yeah.
>
> *RILEY:* Uh-huh. How about giving him the good?
>
> *MOTHER:* OK. I'll excuse him.
>
> *RILEY:* You're proud of what he already done.
>
> *MOTHER:* I'm very proud of what he already done, and he knows that. I guess you can—I don't know—whether you can say you can excuse one time?

RILEY: *(to Linda)* How you feel about it?

LINDA: I can't understand it, that's all.

RILEY: Well, all these weeks I'm showing you right there. *(Points to book with clean urines from previous weeks, which is lying by Riley on the floor.)*

LINDA: I know how to read the sheets and understand. I don't understand last week.

RILEY: How you feel about his goodness?

LINDA: Well, I'm glad he did it.

RILEY: How you feel about him going back into it?

LINDA: I don't. I don't like it.

RILEY: How does it make you feel?

LINDA: How does it make me feel? Disappointed.

RILEY: *(to Ed)* How do you feel about it?

ED: I don't feel nothing. You see, I don't understand it, so I'm feeling very negative toward it. Cause I can justify codeine and the medication that was prescribed for me, but nothing else.

RILEY: Yeah, well I know you were supposed to take some of that medication, right?

ED: So, like, what can I say? I can't say, "Yeah, I was dirty," because I wasn't dirty. In order to be dirty, I got to do something. And I haven't did anything, so what can I say?

RILEY: So, in other words, that medication could have these ingredients?

ED: Well, like, I'm not the pharmacy.

RILEY: Yeah, but the medication you're taking could have these ingredients?

ED: No, not to my knowledge; my knowledge of penicillin and Robitussin—no. You know, that's my knowledge of it. You see, I'm not looking for that as a bypass as to why that's in there, because I don't think it is.

RILEY: Well, let me give you this thought I had.

ED: All right.

RILEY: You have been able to stay clean for X number of weeks. You have been able to even take a decrease in the meth, right? So, I don't need to solve this no more, because you can handle this.

ED: True.

RILEY: I'm not God, and I'm not gonna wipe you clean, because I can't.

ED: That's right.

*RILEY:* Now, you can handle this, the witness is right there. (*points to book*) He can handle it. Now, nothing went different around the house, has it?

*MOTHER:* The same thing. Same as always. So, nothing went no different.

*RILEY:* So, you can master your own ship. I don't have to deal with you and your drug usage, because that could be eliminated unless you want it.

*ED:* That would have to be something that I would have to start back.

*RILEY:* Well, you know how, you know how.

*ED:* And you can do it. Right.

*RILEY:* So that's fine. Now, that's where I got a lot out of it. I know you're strong enough to do it.

*ED:* Right.

*RILEY:* You got the strength to do it. You've got the means to do it.

*ED:* Well, I hope I continue to prove that a . . .

*RILEY:* Well, just say for instance—how would you say—when you go back on it.

*ED:* I can't look at that perspective.

*RILEY:* You can't look at it?

*ED:* That's taking steps backward. I got too much to lose there.

*RILEY:* Well, you gotta think on that then.

*ED:* Regardless of the people around me—how they feel about the situation, I got more to lose than anybody, because their situation is either to accept it or reject it. They're not going to suffer the same as I am. You know, I got more to lose.

*RILEY:* You know, another thing coming to mind now—we're in the ninth week. Time passes. But there's still a lot of pieces that may have to be ironed out. You know?*

*Later in the same session, Riley saw Linda and Ed together. He continued on the theme of Linda's past.*

---

*After the session Riley checked with the Drug Dependence Treatment Center (DDTC) physician and found that he had prescribed Robitussin and penicillin for Ed as treatment for a respiratory infection and cough (possibly caught from Linda). The Robitussin included codeine and this was the narcotic that had been detected in Ed's urine. Thus the group had been reacting to a false alarm.

*LINDA:* (*sighs*) Boy, oh boy, oh boy.

*RILEY:* You know, last week I was putting all those pieces together, or trying to put all your pieces together, and do you know what? I nearly went out of my mind just trying to put them all together.

*LINDA:* I guess you would.

*RILEY:* You know, and—I wonder how it affects you. You know, like, your mother passed away at an early age, you know, and you were no more than five years old.

*LINDA:* That's right. About five or six.

*RILEY:* About five or six.

*LINDA:* I think I had just turned six.

*RILEY:* And the part about it you were five or six, and you said you just left her, and then you got the word that she was dead.

*LINDA:* Yeah, well, I didn't find out until my mother had been dead for three days.

*RILEY:* It seems like you're in the dark in everything.

*LINDA:* Well, why did they never tell me, you know? When she did decide to tell me, she decided one night after we ate dinner to call. We rushed from the third to the second floor landing, sat on the step, and we thought we had did something, and she said, "Your mother's dead," and she turned around and shut her bedroom door and went in her bedroom, and that was it. And me and my brother had to deal with it.

*RILEY:* But you still don't know how she died.

*LINDA:* She died in her sleep. Far as I know.

*RILEY:* And does that sound right to you?

*LINDA:* Well, there was a lot of controversy about that, and I . . .

*RILEY:* Like what?

*LINDA:* My mother had a big house to herself. She had roomers, you know, in the house. She had a few roomers. At this particular time there was this man rooming in there and the way I understand it was this man and my mother had an argument or something before she died. I think the man thought that he was going to take advantage of her because she was a woman; she was the only one in the house other than himself and he was the only man. It had something to do with rent, from what I can understand. He was supposed to pay it. They got into an argument. My mother being the type of person that she was, from what I remember of her, one thing led to another and I think she cut him. I'm sure she did. The last time I saw him the mark was still on his face.

*RILEY:* She cut him?

*LINDA:* Right. Well, he tried to knock her down the steps.

*RILEY:* So, her death wasn't just from natural causes?

*LINDA:* Well, from what I could understand, on the death certificate it said the cause of death was some type of poison; I think it was nickel something. Anyway, my aunt, my mother's sister, said that she believes that the man gave my mother a drink, and something was in it or something. You know, probably some type of poison.

*RILEY:* Like I said before, the women seemed to have some very horrible deaths. Have you thought about yourself?

*LINDA:* I think about it all the time.

*RILEY:* What have you thought about?

*LINDA:* Nothing, really, I just—you know.

*RILEY:* Being another female, when all the other females died at the age of thirty. Thirty-two, at the most.

*LINDA:* Well one of my sisters, she was forty-two when she died. I don't know. Somehow I think I might die early; sometime I say I ain't going to worry about it. When my time comes, I'll just go, that's all.

*RILEY:* Do you talk to Ed about it?

*LINDA:* Not about me dying, no.

*RILEY:* What do you talk to him about?

*LINDA:* Sometimes we may talk about, you know, my parents or my uncle, or something like that. I tell him different things and we talk about it. There are certain situations where I can be at a complete loss as to what happened or how did this happen; I can't figure out why. I talk to him about it because he always seems to be able to give me a logical explanation, and one that I can accept, you know, and I can accept it because I can see exactly what he is saying, that it could be this way. A lot of things I don't understand about, say, my uncle, for instance, I talk to him about it . . .

*RILEY:* The one who raised you?

*LINDA:* Right. He can shed a little light on it sometimes.

*RILEY:* You still don't have a picture of your mother?

*LINDA:* No. His sister.

*RILEY:* His sister has a picture and you don't see it?

*LINDA:* She claims that it fell behind her mantlepiece, and she ain't gonna have it knocked down. I don't believe it's behind her mantlepiece, I believe . . .

*RILEY:* It's like your mother wasn't even there.

*LINDA:* That's right.

*RILEY:* Ain't that kind of mysterious?

*LINDA:* I'm starting to think like my brother; sometimes I find myself thinking like my youngest brother. I don't believe she's dead either.

*RILEY:* You don't believe she's dead?

*LINDA:* Sometimes I don't.

*(later in the interview)*

*LINDA:* So she'd ask me different things, telling me that my mother wasn't dead, right? OK. So I'd think, "Why? How do you know this?" One time I had run away from home, so to speak; I just got really pissed off at my uncle, and I just decided that I wasn't going home, you know; to me, that wasn't running away. And I had stayed around her house. Right? So, she went out, this particular day, my uncle's sister came and knocked on the door, and I was in her house, by myself, and I don't remember exactly what my aunt said to me, through the door, but whatever it was, I must not have been thinking too good anyway, because I let her in and she saw that it was me; and then I had to go with her, right? And they were going to have this lady locked up, and then all of a sudden, they decided they weren't going to do it. OK, so she was asking me some questions, you know, about had they ever told me the truth about my mother? She said that my mother ain't dead. So, if my mother's not dead, why the big farce? Of a funeral, you know.

*RILEY:* Mm-hmm.

*LINDA:* And at this particular time, you remember that I got really upset about it, 'cause I couldn't figure out where I was going. What was really happening, because, OK, I said I had went to a funeral, in Baltimore, that was one of my sister's, the oldest one—she was forty-two—I went to her funeral, so she was saying, "Linda, what did the lady look like?" So I told her. You know, the last time I remember seeing that sister I was about two, 'cause it was when our father died; I don't really remember her that well. Ummm, so I told her what she looked like. She said, "Linda, that wasn't your sister." Everything is very mysterious, you know, and I said, "Well, if it wasn't my sister, who was it?" She said, "That was your mother." She said, "I hate to tell you this, but that was your mother."

*RILEY:* That was your mother being buried.

*LINDA:* Yeah, that I went to the funeral for.

*RILEY:* But when you was thinking that's your sister, but that was your mother.

*LINDA:* Right.

*RILEY:* So they say.

*LINDA:* So they say.

*RILEY:* Sounds like you—it ran you crazy, one way or the other.

*LINDA:* Well, see, that's where I can lean on him because, like, at that time I was . . .

*RILEY:* He can't give you the answers.

*LINDA:* He can't give me the answers, but he can tell me things, where sometimes, you know, you get upset and you don't think rationally, right? OK.

*RILEY:* So, he can help pacify.

*LINDA:* Yeah, well, he can tell me, like, "Linda," like he said, "if that was your mother, then. . . ." That particular sister, she had a different mother than I did, right? And like I told Ed, when I saw— remember I told you, when I went to her house, before the funeral, her mother was there—her mother's still alive, as far as I know; she's still alive, and her aunt, they live together, right? She showed me a letter that my sister wrote to her a few months before she died. You know, they say sometimes people can tell when you're dying, and I don't know if it's true or not, but in this letter, because I read it, her mother told me to read it and then she started crying, and I had to stop reading it because I didn't want to see her get upset because she was a very elderly lady, like seventy-five. In the letter it's telling her, "Mom, I'm coming home, and I want to be with you for a while." Things like this. And then I'm reading this letter, so then I don't have any doubts that this is my sister, but then I seen this lady, she tells me something else. I can't really say I don't believe this lady is really crazy. I doubt if she's crazy; I think she's very sane at the time she told me. She wasn't drunk, so that couldn't have been an excuse, you know? I don't know where she got it from, but wherever she got it from, maybe she had a good reason for telling me, I don't know.

*RILEY:* Have you done any tracking for your mother's name, as far as deceased—all like that?

*LINDA:* No. I thought about doing that, I thought about going down . . . to New York.

*RILEY:* Why not?

*LINDA:* I don't even want to deal with it.

*RILEY:* But you have to deal with yourself, and, uh . . .

*LINDA:* Well, see, I feel like if I thought digging into my mother's death or if she's still alive or what—it's not that I'm afraid that I'm going to find something that I don't want to accept, but right now, I'm just trying to say that my mother [being] dead—that's all I've known since I was what—five, six years old—so I'm going to say she's dead. I don't care what nobody says.

*RILEY:* OK now.

*LINDA:* You could bring a lady in right now and say, "This is your mother." But I'm going to say she's dead.

*RILEY:* OK, you say that she's dead, OK?

*LINDA:* Uh-huh.

*RILEY:* OK. You say that she's dead, OK? And yet, sometimes, you may get a notion, or an idea, or something may make you think of Mother, you follow me?

*LINDA:* Right.

*RILEY:* And, then, you turn around and ask Ed, right?

*LINDA:* Right.

*RILEY:* And Ed sort of gives you some kind of satisfaction, but you are disturbed, you follow me? But, this disturbance keeps coming up sometimes, and it's like . . . by going over the record, how can you get rid of it? Shouldn't you get rid of it completely?

*LINDA:* I guess I should, but you know, I feel like this: whatever the reasons for keeping anything away from me were, they succeeded in keeping it away from me, and I don't want to start a whole bunch of dumb stuff, you know, within the family, because I try not to deal with them as much as I can. So, I'd really rather leave it like it is, because if I started, eventually someone would find out, I guess, and then there would be a whole bunch of stuff. They might try to send me back to a psychiatrist. They'd probably say I'm crazy, then they might . . .

*RILEY:* Did they try to send you to a psychiatrist?

*LINDA:* Huh?

*RILEY:* Did they try to send you to a psychiatrist?

*LINDA:* I went to a psychiatrist when I was six years old.

*RILEY:* Why?

*LINDA:* 'Cause I was really—I guess you could say—well, after my mother died—you know how you stay out of school a certain time for the funeral and burial and everything like that? OK, I went back to school. I've always been very quick-tempered. You know kids have a habit of saying, well, "Your mother. . . ." You know, and I used to get into more fights, and it developed into what I guess they call a behavior problem. Then I more or less—I guess you could say I just went into a shell; I had no interest in schoolwork; I had no interest in nothing. The one interest that I had then, it was my ballet class, and I wouldn't even go to that anymore. I guess they really thought, "Something is really wrong with the child." And I think they went to somebody in the school or were notified by somebody in the school. Well, anyway, they took me to this child psychiatrist or whatever he was.

*(later in the interview)*

*RILEY:* Why don't you find out about it for sure? Why don't you go down to City Hall, and ask if your mother was really dead? Is she dead, or was that your mother that you went to see buried, instead of your sister? You know there's a lot of things . . .

*LINDA:* No, no.

*RILEY:* I want to know how you can—sometimes you can get upset, not knowing who you are, who you come from, where's the rest of your family, and you have to ask somebody, and after you ask them, somebody just to console you for a little while, and then it may come up next week. So, you really haven't buried the dead.

*LINDA:* Oh, well, I'm sorry.

*RILEY:* Do you want to bury the dead?

*LINDA:* Yeah, I want to bury it. I just want to forget the whole thing . . .

*RILEY:* Well, why don't you . . .

*LINDA:* . . . a lot. I can tell you at one time I had completely buried it until things started happening.

*RILEY:* What brought it back up?

*LINDA:* Like I said, this lady started telling me that was my mother buried, and they had told me it was my sister. You see, I had really forgotten it, 'cause if somebody asked me anything about my parents, I said I was an orphan, you know.

*RILEY:* Did they want you to go crazy, or are you crazy?

*LINDA:* No. I believe I'm just as sane, if not saner, than they are.

*RILEY:* Well, why do you keep putting it off?

*LINDA:* I don't know, I guess I don't really want to be bothered. . . . Like I said, I'm not afraid because I feel like if I went down there tomorrow, and I found out that my mother's not dead—let's say on the off chance that she's not dead—and I could locate her in some way or another, I wouldn't be afraid to face it. Because . . .

*RILEY:* You wouldn't be afraid to face it?

*LINDA:* No. Because I have always felt . . .

*RILEY:* Suppose your mother is out there, and needs you?

*LINDA:* Listen . . .

*RILEY:* What would you do then?

*LINDA:* If I found out that my mother was alive today or tomorrow, and regardless of whether she needed me or not, I'd go to her.

*RILEY:* OK. Then why don't you find out whether or not she's dead or not, so you can get it all together?

*LINDA:* 'Cause I want to believe that she is.

*RILEY:* Why don't you find out for sure? What's your fear?

*LINDA:* I don't have a fear. I want to believe that she is because . . .

*RILEY:* Why don't you make sure? Because you've got a daughter now.

*LINDA:* Yeah, I have a son, too.

*Riley continued his efforts to motivate Linda to find out the truth about her mother and her past, meanwhile keeping Ed in a decentralized, neutral position where he simply had to observe. Riley pointed out the effects of this situation on their daughter and on her relationship with Ed:*

*RILEY:* What are you going to tell your daughter when she says, "Where's my other grandmother?"

*LINDA:* Tell her she doesn't have one anymore. She's dead.

*RILEY:* But you'd be lying to her.

*LINDA:* Why is that a lie? That's not a lie! I'm telling her what I was brought up to believe.

*RILEY:* Yes, but you still have doubts! You don't know whether she's dead or not! You don't know where she's at!

*LINDA:* I know, I don't.

*RILEY:* OK, so how are you gonna tell your daughter?

*LINDA:* I'm going to tell her like I . . .

*RILEY:* "Where's my other grandmother?"

*LINDA:* I'm going to tell her exactly what I was brought up to believe, that she's dead. Now if she wants to walk into my life when I hit thirty or forty years old, that's on her.

*RILEY:* That little girl of yours is going to start asking you a lot of questions. How are you gonna deal with that?

*LINDA:* Oh, I'll deal with them.

*RILEY:* You can't deal with your own.

*LINDA:* Yes, I can.

*RILEY:* You have to go to Ed to deal with them; you can't deal with your own.

*LINDA:* You ever start feeling—I don't know—you ever just feel kind of depressed sometimes?

*RILEY:* Yeah.

*LINDA:* And you have to have somebody to talk to?

*RILEY:* Well, there's a lot of things you could talk to him about. But you're talking about something you have no answer for.

*LINDA:* (*sighs*) Maybe I am, but like I said, I don't even want to be bothered. I don't want to find out.

*RILEY:* What are you going to tell your daughter?

*LINDA:* The same things that I've been told. That she's dead. Now if she waits till I'm forty years old, and my daughter is twenty-some years old and she walks into my life and says to me, "I'm your mother," I'm going to ask her, is she crazy! She's gonna have to show me valid proof that she's my mother! And that's it!

*RILEY:* What do little girls ask? . . . They ask quite a few questions, don't they?

*LINDA:* Oh, yes, they ask quite a few.

*RILEY:* And they want some answers.

*LINDA:* Right. And I'll try to answer my daughter, too.

*RILEY:* But just think, every time if she don't get the right answer she'll come back tomorrow, and that sends you into another depression, and you'll go running back to Ed or somebody, because you're going to have to start thinking about your mother, and death, and all like that. You just keep—it's gonna be adding and adding. So when you gonna stop it?

*LINDA:* I don't know. Maybe one day I will see if she's really dead. It's not really important.

*RILEY:* Have you talked to Ed about finding out for sure?
*LINDA:* I think one time I mentioned it, but I never did it.
*RILEY:* What did you tell him?
*LINDA:* I think I mentioned it to him, I don't know.
*ED:* I don't even remember.

(*later in the interview*)

*ED:* That means a mess of confusion for the mere fact that so many things were kept secret from her all her life, you know, and so, there must be some stones they must not want to overturn.
*RILEY:* They don't want to, they don't want to, but the part about it—she has to carry it.
*ED:* Right, but can she?
*RILEY:* I don't know if she can.
*ED:* See, because that might bring more harm than good.
*LINDA:* Yeah, right now I could feel like if I found out she was alive, I could deal with it. Just suppose I found out that she was alive. Right? Suppose I found out that there was nothing wrong with her— then see, I start feeling bitter toward her, whereas I don't want to feel this way toward her at all. You see, if I found out she's in good health and sane mind—say she's not insane, she's just as sane as we are, right? Then I'm going to start thinking, "Well, where were you when they were doing all this to me?"
*RILEY:* When you say sane mind . . .
*LINDA:* "What did they say to you that would make you desert your children—let them bring your children up to live a lie—not knowing if you're dead or alive?"
*RILEY:* Suppose she doesn't have a sane mind?
*LINDA:* Well, if she doesn't, I want to try to find out how long she hasn't been sane. You see, because if she's been sane long enough during the course of the time that all of this was going on—she was supposed to have been dead—I'm still going to feel bitter toward her, because if she was letting somebody tell her children that she's dead, what kind of mother is she? That's not my concept of a mother. I'm sorry.

(*later in the interview*)

*LINDA:* You see—you have to understand—I am tired.
*RILEY:* OK, you're tired.
*LINDA:* I'm very tired . . .

*RILEY:* You're tired!

*LINDA:* . . . of letting people get to me to the point where—
see, people try to do things to you because . . .

*RILEY:* You're not tired. You're not tired, 'cause you ain't closed
the door. You allow it open. Now, why don't you ask your husband to
say, "Hey, let's solve this thing."

*LINDA:* Because I think we've got situations that are more
important to both of us than that.

*At that point Riley shifted direction in order to bring Ed more
actively into the interaction. He wanted Ed to (1) support the idea
that Linda's unanswered question had effects beyond herself, (2) keep
the past from continuing to intrude on their relationship, and (3)
mobilize Ed to provide her with tangible support for getting her
question answered. Thus the couple could be rejoined at a different
level and with a different structure.*

*RILEY:* Umm, not if this is going to make you emotionally
upset! Why should he have to go through all of this? (*to Ed*) How do
you feel when she goes through this situation?

*ED:* Bad. 'Cause it does affect everybody around her that cares
about her. You know. In many ways. It might be hard for her to
understand how it really does affect, you know, people close to her.
It's like coming in here is a thing of protection: "I don't want to see
that, because you see, I know the good things," and that's what I want
for her. I don't want the bad things to be an influence on her, or our
relationship, and sometimes those problems tend to influence a
relationship a helluva lot.

*RILEY:* It's like you're fighting an invisible army.

*ED:* Right, you can't win. Regardless of what you put up to
defend yourself, it's not anything you can do. You just keep putting up
a fight, 'cause if you give up there's always that aspect that you don't
care.

*RILEY:* If you love your husband, how come you keep him in a
fight?

*LINDA:* I don't know.

*RILEY:* Do you love your husband?

*LINDA:* Yes, I do!

*RILEY:* Do you want to see a burden on him?

*LINDA:* No, I don't!

*RILEY:* OK, why don't you relieve the burden, because he's the one that you have to talk to, and he's the one who has to come up with some kind of a way of satisfying or easing the tension that you're going through.

*LINDA:* You know, when I go through tension about my mother, or stuff like that—suppose somebody throws it up in my face, 'cause ordinarily I don't really think about it.

*RILEY:* That could be thrown up anytime.

*LINDA:* Yeah, well . . .

*RILEY:* So, the door could be opened any time.

*LINDA:* A lot of times people will throw it up in my face and I won't even pay any attention.

*RILEY:* Yeah, but when you was here by yourself, here it comes.

*LINDA:* Not all the time. It's not all the time!

*ED:* It's like the situation we're at, that particular thing isn't outwardly done, but it's really what's cooking up the situation anyway. If that was out of the picture, those situations wouldn't come up, because you wouldn't have that inward feeling.

*LINDA:* I don't know . . .

*ED:* You knew with that down there constantly growing in the fire, you got that little spark; anything could ignite that spark, it doesn't have to be pertaining to it, but it just brings it on up because it's there.

*LINDA:* That might be right, I don't know.

*ED:* If it wasn't there, you know, you wouldn't have to deal with it.

*LINDA:* You know, I just can't see myself . . .

*ED:* Like with the thing of deceit. Not thinking in the prospect that people, you know, are honest for what they're doing. You'd be thinking, "Well, there's a catch to it"; there's a reason, you know, other than the reason that is sincere.

*LINDA:* Yep. I do that.

*ED:* Right.

*LINDA:* It's not funny, but I do. (*to Riley*) Now what he just told you is really the truth. You can sit up here and tell me something but I might look at you as if I believe it, but going through my mind is "Yeah, right." I believe you no further than I see you sitting there.

*RILEY:* No farther than that.

*LINDA:* That's it. You have to show me. You cannot just tell me something, and I'm gonna believe that it's true. You have to show me . . .

*RILEY:* Well, you tell me something.

*LINDA:* OK, what?

*RILEY:* If I have to show you, well, you show me something.

*LINDA:* As far as if it's true or not, yeah.

*RILEY:* OK. You said you love your husband.

*LINDA:* Right.

*RILEY:* OK. And you know that you bring him—sometimes you bring problems to him that he cannot solve, but he tries to pacify. So, in other words, you said you love him, and you are supposed to help him.

*LINDA:* Uh-huh. So what you want me to do?

*RILEY:* So, why don't you and him find out what took place, and end it? And then we could go on, to the future, and keep things in the past.

*LINDA:* (*to Ed*) You want me to do that?

*ED:* It would be a good idea.

*LINDA:* You want to do that? I mean, if you want to, I will do it. Because I didn't think it was a burden on you, but if that's what you want me to do, I'll do it.

*ED:* It would be good.

*LINDA:* All right. So, in other words, you just want to air the whole house, right? Open all the doors and windows and find out what's inside, right?

*RILEY:* No, you don't have to open all the doors and windows. There's just one thing, or two, that you need to know. That's is your mother alive or dead?

*LINDA:* But you see, if I find out if she's alive or dead, well—let's say I find out she's alive—that's not going to be enough for me. If I found out tomorrow that she was alive, you see, then that's gonna make me want to go to each and everybody and I'm gonna want some answers. See?

*RILEY:* If she's alive, and in good mind. OK. Suppose she's already deceased?

*LINDA:* Uh-huh.

*RILEY:* Now, them other people, they have their sickness; you don't need it! You follow me? You don't need that.

*LINDA:* Right.

*RILEY:* Now, if she's alive—hey—you try to find her.

*LINDA:* Well, see, that would be my next step, anyway.

*RILEY:* So, you don't need them other people. You need to get up and find out you don't need them.

*LINDA:* They wouldn't care if I was dead in the street.

*RILEY:* Right. So, all you want to do, you don't even need to touch base with them. And all you have to do is find out if she's alive or dead. Then you can go through other channels. 'Cause I want you to be able to give your daughter an honest and straight answer, which your mother wasn't around to give you yours, but you're around to give your daughter. And you said you want your children to have better than what you had, so I think it's time.

*LINDA:* Not only that, I don't want my daughter or my son to grow up and be that sheltered from anything.

*RILEY:* OK, so you've got to start working on it.

*LINDA:* All right. I'll do that.

*RILEY:* No. You both will do it.

*LINDA:* Well, we'll do it together. I guess my first step—I'll go down to City Hall.

*RILEY:* OK. I'll leave you until next week. Let me know how you made out. OK?

## ELEVENTH SESSION

During the following week Ed and Linda visited both the city morgue and City Hall to ascertain, through the two women's birth certificates, (1) whether her ostensible mother was her biological mother, and (2) whether and when Linda's mother had died. Riley met with them immediately following their second (posttreatment) Family Evaluation Session. They reported that they had confirmed that the woman in question was her real mother and that she had indeed passed away when Linda was 6 years old. A ghost had been exorcised.

## TERMINATION

In the 12th session, Riley saw Ed alone to terminate with him. Ed was doing well in staying off drugs and was also experiencing success in his college courses. Riley showed particular skill in acknowledging these positive changes and giving credit to the family, yet leaving the responsibility with Ed. He was also quick to counter Ed's assertion that he had wasted a lot of time, since that would minimize Ed's accomplishments. He relabeled Ed's past experiences as an asset, and implied that Ed could continue to make progress long after therapy was over.

> *RILEY:* You know, you're looking good.
> *ED:* I try to. The trouble is, now . . .
> *RILEY:* Like what?
> *ED:* Christmas is coming up, you know.
> *RILEY:* Oh, is that all. (*laughs*)
> *ED:* It bust a hole in my pocket today, man. I seen all of it go, ain't nothing coming my way—everything is going out.
> *RILEY:* I want to know how you feel about Christmas coming and. . . . About how much were you making a day when you were dealing?
> *ED:* It would range from seventy-five dollars, maybe, to one hundred fifty dollars.
> *RILEY:* About a bean and half a day? So it wasn't nothing for you to clean, in a good week, to clean about one thousand dollars?
> *ED:* No. I could do that in a couple of days, really, depending on how it was.
> *RILEY:* But on a normal week . . .
> *ED:* Right, you know, subtracting myself and little odds and ends—yeah, you know, in a week's time, I could clean a bean, it would be no problem.
> *RILEY:* That's the part that—how you say—that gets touchy.
> *ED:* Well, it had got touchy before, a little before I came to the program. You know, things started to fade out a little bit. I was getting bad packages and so forth, you know, little run-ins with people, you know; then things started to decline a little bit, which— that's in the business, but it just so happened, I stepped into the program at this time and I never tried to regroup and pull everything back up. 'Cause when I left, I left on a low level. I didn't leave on the high level I was on.
> *RILEY:* Well, maybe what I'm thinking about is what cash you had, you blew, and Christmas is like a wedding: you never really have enough. You understand? And knowing you were in a position to have more, before—now, does that have any thoughts with you?
> *ED:* I'd say in the last couple of weeks, right, I've been thinking about it more and more, you know, for the mere reason I've seen things that Linda wanted and I've seen things I want for myself,

right? You know, for the children, I've already put aside; I know what they need. That's a must. I know they're gonna get what they need. But say for us, you know, the things that I see that I might have to wait until afterward. Pick up a piece here and there. Other than that, there's no real problem. Say like today—I took my daughter downtown and picked up some shoes and boots for her and a few things for Christmas. I felt good about it, even though I didn't get myself anything. And today is my father's birthday and I picked him up something. It looked pretty good even though when I was finished I didn't have any finance for myself, so to speak, but it's just the idea that I seen something good getting into it.

*RILEY:* In other words, you spent this from the heart, not from the pocket.

*ED:* You know, this didn't really come out of the pocket 'cause I really didn't have to do it, you know. It's just the thing I felt—I want to get this, so I'm gonna go ahead and do it.

*RILEY:* That sounds good. The reason why I say this is that you suffered in a way. Suffering, how would you say, you've come from here to there as far as finance. You was able to get all the material things that you wanted. So you have to suffer a little and do without it.

*ED:* I'm not saying—as far as material things, I have a little reserve, so to speak. If I had to, I could hold out the rest of this year and on to next year and still be in good shape. You know, that's material as far as what I need—you know, shirt on my back and so forth and so on. You know, I wouldn't have to deal with anything [drugs]. It's just like, well, I can pick up a piece here and there, when I see something, you know. But just to have—I'm not in the position now where I really need, so anything that comes my way I could scatter to the family more so than to myself.

*RILEY:* You're doing well. As a matter of fact, it seems like you were prepared for this.

*ED:* Not really, it's just the way my mother brought me up. You know, as far as having things. The value of one thing is just the same as the other to me. I don't have anything that's a favorite, do you know what I mean? Everything is as good as the other. So, I take care of my stuff, you know. So, it's not an issue whether or not that I have to have it, 'cause I didn't abuse what I got because I have so much, you know. I just take it all as one thing and use it that way. So, it will last me longer.

*RILEY:* How's school going?

*ED:* Pretty good, now. Mainly, I got what I wanted for next semester.

*RILEY:* Oh, you did?

*ED:* I preregistered; my bill is paid. I'm just biding my time now. I just about know my grades.

*RILEY:* So when you did see that counselor, you came out OK?

*ED:* Yeah, we had a good time. We talked for a couple of days as a matter of fact. I kept going back to see him, plus I took this evaluation test. It wasn't like an aptitude, it was just what my main interests are, you know. Everything fell into place as to what I wanted, you know. We worked out a system for me that seems to be pretty fair as far as I can see. Something to give me a chance to get into school. Since that period of time I've been out, you know, it will give me something to work with as far as studying, 'cause that was my main problem. I don't have any study habits. I don't know how to study. It was doing something to me 'cause, like, I would put out so much trying to learn and when it comes time to execute, all of it was locked upstairs. You know, and then when I don't need it, it comes out. It's like the night before a test, I crammed the book and I shouldn't. I get in front of a test paper and it's like I don't know nothing. Class is almost over, the test period is almost over, and then everything starts to come out. I had to rush to finish up. It leaves me incomplete sometimes. I see it's just to take it every day, with the class, you know. What I pick up today in notes—to go over that. What I pick up tomorrow, I'll go over that. With cramming, you don't know nothing. I should have judged that from my first test, but with the first test, I really tried to study; I got a "C" but I felt I could have got a "B" or an "A" out of that.

*RILEY:* You did a lot of mastering.

*ED:* I'm so far behind that all I can see is catching up.

*RILEY:* No, you're not behind. You got to stop thinking that you're behind; you're looking at age and you're looking at time. Now, let's face it; you're not behind because there's certain times in a person's life when they want to do something, certain times they don't want to do something, certain times people want to make something of themselves. There's people who get to be thirty-five and are in the same spot hanging on the corner. Something turns them—something turns them around; you understand. There's certain times people have to leave home, or don't leave home. So, this is just your time. Some people's time comes sooner, some people's time period comes later. So, you're not behind.

*ED:* You know, I can understand that while you're talking to me, but it's just the idea, Paul, you know, like in the period of a day, since I don't stay in the neighborhood as I used to, I spend a lot of time, back and forth, coming out here, you know. I might stop in town, first I go to school. I travel around; like I go down to Lombard Street, around all the condominiums. And I see that those are the type of things I feel as though I could have had that, you know, and I didn't. It's the kind of things I be striving for.

*RILEY:* Maybe I can speak to you a little better. I'll use me. It took a time for me to really know what I really wanted to be. I am many things. I'm a licensed hairdresser; I'm a pool shark; I'm an artist. Follow me? But all of these things was part of a life that I came in touch with, right? Now, what happened fifteen years ago was that just out of a clear blue sky, out of the clear blue sky, it wasn't planned or nothing, there was an opening at the Rebound Health Center, and they needed another man. I belonged to a surveying team. I went to the top of the class there. Then after that, it was Neighborhood Aide. I went to the top there. Then I turned to being a community organizer. Now I was in the position of helping people. And, I liked it one minute and one minute I didn't. Then I come to Child Guidance and took up the training of counseling. And I felt this was the same connection as the community thing because this way, in the community thing, I was giving; now at Child Guidance, they give, I refine it and give it back. Now here I am late in life, where way long ago it wasn't there and wasn't even in my mind. So, it took a time and then the opportunity is there. So, you can't look and say, "Hey, I'm starting now, I should have been." There ain't no "should have been." You had your head in something else. You can't wipe that out, 'cause nobody could have told you five or six years ago you would get into this. It wasn't your time. Sometimes it's a crisis, sometimes it's just boring. And then you say, "Hey I'm going this way." You have to choose your own destiny. Now what time you take to choose it, it isn't set. Now you may be set right here now into something you like. Who knows, two or five years later, you may see something better. It may be an extension from what you're in. Who knows, you may want to be a lawyer.

*ED:* Very true.

*RILEY:* So don't feel that you've lost anything; you haven't lost anything. Because all that was the training; you had to learn to deal with lower, middle, upper, business—all types of people. Now that is an asset.

*ED:* Yeah, that is experience.

*RILEY:* That was training. So, you are right on time. Right on time. Since everything is going OK, you got your thing together, I guess you and I be parting company.

*ED:* Who do I have to, you know, deal with then?

*RILEY:* Well, you'll be with Elton.

*ED:* Elton?

*RILEY:* Right.

*ED:* OK.

*RILEY:* I'll still be here if you feel you need to get in touch with me. Feel free.

*ED:* OK. Because a few things might be coming up and I might need some advice on. I don't know as of yet; I'm trying to find out everything I can about it and see exactly what I can do and what I can't do.

*RILEY:* Pertaining to what?

*ED:* Employment, more or less. You know, certain situations you might be able to help me more than anybody else. 'Cause you know my situation better than anyone else right now.

(*later in the interview*)

*RILEY:* We'll see how things make out and I'll give you a call in a couple months or so. It's like we tightened up; now we're going to get loose. Because you know how to handle the drug situation.

*ED:* I feel as though I can.

*RILEY:* You know how; you all got together on how each person can be involved. So, you know the system of handling that. So, I don't need to help you on that, right? And right now you even got into school, and you're doing good with that. But the part about it—I don't like to praise a person unless I explain the praise. If I praise you, that makes you way up there and it doesn't give you room to fail, like you would let me down. You follow me?

*ED:* Yeah, but then I look at it as if I am also letting myself down.

*RILEY:* That's it—I want you to praise yourself. I don't need to praise you. You praise yourself, because you did it.

*ED:* You're my counselor, right. I have gained a certain respect for you as my counselor and as a man in general. But I can't base what I'm doing simply on the fact of how I feel about you. You know, it's got to be me—what I want out of it. If I'm dirty, I got to suffer. You're not going to suffer for me being dirty in the sense that I am; you might be let down . . .

*RILEY:* Right.

*ED:* But you're still not going to feel the same as I because you're not going to be subjected to that. So, I always feel that I have more to do than anybody else that I'm dealing with, you know, and I do try to keep the faith, so to speak, somebody has a certain trust in me; I try to keep that, 'cause I feel like you got to have somebody on your side, you know; you can't fight any battle alone.

*RILEY:* You have people on your side. You found out how close they are.

*ED:* True.

*RILEY:* Since we've been coming here, how close they are. They're right on your side.

*ED:* In a sense we became closer, the whole family, you know; I've noticed the change. Especially with me and my father, because we were distant.

*RILEY:* Here you're buying him a present already.

*ED:* It wasn't a thing that I didn't respect him or love him, because he was my father; it was just that we never had any binding relationship. He was always working, so to speak. So, it was never a thing where you can take your son to the game. My father didn't take me to the game; if I went it was by myself. He didn't have time. I don't think it was because he didn't want to. It was just what he was doing and how he had to do it, the schedule wouldn't fit in.

*RILEY:* I think it's a two-way street. You have to be part of the joining also.

*ED:* Right.

*RILEY:* Since you and your father have been coming here, you and he have got more close, because he was involved with what's happening.

*ED:* Yeah, he knew exactly what was going on, whereas before he didn't.

*RILEY:* Now, this way can continue; it doesn't have to be on that, it can be on any other thing, you see. And, just like you say, the relationship has gotten more close and I know you learned something from him as well as him learning something from you. So that's a whole structure that you can use in other things, the same way like you feeling good. I want you to be feeling good like you're feeling good right now. You could feel good better than me. 'Cause you're the one that's in it. So you look to yourself for the praise. Praise yourself, not me praise you.


## EPILOGUE

By the conclusion of therapy Ed had been free of illegal drugs for 9 weeks and was continuing his studies—the two primary goals of treatment. After a lapse of two or three sessions, the father had returned to therapy and had been attending regularly ever since; he and Mrs. E were spending more time together and their relationship was less stressful.

If the treatment paradigm had allowed Riley to continue a bit longer, there were three issues that he would have liked to have worked out more definitively. First, he would have implemented a procedure for Ed to detoxify from methadone.* Second, he would have clarified and set in motion a specific plan with the family as to when Ed and Linda would move out of the parents' home, as well as the issue of which couple Tina would continue to live with. Third, Riley would have spent more time on the relationship between Ed's parents, in an effort to bring it to a more functional level—to help them through the transition from being parents to grandparents and to bring more rewards to their marital union.


### FOLLOW-UP

Posttreatment follow-up information has been gathered on this family over the 3 years since the end of therapy. Ed continued to be enrolled at the DDTC for 8 more months and was on methadone for most of the time. In the eighth month he initiated and completed outpatient detoxification from methadone. He used marijuana regularly off and on during this period and also supplemented his methadone with illegal opiates at various points during the first year. During the second and third years he did not use illegal drugs except for recrea-

---

*This was a fairly early case, and at that time methadone detoxification was not approached as boldly as it was in subsequent cases. Instead, the tendency was to focus on getting the index patient (IP) to refrain from taking illegal drugs, and to deal with methadone detoxification primarily if the IP and parents were strongly inclined toward it (see Chapters 2 and 6).

tional smoking of marijuana (once or twice a week), was not on methadone, and had not returned to pushing.

Mr. and Mrs. E continued to engage in outside activities together, although during the first year these frequently included their granddaughter, Tina. At some point during the first year Linda and the children moved out of the home. Ed continued to live in his parents' home during the 3 years.

Upon completion of his academic year at the community college —which ended 7 months after termination of family therapy—Ed obtained a full-time maintenance job with the city. He continued to hold this job throughout the 3 years.

# 11

# FACING RETIREMENT: *WORKING WITH ELDERLY PARENTS*

JOHN M. VAN DEUSEN
PETER URQUHART

IN PREVIOUS CHAPTERS it has been made clear that the course of drug addiction is strongly linked to certain characteristics of family life experience. Age is one such factor. A drug problem frequently emerges at the time in life when a passsage is anticipated from the dependency of youth into the self-reliance of adulthood. The integrity of the family of origin may be threatened by a member's shift toward autonomy. In such families, the onset of a symptom that postpones this passage may constitute a "solution," postponing or avoiding the greater family crisis (see Chapters 1 and 4).

An addicted eldest child presents a powerful example to his younger siblings of the "dangers" that lie beyond the family circle. On the other hand, should the first child manage the transition to adulthood responsibly, increased pressure might come to bear on the second and later children. The youngest child may be forced to travel the hardest route of all, becoming the final link in making or breaking the future viability of the family—now reduced to the husband–wife dyad.

While the age configuration among siblings is an important factor in determining which child becomes addicted, the effect is mediated by the *age of the parents*. Parental age warrants deeper consideration in clinical diagnosis and treatment than it has received from many family therapists. Any strategy adopted by the therapist will either support or undermine the plans and ambitions of the parents for their children, the children for their parents, the parents for themselves, and the children for themselves. If the therapist is insensitive to the fact that not only the addict but the entire family experiences critical life cycle transitions, his approach may blindly ignore the relative needs of some family members, or set off their needs against those of others (see Chapter 4).

In contrast to the extensive clinical material of the other cases in this book, the present chapter is more narrowly focused. Emphasis is predominently on issues pertaining to parents who are elderly and the difficulties involved with the addict's leaving home under such conditions.

Implicitly or explicitly, parents who are left with an addicted adult child at home usually indicate discomfort at the prospect of that child's departure, despite his age. The operations of the therapist must give credence to the parents' hesitancy, without giving them the impression that their reluctance is right or wrong. While their expressed concern is for their offspring, the underlying issue is commonly protection of their own interests. However, this is usually outside of their awareness and they focus instead upon the addiction. The parents' point of view is that it would be irresponsible for the child to leave home before he is fully "responsible" for his behavior.

The parents' position constitutes a contradiction, or paradox, that severely limits the child's chances of attaining independence, though it is rarely recognized as such by any member of the family. In effect, the admonition keeps the child from acquiring the conditions or status needed to exhibit responsible behavior, or to have the parents perceive it as such. The addict is in a bind in which it is impossible to leave home responsibly or to demonstrate responsibility at home (see Chapter 1). Therapy with families of this sort must seek to change the conditions that keep the child and parent bound in interdependent positions. The paradox must be broken before a new manner of relating can be established between family members. Following one case through the course of therapy, we can see how the therapist moved toward this objective of breaking the paradox, and how the factor of the parents' advanced age was handled in relation to this task.

## CASE EXAMPLE

### INDUCTION

The addict, Paul, was the only son in this Black, middle-class family. He was age 25, had served in Vietnam, and lived at home with his mother and father. An older sister was not living at home, but had regular contact with her brother and parents. The addict had begun drug use as a business venture (i.e., dealing) after leaving the service. He was successful, and increased his personal use of heroin. After several years, he began to see the habit as harmful and tried twice to detoxify, unsuccessfully. He had had several arrests, one of which was pending trial at the time that therapy began. He said that he was now motivated to detoxify and intended to enter school and find a job as soon as he finished.

In the first interview between the client and therapist (Peter Urquhart) the client indicated that his home life was good. He felt his parents were a strong, positive influence on him, and saw no problem in having them enter therapy. Throughout this interview the client presented a tone of cooperation. Urquhart did not attempt to persuade; rather, he conveyed the idea that the requirements of therapy were few and obvious to both him and the client. These were: the management of medication, gradual detoxification, and active involvement of the family. The therapist's manner dovetailed with the client's stance of cooperative, responsible participation: there was no confrontation, no question that the therapy should proceed any differently than the therapist had described it. Following through on this continuity, the therapist obtained the client's assurance that he would be responsible for bringing his parents in for the first family session—which he did within the week.*

### FIRST FAMILY SESSION

The therapist began therapy with the family by asking the client to discuss his personal goals (described to the therapist the previous week). The client specified two goals: (1) detoxification, and (2) completion of a correspondence course, to obtain a decent job. In keeping with the earlier spirit of cooperation and responsibility, the client said that he believed he could finish the course ahead of schedule and be employed within several months. At the outset of therapy, then, he was already presenting a fairly specific set of goals. However, means for accomplishing these goals remained undeveloped at that point. (Getting the client to articulate such goals will take

*Editors' note. This was one of a very few cases in which the therapist did not have to contact other family members directly in order to get them to come in (see Chapter 5).

more work in many families, but needs to be accomplished as early as possible in the therapy.)

When the therapist asked the client's father and mother, respectively, what their goals were for the family, neither could respond other than to say that they wanted to see their son "straighten up" and stop "sliding back." They clearly had not thought or talked about what life on their own would be like after their son left home. Their attention had become fixed upon the son and his drug problem. Yet, they had difficulty defining this problem in terms that could be adapted by the therapist into goals supportive of the client's own plans.

Two key transactional problems were manifested during the parents' discussion of goals. First, it was learned that the father had recently retired. He was presently spending 4 to 6 hours a day in the company of his son, even driving him to the drug-treatment program to pick up medications.* Second, the therapist observed that the mother cut in on the father's communications with the son (in the session and at home), redirecting it toward the drug problem. The therapist asked the client how he felt about these tendencies of his parents. The client responded that he saw them as positive—as signs of concern and caring in a close-knit family. This clarified that, at least on the surface of their relationship, the mother, father, and son had evolved a durable status quo with one another since the onset of the son's drug problem. The son recalled that his parents had been steady and helpful all through his life.

Further inquiry by the therapist brought out that the household rules were set by the mother: both the father and son stated that she permitted no fighting or other bad habits in the house. The mother confirmed this, and indicated pride in having maintained *order* at home. There is an irony implicit in this statement, given the nature of the client's drug problem, that became explicit slightly later in the session, when the therapist asked the parents how they adjusted to life without children when the son was in the service. It seems that the father at that time worked two shifts daily. He was almost never at home during the day, and the mother was quite lonesome. She indicated that the experience was not at all pleasant. To establish a base for the client on the issue of leaving home in the future, the

---

*Editors' note.* This was father's new "job," replacing the one from which he had retired.

therapist stated that he assumed this would be a goal after the detoxification was completed, something the parents would have to consider more carefully. The client agreed, adding that he wanted to get married, too. The father's response was critical; he indicated that the son needed to be able to take care of himself before he could even think about leaving. The father recalled that in his own life he had carried this kind of responsibility for 35 years.

The paradoxical nature of this criticism is apparent: the son should not be permitted to take care of himself, says the father, until he is able to take care of himself. Yet, the father gives no indication of how the son could demonstrate this competency. Nor does the father indicate that he should offer guidance to the son in this matter, despite his own wealth of experience.

Mother's statements in this same discussion revealed further aspects of the paradox and its function in family relations. When the therapist asked if the closeness among family members would present a problem in the client's leaving, she stated that she saw her son's goal as fine, that she would do everything she could to help him leave: give him money, food, clothing, and so forth. The strings implicit in her "good will" were not apparent to the mother or the father. The parents revealed that the client did not presently have to pay them room or board, just "take care of himself" (another facet of the paradox). This arrangement effectively deprived the client of any opportunity to demonstrate responsibility: the parents' accommodation of their son was warm and loving, yet it provided no area where independence or personal success was sanctioned, and placed no obvious values on autonomy. So long as the son cooperated with this complacent ethos of the parents, the status quo would remain. Neither he nor they would grow, and the family system would remain at its present life cycle stage.

The atmosphere of the discussion changed sharply when the therapist informed the client that his urinalysis for the past week had come up dirty (indicating illicit drug use). The parents did not understand what this meant and the therapist asked the son to explain it to them. The client equivocated—blaming it on the treatment system. Since his own urines were surely clean (he asserted in a "cooperative" tone), another patient's urine specimen must have been confused with his. Here, the theme of goodness and cooperation, so carefully nurtured elsewhere in the client's relationship with his parents and the therapist, was breached. If appropriately followed through, this topic area could be used by the therapist to demonstrate to the parents that the son's expression of good intentions is not always to be believed, leading them toward a better grasp of how to evaluate his problems and how to respond to them. The therapist, working from the strength of the cooperative spirit developed up to this point in the therapy, could now be explicit without being confrontative. In this first session, however, he merely indicated the discrepancy between the urine report and the client's story, and let the client's explanation stand. In later sessions, should the urines remain dirty, he would still be able to come back to this discrepancy and use it further.

## PROGRESS OF THE THERAPY

The therapy proceeded regularly for 10 sessions, the parents and son attending faithfully each week. In these sessions, the therapist's strategy became one of gradually and quietly setting the conditions needed to disentangle the client from the confines of the paradox demonstrated in the first session. This required getting the parents to do two things: first, to agree with their son that detoxification and leaving home were reasonable goals; second, to support these goals, at least in principle. The paradox had until now prevented the parents from agreeing with each other that something could and should be done by them. To change this situation, the therapist obtained an explicit statement of support-in-principle from each parent, leaving aside all issues of how the principles could be translated into practice.

Once the support had been expressed by each parent, the therapist carried it a step further by getting each parent to agree that a real expression of support for their son's goals required that they take a *stand* with him, drawing the line on certain matters of consequence to them (and thereby drawing explicit boundaries in their relationship with him). In this particular family, the therapist was at a definite advantage, since there was already expression of concern from all three members around the single issue of drug use. The lines could thus be drawn around this issue, starting from the addict's own commitment (stated in the first session) to completion of detoxification within a specific interval of time. In other families, where members are not in consensus about the immediate importance of the drug problem, the therapist may have to lead the therapy *gradually* toward work on that area, focusing first on other, smaller issues as a way of guiding the family into the desired kind of interaction.

In this family there was little evident change, week after week, despite the early success in getting the father and mother to agree to a common stand against indefinite acceptance of the drug problem in the future. In a more acute inquiry into the parents' own expectations for themselves, the therapist found no evidence that husband and wife had any sense of a life of their own, apart from the son. Their commitment to a stand against the problem was thus an empty one; it could not be enforced by the parents until they had developed some image of a future worth looking forward to.

The empty quality of the parents' commitment was most obvious in their complete disorganization and confusion on how to deal with the drug issues if confronted with a crisis. The therapist asked about various crises in a hypothetical manner, with several examples that the parents had not been exposed to previously. He added realism, however, by discussing in the same sessions the continuing actual problem of dirty urines from the client. From week to week, the addict repeated his explanation of a mix-up somewhere in the treatment system. Over time, this story lost its credibility with the parents, and as it did so they became less helpless in relation to the drug problem.* Their increasing doubts were shaped by the therapist into a more productive form: taking a stand and staying firmly with it.

> URQUHART: What if your son were to continue using drugs in the future?
> FATHER: Well, I couldn't just cut him loose.
> URQUHART: I agree, but how far would you carry him? A year? . . .

In the middle sessions, the therapist alternated this redirection of the parents' understanding of and response to the issues of drug use with discussions focused on the issues of how they were going to live, day to day, once the son was gone. He helped them plan for the future.

*Editors' note. One might say that their increasing anger at being "conned" helped them to distance themselves from their son, thus fortifying the generational boundary.

## TERMINATION

By the time of the last family session (about 3 months after the first), the client still had not completed detoxification, but had reduced his medication to a low dosage. He had also completed most of the correspondence course, and the therapist made sure the parents recalled the son's early prediction that he would make rapid progress with this training program. He encouraged the parents to congratulate their son on this demonstration of success. Earlier, when the son had described his financial skills in drug dealing, this was also pointed to as an area of success, but the parents accepted it only half-heartedly.

The son expressed an intention to finish the detoxification in the next several weeks, and the therapist asked the parents if they were set in their expectations for the son in this regard. He asked what action they would take if the son did not follow through. As in earlier discussions of this issue, the father was hesitant. He said that it was hard to define things sharply, that so much depended on the circumstances. The father hoped it would work, though, because he was "fed up" with the problem. To strengthen this commitment, the therapist asked the father if he were definite about that (i.e., about being fed up). The father replied that he was, and the therapist asked him why, then, it was so hard for him to take a stand.

The father disagreed vehemently.

FATHER: It's *not* hard to put my fist down!
URQUHART: But you haven't smacked it all at once.
FATHER: I feel, give a person a chance.
URQUHART: You know, when my father put his fist down I remember him saying, "This is for your own good."

*At this point, with the father nearly fixed in his commitment, the mother introduced qualifiers ("circumstances") that muddled the issue once more. This repeated the pattern she had taken earlier in therapy, whenever father, son, or therapist were on the verge of commitment. Mother's rationalization in the present discussion was an assertion that the son must have a job before he could have money to be on his own. She added that all the good jobs were taken, however, and that it would be pretty rough to put the son out on the street without a job. The therapist knew that the parents' commitment would remain empty until this pattern of interference, which amplified confusion and maintained the status quo, was eliminated from these interactions. He returned to the issue at hand: the son needed to know the consequences that would follow if he kept using drugs. The father hesitated one last time, but the mother then urged him to be firm.*

*MOTHER:* Sticking with Paul won't make any difference; we need to set a limit.

*FATHER:* True, but sometimes there's no limit to life.

*URQUHART:* We're not saying there's a limit to life.

*MOTHER:* I can't go through it again! I stay with Paul at home all day. My nerves are on edge!

*The therapist at this point urged the mother to tell her husband how she felt when her nerves were on edge. After the mother expressed to her husband how much worry and difficulty the son caused her—the first time in the therapy that she had openly stated how she felt—the therapist turned to the son and asked him if he was ready to lick the problem now. The son said he was, and the discussion ended with the therapist, parents, and son laying out details for finishing up the detoxification.*

The parents were not seen again after this session. The son was seen three more times, alone. There was no formal end to the detoxification, but the son did stop going to the treatment center for medication, and shortly thereafter moved out of state. He completed the correspondence course as planned, and found the job he wanted. A number of follow-up contacts with the family and client over the next 4 years revealed that the son had kept a steady job, gotten married, become a father, and not returned to drug abuse.

## SOME GENERAL POINTS

Experience with several other families having this same general constellation—youngest or only son still residing with his parents—shows a remarkable consistency of qualities, illustrating variations on common themes. The status quo, or "stuckness," induced by paradoxical entanglement of parents and son in the drug problem is recurrent. In some families it is expressed less directly, often in the form of proverbs that rationalize failure and keep the conflict at an impersonal plane, free of affect. In line with these aphorisms, the family's sense of time is indefinite, making "future" and "progress" vague concepts. The therapist's best means of devaluing the aphorisms of the parents is to have at hand a stock of counterepithets.

In contrast to the looseness and vagueness of goals in these families, there is a consistent expression of closeness, with reciprocal concern and "care" between parents and son. Sometimes this is literally symmetrical: the parents care about the son because he is sick; the son cares about them because they could become sick (alluding to such physical symptoms as hypertension and heart disorders). Sons do not confront their fathers and mothers, but describe home and family as solid, positive forces in their lives. Parents describe their sons as "good boys."

The issue of impending or current retirement is usually hidden beneath the family's veneer of closeness and concern. Where a working parent is about to retire, the shift that this will create for the other members' daily living patterns may induce a crisis in the marriage or the drug problem. Long-established roles are called into question; the matter of replacing the breadwinner function can be especially problematic. Where the working parent has retired and begun adjusting to life at home, his presence may already have induced the crisis, as in the example given here of a father trailing his son all day long in search of companionship. The most prevalent times and places of stress are likely to occur at meals—when the whole family is together—or on occasions when the son actually desires privacy. Even at these times, the family's style is apt to be quiet and careful, without outbursts of anger or other emotional peaks.

A final consideration of importance in working with elderly parents is the influence the therapist's *own age* has on the way he is perceived by the family. The therapist cannot effectively commence work on the main objectives of therapy until he is recognized as someone who is appreciative of their views. A younger therapist's credibility may be immediately discounted by elderly parents. When this occurs, it can best be countered through establishing the therapist's specific competence concerning problems of addiction, accompanied by patent "common sense." Explicit agreement with the parents is not always necessary (or wise). A sense of appreciation can be conveyed by the therapist simply by listening, without an outright commitment to anyone's views.

# 12

## DETOXIFICATION AT HOME:
## *A FAMILY APPROACH*

SAMUEL M. SCOTT
JOHN M. VAN DEUSEN

A CRUCIAL MATTER in conducting therapy with families of opioid addicts is the plan for withdrawal from dependency on heroin or methadone. One approach to this is to enlist the cooperation of the family in creating an atmosphere for the addict to detoxify in his own home. In the therapy model presented in Chapter 6, a rationale for home detoxification is given, along with a number of applicable guidelines and techniques. It is the purpose of the present chapter to expand on several aspects of these guidelines, presenting more detailed information on the therapeutic process and many of the "micromoves" involved. Emphasis is on the use of family members' competencies toward the accomplishment of certain therapeutic tasks. The tasks are designed to alter family system functioning and to develop or shape new competencies en route to the ultimate task of detoxification.

It should be understood that home detoxification is an experimental paradigm. As noted in Chapters 6 and 18, the methods are still undergoing expansion and refinement. However, many of the principles and procedures discussed below have more general application than just home detoxification. They are applicable in almost any detoxification schema that involves the family of an addict, as well as many other situations that occur in family therapy.

The chapter first describes a number of principles of treatment strategy pertaining to family involvement in the detoxification of an addicted member. It then presents material from a clinical case that both demonstrates some of the techniques emanating from the principles and provides pointers on undertaking a home detoxification. The text concludes with a summary of the major components of the therapeutic process.

## PRINCIPLES

Family therapy is a mode of treatment in which family members directly concerned with a problem work collectively to resolve it. Whatever the symptom and goal, certain themes must be activated from the outset of therapy if it is to proceed smoothly and steadily toward desired change. Each family has its own intrinsic patterns of thinking, speaking, and acting that it brings to therapy and that affect what can be usefully accomplished in treatment. The therapist must find a way to achieve therapeutic goals within the unique situation and value structure of the particular family. He takes these as given and then designs his interventions within the constraints delineated by them. (For example, a therapist would never ask a family to eat meat on Friday if the family would not, for religious reasons, eat meat on Friday. But he could ask the family to change the type of nonmeat food for a Friday.)

The therapist's relationship with the family is always a major concern. To be effective, he must win the trust of the addict and the family. As noted below, selling the idea of detoxification at home is difficult at best; without trust it would be impossible. With trust, it can be made to sound like a reasonable and realistic alternative.

### ACKNOWLEDGING THE PROBLEM

A common pattern in families containing an addicted member is the extremely superficial way in which family members acknowledge that drug abuse is problematic or debilitating. Members may voice strong concerns over the problem, but when their statements are added together, they give no sense of a crisis at hand and they do not show any active movement toward change. The family has become "addicted" to the addiction—they may despise it, yet they tolerate it. Few methods of treatment acknowledge that the family has become accustomed to addiction. One typical modality involves the physical isolation of the addict. He may leave home for several weeks to enter an inpatient program to withdraw from drug dependence. On his return home, he may not be "dirty," but the forces in the family that maintain the addiction (which have not been affected by his treatment) tend to set him up for a return to his former habits (see Chapters 1, 7, and 9).

The idea of detoxifying at home brings the treatment plan into direct confrontation with the family's idea of what should be done about addiction. Family members no longer can sit on the sidelines saying, "We've done all we can." They are called on for active participation. In fact, the very mention of this idea is sometimes enough to induce a crisis, thus disturbing the stability of the addiction within the family system. Consequently, the attention of the addict and other members is diverted away from the standard, expected features of medical treatment. The usual counters and avoidances to treatment, such as noninvolvement and relying on professionals, are thus unseated. The matter of who is treating whom becomes purposefully obscured. This places a demand on the family members to organize. They must decide what their responsibilities are and how to mobilize to carry out these responsibilities with regard to treatment. Implicit in the theme of detoxifying at home is the message that responsibility for the problem and its resolution remains with the family and not the therapist (see Chapter 6). Once the family begins to accept responsibility for the problem, the goals and tasks of therapy are immensely simplified.

## ESTABLISHING TRUST

The first requirement in working toward detoxification is trust. This must be initiated early and continually expanded. To engage the family's trust, the treatment plan and therapeutic strategy must be built on the strengths and limitations of the family. These qualities are revealed in the family's responses. From the beginning, the family should be given alternatives and the right to make decisions from those alternatives: "How do you feel about him [the addict] detoxifying immediately, as opposed to two weeks from now?" This kind of a question focuses on procedural issues. The more basic issues, such as whether detoxification is to occur at all, are put to rest by implication, as the tactical needs are discussed. A lack of consensus by family members should signal the therapist that the discussion is still too intense; he needs to move more slowly, shifting to more superficial issues. Intense confrontation at such an early stage would create a negative attitude that would be difficult to change. Questions such as whether the addict's medication dosage should be increased, reduced, or kept stable permit the family to voice their general feelings, revealing to the therapist what level they find most comfortable in discussing these issues.* By channeling discussions to this preferred level, the therapist accedes a certain degree of authority to the family, without having to lose his hold over the content or progression of therapy. By adopting a manner of acceptance, he expresses respect and support for the family's own qualities and capabilities. Once a basic mode of working with the family has been established, repetition of this pattern in various forms creates a ritual wherein the family follows the therapist's lead almost automatically.

## ASSESSING COMPETENCIES

The personal experiences, competencies, and ambitions of family members are important both for building trust in therapy and for giving the therapist clues as to the most appropriate direction to proceed. The therapist can use his knowledge in these areas to create arguments in favor of home detoxification and to develop goals of treatment that are tailored to the family. The basic idea is to make use of what the family members know already, whatever skills they already have. This allows therapy to be based on success and strengths.

Strategy evolves by observing the family's reaction to new information. Such new information might be drawn from the addict's knowledge of drug pharmacology and drug use (such as with the cases in Chapters 7 and 10). He is asked to share his expertise with the family. This could show the addict in a competent light, which can create trust between the family, the addict, and the therapist. The therapist's view that the addict is competent reflects favorably on the family's competence. The therapist can point out that in order to obtain street drugs consistently and successfully, the addict must be competent in acquiring and handling money. Discussions exploring this topic can make the addict more competent in his parents' eyes, and this competency reflects back on their skills as parents. Meanwhile, the addict's competence on these topics is also being transmitted to the family as they become acquainted with the variety of alternatives the addict has at hand to obtain and use drugs. This knowledge places the family in a better position to understand the addiction and consequently help the addict to detoxify at home. It also

*Editors' note.* However, in Chapter 6 it is cautioned that the therapist must remain aware that by discussing methadone dosages and so forth he is implicitly reinforcing the family's perception that the addict is a handicapped person.

shifts the structure and power balance from addict to parents; his authority is decreased as they become more knowledgeable. The confidence and expertise elicited through such discussions should be continually acknowledged, labeled, and reinforced by the therapist.

## CHALLENGING THE FAMILY TO ACT AND ORGANIZE ITSELF

Challenge can take place once trust has been established. The process of challenging should take place in small steps. The therapist's suggestions may come in small doses, usually framed in terms of the competencies that family members have already shown. By first noting that they are competent, he can more easily move toward testing their responses to his suggestions. The notion of home detoxification should not be addressed in an explicit, direct manner until the family members are able and willing to discuss the implications of the challenge. Again, this requires a cultivation of confidence between family and therapist. In some families, this kind of affinity will come early in the course of therapy, almost without effort or awareness. In most cases, however, establishing such a rapport will entail a combination of patience, persistence, and modeling by the therapist, so that the tasks he eventually presents can be viewed as feasible by family members.

The process of challenge is started by getting the addict and other family members to commit themselves to performing, on a "practice" basis, a small task or project. The task should address some problem that they are not only capable of working on but, more important, one that they are willing to do. The tasks may be performed either within the session or at home. A task in the session should be a representation of what is to take place at home. For example, if one member of the family is to be an observer at home, that person should also observe in the session (i.e., "enactment" of the task).[100] Instructions should be concrete, clearly focused, and *absolutely understood by the entire family*. The therapist should confirm that all members accept their part of the task as reasonable, even if they do not entirely accept the overall plan. A commitment by each person only to his part is quite acceptable. Each item must be negotiated, so that all members are aware of their own and others' parts.

By focusing, at least initially, on a minor rather than a large-scale task, the therapist increases chances of success later on. A small task is more likely to be handled competently by the family. This facilitates further success in subsequent tasks and increases the family members' trust. A narrow focus also steers the family's expectations away from misinterpreting the single task as a panacea or cure-all. At this early stage in therapy, the therapist should not allow the family to expect that detoxification will come quickly or easily.

When the therapist sets up an initial task, it is not overly cautious for him to predict failure. Doing so ensures that the outcome, whether success or failure, has further use in the therapy. If there is failure in performing any aspect of the task, the therapist focuses on this in reviewing it—exploring with the family how this may resemble other ways in which they have been unsuccessful. The discussion should then proceed from such "weaknesses" into areas where more positive approaches and solutions can be developed. Successes and recoveries have taken place somewhere in the family's experience; these must be elicited, cultivated, and brought into the service of therapy. This exercise of analyzing an initial failure can produce a considerable saving of time and effort in implementing the actual detoxification plan.

## EXPANDING CONFIDENCE AND COMPETENCY

As predicted, a family will typically fail to do all that is required in an initial task. A partial success can still be built upon by the therapist in a variety of ways. The family's admission of failure gives the therapist tactical leverage: he can use it as a contrast to their successes in other areas, thus magnifying these successes. It may also be treated as competency of a different order—the therapist relabels the family's "failure" as a skillful monitoring and self-evaluation of their task performance. Defining their failure as successful "practice" expands the area of trust between the family and therapist. The therapist may use this base to launch another challenge aimed at improving the performance. In this manner, tasks proceed toward the point where implementation of actual detoxification is likely to meet with success.

In those instances where the family has met with total success in the first trial, the therapist may express surprise and a continued prediction of failure: "This must have been a fluke." This reminder to the family that it has failed before, that failure is one of its patterns, publicly asserts a specific level of expectation. The assertion helps to extend the task's usefulness, challenging the family to improve or repeat their performance. Strategically, the first success is considered as happenstance. A second occurrence may be coincidental. After a third success, the therapist might agree that something is indeed going right. In some families, it will be necessary to go through this ritual explicitly, pointing out to them what improvements have been made each time around. In others, it is sufficient to prod them into self-discovery and confirmation of their own failure or success simply by recounting the details of their involvement.

## ADDRESSING OBSTACLES AND CRISES

Obstacles and interferences that might affect the detoxification strategy can emerge at any time during therapy. They may come in the form of trivial matters, or as major crises. The meaning attached to this information by the therapist must be incorporated into the frame of what the family is doing and how they are going about each step they have decided to take. When the information is in this form the questions "What was done?" "Who did it?" "When?" and "How?" can successfully be absorbed into the larger strategy of the detoxification process. On the other hand, crises are more difficult to define, and need always to be viewed in the larger context of their occurrence: What function does a crisis hold—in relation to a specific situation— for the addict, the family, and the treatment plan (see Chapters 1, 4, and 8)?

Stress is a normal life occurrence and therapy a normal context for dealing with it. A variety of concerns or discomforts experienced by family members during treatment may be reported, whether or not they directly relate to the original problem of addiction. These should be dealt with during the early and middle stages of sessions. However, early in the course of treatment, sessions should end on an "up" note (even if it is unrelated to treatment goals or content), since the "last impression" counts for much in deterring anxiety between sessions. An especially common concern regards the physical health of the addict. As medication levels are reduced, the therapist may point out to the family that the patient will express some level of discomfort, but that this is normal and not serious. The patient may be called on to confirm this and describe what kinds of behaviors the family may expect from him. His experience and knowledge are again interpreted as competency, diminishing the likely emphasis upon crisis and dependency in later periods of discomfort.

## INITIATING THE DETOXIFICATION

Whereas the general goal of detoxification, per se, should probably be established at the outset of therapy (see Chapter 6), the notion of actually doing it in the home may be broached at a later point. As the therapist creates the right set of conditions during the process of therapy, he continues to get information concerning the family's ambition, abilities, and opportunities. When he determines that the time is right, home detoxification can be introduced in a way that seems natural and fitting. This can occur at any point during treatment. There is thus no single method or protocol for the introduction of such a plan. Instead, a broader plan is needed that develops trust in the therapist and elaborates the specific patterns of competency that appear naturally in each family. While this is a focused strategy, it is not a fixed one.

The steps leading to an actual detoxification exercise, including the groundwork for probable success, usually constitute the larger part of treatment. Administration of the actual plan may require little time or effort once trust and competence have been established. During therapy, issues relating to the detoxification plan may come into discussion without the therapist suggesting them. Once posed, such questions allow further discussion of the logistics of detoxifying. The therapist's primary function at this time is to transpose such discussion from speculative ("if") concerns to procedural ("how") ones, making the planning more certain and specific. For many families, the discussion of detoxification may culminate in plans for detox over a "long weekend," with a clear strategy and plans for dealing with potential problems.

One unexpected but possible occurrence is an assertion by the addict that he has covertly detoxified already, circumventing the necessity of further planning for home detoxification. This should be checked out by the therapist. Family members will undoubtedly have their own thoughts as to how to determine if the addict has indeed detoxified, since by this time the family has already been exposed to what can be expected of the addict during such a process. The therapist may aid them in testing this information, using his technical knowledge and resources.*

*Editors' note. It is usually wise to view such a revelation, or "flight into health," as a resistance move by the identified patient (IP) designed to undercut attempts by the therapist to bring about family reorganization.

## COMPLETING THE CYCLE

The goal in detoxification is not simply withdrawal of the addict from a dependent state, but alteration of the larger family cycle of addiction and withdrawal (see Chapter 1). Successful detoxification helps to counter this cycle by providing a shared experience that includes the realignment of family structure and the mobilization of family resources. The individuation of the patient from the family of origin may remain an issue; improvements in the parents' marital relationship may be another. The detoxification typically changes circumstances to a point where these problems may be worked upon directly, but this is a matter to be decided by the family members and therapist at the appropriate time. Specific strategies for individuation, marital counseling, and so forth, are described in other chapters.


## IMPLEMENTATION IN A CLINICAL CASE

This section presents techniques derived from the foregoing principles through use of material from a case example. This case was our first attempt to actually implement a home detoxification. Although the treatment of this family proved to be exceedingly difficult, partly because every member was found to have a serious problem with substance abuse, the case was chosen because, at the time, we were beginning to look for new ways to create a therapeutic family crisis by intensifying the detoxification process. Home detoxification allows containment of the crisis within the family and provides the family with an opportunity for its natural healing forces to be actualized.

The therapy done with this family was definitely experimental. From it we learned lessons that have helped to set the direction for later work within the Addicts and Families Program. The case demonstrated to us both the potential of the home detoxification paradigm, and also the limitations of a rigid, 10-session treatment contract.

This family was intact, blue collar, and Irish-American, with two sons (ages 23 and 20) and two daughters (ages 21 and 16), all living at home. Both parents worked, but none of the children were employed steadily. The younger son, Tom, was the IP and had been addicted to heroin for several years. He had not been able to detoxify successfully previously. The older brother and sister were also heroin addicts, while the younger daughter was using "soft" drugs regularly. All three heroin addicts were enrolled in some form of treatment program when family therapy began. The father and mother were later found to be heavy drinkers as well—the mother to the point of alcoholism. Eleven sessions were conducted with this family, over a period of 5 months.

## COMPETENCY AND TRUST

*In an early family session, the patient told the therapist (Samuel M. Scott) that his desire to use drugs was very strong most of the time. The therapist then directed the discussion toward ways that the patient used to control or overcome this urge.*

*TOM:* I don't know what the hell I want to get from it, but I'll just get the urge to cop all the time—a lot—you know. I always want to go out and get high.

*SCOTT:* And how do you stop yourself from doing it?

*TOM:* I never really did stop yet.

*SCOTT:* OK, let's do it this way: this past week, how many times did you have the urge?

*TOM:* Every day.

*SCOTT:* OK, every day.

*OLDER SISTER:* On Friday he told me he wasn't going to.

*SCOTT:* OK, that's cool. Now, having had the urge, how many times did you do it?

*TOM:* See, I don't want to here—I don't like saying it in front of my parents.

*SCOTT:* Well, this is the toughest thing in the world for you, next to kicking. This shows just how much you love your parents, next to kicking it. I guess what I'm saying is, if you've got a way of getting around it when you get the urge, that's what I want to know.

*MOTHER:* You're trying to say, where there's a will, there's a way.

*SCOTT:* No, I'm not trying to say that at all. I think you have a way of getting around it.

*TOM:* Yeah.

*SCOTT:* What's your way?

*TOM:* Stay in the house all the time.

*MOTHER:* Yes.

*SCOTT:* What?

*MOTHER:* He stays in almost every day.

*SCOTT:* OK. Then you do have a way, right?

*TOM:* Yeah.

*OLDER SISTER:* There ain't no way he can get it, though.

*SCOTT:* Yes, but it's a beginning, you see. I know why he's staying in the house, because if you go outside the house you're going to run into a familiar face. A familiar face is going to have something to offer you, and you're going to get it.

*Here, staying at home is relabeled as a competent, responsible action on the part of the patient. It is thus categorized as an area of success in dealing with his problem, making it potentially useful to a detoxification strategy. Obviously, it is especially congruent with the notion of detoxifying at home.*

The competencies of other members should also be explored early in therapy. This can be done without saying directly, "See, you are competent." Implication and allusion can be used to help the family identify its own competencies. Initially, the therapist may be needed to draw these out, but eventually he tries to enable the family to continue doing this work on its own.

*The younger daughter did not attend the first family session despite the therapist's instruction that the whole family should come. It seemed that the parents were not in agreement that she should come to future meetings, either. The therapist proceeded to tap the mother's and father's competence as parents by getting them to unite in their response to this issue.*

*SCOTT:* Will you see to it that she is here next week?

*FATHER:* I'll do my best.

*MOTHER:* She'll say yes; she'll be here.

*FATHER:* I'm not going to drag her down here by the ears, but I'll sit down and talk to her. It would be very nice if she came, I'll tell her that.

*(later in the interview)*

*SCOTT:* What would happen if the two of you said she had to come?

*MOTHER:* I think she will.

*SCOTT:* Would she if the two of you just decided that she should come?

*MOTHER:* I think so.

*SCOTT:* How about you?

*FATHER:* I don't know. I'll be honest with you—I don't know.

*SCOTT:* I'm going to have some problems here. You're going to have to help me now. This is a rule now.

*MOTHER:* I can talk her into it.

*SCOTT:* This is a rule now. We're going to set a rule up.

*FATHER:* She's funny as hell, that girl. I think she needs a little working on, myself.

*SCOTT:* Well, the two of you are going to have to decide whether or not she's to come in or not.

*MOTHER:* Yes.

*SCOTT:* OK, you two are going to have to make that decision.

*FATHER:* I can make it.

The therapist uses the data he gathers while observing the family's structure—and testing its capabilities and limits—as a means for developing trust. This is crucial business, because trust may be all that carries the treatment through instances of misunderstanding and confrontation.

*At a later point in therapy, the addict (who earlier stated that staying at home helped him to overcome his urge to take drugs) expressed concern that he would go out after the session. The therapist cast this problem back onto the family by asking the addict how the whole group could help.*

*SCOTT:* You all know that he's going to go out and he's going to shoot up. He says he doesn't want to. (*silence*) Let's deal with the question. Come on.

*MOTHER:* What can we do to help you, Tom? You don't want to do it and we don't want you to do it. What can we do to help you? Well? Tommy?

*TOM:* What?

*MOTHER:* You have to give us an answer.

*TOM:* (*pause*) Keep me from going out.

*This response reiterated the previous idea that home was a safe place, a theme that would be useful throughout the treatment. It provided a concrete solution to the present crisis, that is, for the family to help the addict by keeping him at home. Most important, the suggestion came from the addict and the family was probably capable of fulfilling it.*

## SETTING THE GOALS

The therapist should move quickly to obtain a stated consensus that the primary goal of therapy is successful detoxification. The credibility of the addict's desire to detoxify is less important than obtaining a statement to this effect in the presence of the other family members. Their acceptance of his credibility is less important than their agreement that detoxification is preferable for them, also. The therapist's task is then to reaffirm that the detoxification is indeed a central purpose of the therapy, and that the presence of the entire family is essential to fulfilling this goal.

Once the primary goal has been established, the next step in therapy is to negotiate *when* and *how* the detoxification will be accomplished. While home detox represents an optimal solution, it is by no means the only path available. Concrete plans are shaped by the expressed strengths and commitments of the family, and must be commensurate with what they can indeed do. One means of assuring that the objectives are achievable is to keep them implicit, that is, relative rather than absolute. This requires that the therapist understand what the members are currently capable of doing and willing to do. For example, to say that this or that member should separate from the family is abrasive and probably aligned with one faction within the family. A more balanced, productive statement is to say that these members can separate in this or that way. Once the goal is set in a form that is agreeable to all, the tasks necessary to achieve it will follow easily. Where separation is the goal, one acceptable alternative might be to have the member move in with a grandmother or other relative. Similarly, where the goal is to have a member detoxify, efforts to this end can be activated through the listing of options. In some families, the detoxification may begin with gradual decrements. In others, it may occur over the course of a weekend or an entire week. The important thing to remember is that the family be successful. If unrealistic goals are set, the family can never achieve them and can never be successful. Success breeds success, in therapy as elsewhere in life. The feeling of failure does not bring success.

*In the session where the patient expressed concern about shooting up after the meeting, the therapist directed the discussion to address this problem.*

*SCOTT:* Let's stay with tonight. You're going to go out with your girlfriend and what?
*TOM:* Probably go out and eat.
*SCOTT:* And what?
*TOM:* Or stay in.
*SCOTT:* And what?
*TOM:* I'm coming home.
*SCOTT:* And what, though?
*TOM:* Go to bed.
*SCOTT:* I understand that, but you know what I'm driving at.
*TOM:* No, I ain't getting . . .
*SCOTT:* What?
*TOM:* I ain't getting off, if that's what you're driving at.
*SCOTT:* You ain't getting off. Do you mean you're not going to shoot up?
*TOM:* No, no.
*SCOTT:* What?
*TOM:* I'll try not to.
*SCOTT:* That's not the same as will not.
*TOM:* I don't think I will, honest.

*(later in the interview)*

*SCOTT:* What's the answer again, now? Let's do it again. Tonight?
*TOM:* Go out with my girlfriend, and go out and eat, take her home . . .
*SCOTT:* And what?
*MOTHER:* Come home.
*TOM:* Come home and go to bed.
*SCOTT:* *(to father)* No, you ask him what the question is.
*FATHER:* Are you, uh . . .
*TOM:* What?
*FATHER:* . . . going to buy anything?
*TOM:* I—I won't.

*Here, the focus has been scaled down from eventual detoxification to the interval immediately following the session. The decisions, measures, and commitments needed to help the patient stay straight are drawn entirely from the patient and other family members, rather than being imposed upon them by the therapist.*

Adjunct goals, such as returning to school or work, or moving out from the parents' house, are generally deferred until later in the treatment. The exceptions to this are where they happen to fit in with a useful rationale for the detoxification plan (see Chapter 6), or where they become the content of discussions or tasks to elicit competencies. In any event, the primary focus should remain on detoxification, keeping the issues in therapy simple.

## THE USE OF TASKS

Tasks are projects conducted in the session or at home between sessions. They are concrete challenges, used to begin organizing the family in the areas of competence needed to complete the detoxification plan.

*The therapist learned that one problem occurring in the family was that the mother screamed at the other members. This frequently caused the addict to leave the house, despite his feeling that he would probably shoot up after he left. The therapist asked the mother if she could stop hollering for 1 week, which she agreed to try. In the next session, the therapist inquired casually about her performance of the task.*

*SCOTT:* How did we make out last week? I mean, you couldn't stop hollering, right?
*YOUNGER SISTER:* Yes, she did.
*SCOTT:* Get the hell out of here; I don't believe it.
*MOTHER:* They all hollered at me.
*TOM:* I didn't holler.
*FATHER:* She yelled at Tommy yesterday for spitting in the trash can.
*MOTHER:* I didn't raise my voice. Everyone . . .
*TOM:* . . . spitting in the trash can; you yelled at me.
*SCOTT:* Hey, wait a minute! (*whistles to get the family's attention*) How many times does she usually yell in one week?
*FATHER:* A lot. A peck—a thousand [times].

*SCOTT:* Is that any better, once?

*FATHER:* Oh, yeah, a lot.

*SCOTT:* Did you tell her that?

*FATHER:* Oh, yeah.

*SCOTT:* When did you tell her?

*FATHER:* I was telling her all week she was doing good. Didn't I?

*MOTHER:* Yeah. Screaming. They started hollering at me and I was just as calm as could be.

*(later in the interview)*

*SCOTT:* I congratulate you for not shouting.

*MOTHER:* It's almost impossible to live with these kids without shouting.

*YOUNGER SISTER:* That's what I was trying to say before. My brother almost had her crying the other day, yelling, and she wouldn't yell back. That surprised me.

*Although cessation of mother's screaming might seem to be a minor, or even irrelevant event, it was in fact an important change. An irritating and seemingly immutable family sequence—involving all members—had been altered through a change in the behavior of one member (the mother). Its positive effects were considerable, including (1) increased flexibility in the system, as members became open to the possibility that other patterns might also be amenable to change through their own individual actions; (2) the mother gained a greater sense of mastery or competence, which was reinforced by both family and therapist, thus increasing her strength and ability to make future changes; (3) related to (1) (above), the family's notion of hopelessness was challenged; that is, their experience brought them to the realization that change was not a lofty ideal but a true possibility.*

The mechanics of administering tasks include allocating responsibilities in a reasonable fashion. This idea is built on the fact that when a family comes for treatment, each member already has a set of responsibilities, each of which may be identified as being positive or negative. The assignment of tasks to each member of the family only expands what already exists. When every member of the family has been involved, commitments should be obtained from them. When there is difficulty in obtaining commitments, the therapist should try to frame the tasks as situations or exercises that will call on members' prior successes, individually or as a team. Perhaps the family members have had other experiences in the past that were similar to the discomforts of detoxification (e.g., athletic training, a broken arm, childbirth, etc.). Recounting how these were performed lends competency to the tasks. The detoxification can then be framed in the same manner, as a positive effort requiring some kind of input from everyone—even if it only means "staying out of the way" for a period. If all are involved, it becomes natural to use the home as a base for the detoxification.

Actual results might be quite different from what the therapist originally expected from the task. If there is a half-hearted attempt, or none at all, no one should be blamed, however. Nor should anyone in the family be put in the position of blaming another member. The usual pattern of blaming is what the therapist wants to block and change in conducting the detoxification. Failure in completing the task allows the blaming pattern to emerge in therapy, making it available for intervention. The family is used to failing, and the therapist's having predicted it makes the occurrence acceptable. This acceptance certifies trust and provides the basis for trying to move beyond failure in the future.

It is important to recognize that even a faked attempt at the task is an expression of *compliance*, representing a different behavior from what the family has done in the past. Family members have begun to act differently toward each other, even if only to collude together. These organizational shifts can be cultivated and adapted to positive uses in other tasks.

A faked attempt or outright failure can also be interpreted as indicating that the family needs the therapist's help in dealing with the task and, by implication, with the drug problem. In the detailed review of the task, whether it was completed or not, it is important to ascertain where each member of the family was successful or failed in his part. There should be a review of the role that he was assigned and had agreed to perform. The framework is continually refined in this manner, with an expansion of strong points and elimination of weak ones. By stages, the therapist can thus use the tasks to set up the framework for a successful detoxification plan.

*The addict had expressed, on several occasions, his conviction that staying home was the surest way to avoid shooting up. Mean-*

*while, talk of a conventional detoxification schedule had gone no-
where with the family. At the point where he felt they were prepared
for it, the therapist transformed the "stay at home" theme into an
explicit framework for conducting the detox.*

*SCOTT:* Yeah, well, now look. You've got your education com-
ing your way. I've got a faster way of detoxing if you want to do it.
*TOM:* How long?
*SCOTT:* I mean real fast.
*TOM:* What?
*SCOTT:* Well, it would require you staying home (*points to
patient*) and you staying home (*points to father*) for three days and
you staying home (*points to mother*) for three days . . .
*TOM:* I'm not staying home more than three days. I'd end up
getting fired.
*SCOTT:* You could do it over a weekend, a long weekend. If you
really want to detox, you know.
*TOM:* That wouldn't be a long weekend.
*SCOTT:* How long would it be?
*TOM:* Three or four days. I can take that.
*SCOTT:* Huh?
*TOM:* I can take that.
*SCOTT:* What?
*TOM:* Quitting.
*SCOTT:* You could?
*TOM:* Probably. I don't want to though.
*SCOTT:* You could and you don't want to. Well, how can we
help you want to? How can you (*to parents*) help him to want to?
You know, I don't understand what you just said.
*MOTHER:* He sounds like he's contradicting himself. Like, he
can do it. If you can do it, do it.
*SCOTT:* Well, how can you help . . .
*MOTHER:* Why don't you want to?
*TOM:* I don't want to get off it [methadone].
*MOTHER:* Why?
*TOM:* Because I don't want to.
*MOTHER:* Well, what's your reason?
*TOM:* I want to stay on it.
*MOTHER:* What's your reason? You have to have a reason.
*TOM:* I just don't want to get off right now. I'll detox, but I just
don't want to be off it right now.

*FATHER:* You want to go with graduation. Is that what you mean?

*TOM:* What?

*FATHER:* You know—cut, cut, cut.

*TOM:* No, I'm not worried about getting sick, it's just that I want to stay on the methadone for a little while.

*MOTHER:* Why do you feel you should?

*TOM:* Because I want to, Mom. So I don't go out and get high, all right?

*SCOTT:* So what?

*TOM:* So I don't end up going out and getting high or something. I think I'm at the stage where I won't do any more heroin because of my girlfriend.

*SCOTT:* So, what was the reason again? Because of what?

*TOM:* Because of my girlfriend.

*SCOTT:* Marie.

*TOM:* Yeah.

*SCOTT:* I see a smile over there.

*MOTHER: (to patient)* Don't you want to take your coat off?

*SCOTT:* It's kind of a damp night—like it goes through your body, you know?

*TOM:* Yeah.

*SCOTT:* I feel that way right now.

*TOM:* Yeah, it is kind of cold.

*SCOTT:* Listen, if I say something and—boy, you can just jump down my throat if you want to—but you want them to take their coats off, and she wants you to stop biting your nails—everybody is checking on everybody else around here. Listen, you got a damn good reason to give it up right now. And if you've got a damn good reason to give it up right now, I'll tell you, if it were me, I would take my family right into the house and I would say, "OK, I'm going to quit. In a couple, three, four days, I'm going to go straight downhill, clean up my act one hundred percent," because you've got something to work for. You said you can do it. You said you've got a reason to do it, and shit, I'll tell you, man, I'd want to get off of methadone so fast. . . . You know, when I first talked to you, you talked about suicide. Are you talking about suicide now?

*TOM:* I think about it once in awhile.

*SCOTT:* I know you do, but you don't think about it like you did before.

*TOM:* No.

*SCOTT:* You've got a reason to live and, to me, any form of playing with dope—I don't give a shit if it's the government's methadone program or not. . . . (*Looks at parents, addresses them.*) Will you?

*FATHER:* What?

*MOTHER:* What do we have to do?

*SCOTT:* Stay home with him.

*TOM:* Yeah, you have to stay home with me. Next week . . .

*SCOTT:* I'd like him to.

*TOM:* There's always somebody home anyway.

*SCOTT:* But, I think it has to be structured.

*MOTHER:* Well . . .

*SCOTT:* I'll tell you what I'll do, as a matter of fact . . .

*TOM:* Friday and Saturday—I mean Saturday and Sunday—I'm staying in and I'm going to work Friday and Monday.

*FATHER:* Who'll give it to him?

*TOM:* Give? Shit, I can go to work . . .

*OLDER SISTER:* What's he going to do? I don't understand.

*SCOTT:* Well, ask him.

*OLDER SISTER:* What are you going to do?

*TOM:* Just quitting.

*OLDER SISTER:* You mean cold turkey?

*MOTHER:* You're just going to quit. Nothing. That will be good.

*FATHER:* Next weekend, right?

*TOM:* I'm not quitting now because I'm going to work.

*SCOTT:* I hear you. I hear you. I hear you.

*TOM:* If I'm sick Monday, I'll take off Monday.

*SCOTT:* I'll tell you what I'll do . . .

*TOM:* Just give me enough doses up until next Friday.

*SCOTT:* I'll work out a deal with you. I'll work it out so that you don't have to pick anything up next weekend. I mean, I'll work it that you have straight dosage until Thursday. You don't have to come in on Wednesday.

*TOM:* Until Friday.

*SCOTT:* Until Friday.

*TOM:* Yeah, I want it for Friday, too.

*SCOTT:* All right. That means that you two (*to the parents*) have to stay home Saturday, Sunday, and Monday, if necessary.

*TOM:* No—if necessary, I'll . . .

*SCOTT:* If necessary, right? Do you all agree?

*TOM:* He ain't saying nothing.

*FATHER:* I can't just stay home.

*SCOTT:* Whoa, whoa, whoa! Do you want him to get off?

*TOM:* He can't take off.

*SCOTT:* No, wait a minute, Tom.

*TOM:* I don't want him to take off. He hasn't missed a day of work since he's been there. I don't want him to take off.

*FATHER:* I don't mind taking the work off, but my job ain't as simple to get off as his—I drive a milk truck.

*SCOTT:* Right.

*FATHER:* Who the hell is going to take my route? They ain't got enough guys to run the damn routes and they got all the supervisors . . .

*OLDER SISTER:* Yeah, he can go. He's home early, anyway.

*YOUNGER SISTER:* He's home at two o'clock, and we'll take off school.

*FATHER:* I'm home at noontime.

*MOTHER:* Can he go in the hospital?

*TOM:* I don't want to go in the hospital! Damn it! All that shit, I'm going to stay on it.

*SCOTT:* If he wants to do it at home, it makes sense to me. It really makes sense to me to do it at home.

*TOM:* I was thinking about doing that anyway . . .

*SCOTT:* How is this—am I reading your mind or are you reading mine? You're way ahead of me. You're always ahead of me.

*TOM:* No, I was thinking about doing that for Marie [girl-friend].

*As in earlier taskwork, the plan was developed by incorporating the family's expressed capabilities within the basic requirements of the detoxification.\* In this particular family, an agreement was also negotiated with the mother—who had a drinking problem—to drink no more than a glass of wine a day during the detox period (see Chapter 6).*

*\*Editors' note.* As described in Chapter 6, it is advisable for the therapist to establish therapeutic and medical backup during the detoxification period that can be responsive to the kind of physical and emotional crises that can occur. This may include home visits by the therapist, an on-call physician, education about emergency facilities, and the like.

A number of contingencies are likely to crop up as the detoxification plan is administered. As in earlier tasks, these can be predicted and discussed with the addict and the family beforehand, lowering the probability that they will occur or reducing the negative impact on the detoxification if they do occur. Most often, a task fails because the addict leaves the house during the detoxification, or because someone brings drugs into the house for him. If the parents relax their vigilance, one or the other of these acts may occur without anyone but the addict knowing about it. The ideal counter to such difficulties is to enforce one-on-one supervision, with the parents agreeing on shifts. If they cannot manage this for the entire duration of the detoxification, it may be necessary to work up incrementally from shorter durations. Again, as in earlier tasks, failure is interpreted as partial success and used as a milestone for further progress.* Ideas as to other possible contingencies should be solicited from the addict in the course of establishing a detoxification plan. He is also the best source of ideas as to possible counters to such contingencies. Most will involve some form of *securing of boundaries*, including roles, areas, and schedules.

*The initial attempt to detoxify at home in this case proved unsuccessful. The mother held to her agreement to minimize drinking and remain vigilant, but the father let his son go out to the store for a pack of cigarettes, at which time the son shot up. A second trial was also unsuccessful. Although the parents were more watchful and did not permit the addict to leave the house, his sister (also an addict) covertly brought drugs to him.† It became apparent to the therapist that the drug problem in this family could not be viewed as limited to one member, but was shared in one form or another by everyone. Under these conditions, the necessary roles and commitments could not be adequately differentiated. The therapist suggested, half-seriously, the idea of the family undergoing a "group" detox.*

---

*Editors' note. This is not just a therapeutic "ploy." Even if only a partial attempt is made, it is still a change from what was. A partial attempt means that someone, or everyone, did something a little differently. These efforts to change should not be denigrated by the therapist. Like a locomotive that slowly gains momentum, a gradual but building process has been put in motion.

†*Editors' note.* As noted in Chapter 6, the likelihood of success on the first attempt may be increased by obtaining an agreement with the family *beforehand* that they will attempt the home detoxification a *second* time, should the first try fail.

*SCOTT:* It just seems to me that this family ought to pack up—the whole family—and go up into the mountains about fifty miles from nowhere . . .

*MOTHER:* Yeah.

*SCOTT:* . . . in a cabin for about one week. No dope, no methadone, no drinking, and see whether or not you'd like to talk to each other a little bit. Because that's what it comes down to right now.

*MOTHER:* That's what it sounds like to me.

*SCOTT:* But, I guess that's impossible. (*to father*) It would be a good time to do it, because you're out of work right now.

*Soon after, the family in fact carried out this directive, although it was not given to them as an explicit task.**

## FINISHING UP

Upon completion of a successful detoxification, the therapist still has some important work to do with the family. The essential component in success is not the *reduction* of drug use to nothing, but the *deterrence* from returning to active use. If detoxification occurs, the family has demonstrated the necessary competencies to also deter addiction. These skills need to be made explicit, highlighted, and reinforced to assure that they are sustained. This is done by reviewing with the addict and other family members each aspect of the detoxification process: Who took what role? What problems came up? How were these handled? How did the addict feel physically? How did he

---

*\*Editors' note.* Despite several potent factors mitigating success, notably the substance abuse of every family member, the outcome initially appeared favorable in this case, since the IP detoxed successfully. It is important to note that this occurred at the end of therapy and the therapist was unable to follow through because of the research design. Within a few months, however, Tom returned to methadone maintenance for 2 years, and during the first of these years also used illegal opiates weekly and engaged in criminal activity. In the second year he essentially ceased his use of illegal drugs and detoxed from methadone by the end of that year. Since then, or at least through the follow-up period of 40 months posttreatment, his use of drugs was very slight, although he was drinking up to two six-packs of beer a day. He maintained a fair job-adjustment over the follow-up period, working somewhat more than half the time, including two jobs that he held for 1 year each. After treatment he moved out of the parents' home, living with his sister and a girlfriend. After 3 or 4 months he moved back with his parents and remained there, with occasional departures of a month or so at a time to live with a girlfriend. At the last follow-up his parents were reported to be pressuring him to move out for good.

feel about his parents? and so forth. The tone should be positive, stressing the "1 in a 1000" nature of this accomplishment.

Reviewing the detoxification experience also constitutes a disengagement process whereby the therapist helps the family become aware that the success has been theirs, and that he is no longer needed in relation to the presenting problem.[160] If appropriate, there may be a shift of focus to other problems, particularly when the loss of the addiction creates a gap in the addict's (and family's) life. Or, therapy might next deal with the relationship between the parents and the addict. Here, other competencies can be elicited, explored, and mastered through the use of tasks. The procedures are similar to those above. In any event, it is essential that the family make the decision to either work on additional issues or to discontinue therapy. As before, the family either enters this path voluntarily, or not at all.

## SUMMARY

This chapter, in conjunction with the additional material on home detoxification in Chapter 6, provides the basic elements for undertaking a home detox, at least to the extent that the paradigm has thus far been developed. Major components of the therapeutic process are as follows:

1. *Establishing the therapeutic system*
   - Therapist obtains acknowledgment of the problem by the family.
   - The primary goal of therapy—in this instance, detoxification—is agreed upon.
   - The rules for sessions are set (who shall attend, dates, etc.).
   - Family structure and themes relating to the problem are explored.
   - Rules around medication dosage and other aspects of treatment are established with the addict.
   - The addict's drug history is explored in the presence of the family, both to obtain data applicable to the primary goal and to sophisticate the family.
   - Family rules and interactions are restructured, engaging the patient and family in a basic therapeutic system aligned

toward the primary goal. Basic lines of communication and authority are set in place; positions are coordinated.
- "Stress" is dealt with at each session, as it occurs.
- "Red herring" issues are dealt with at each session, as they occur.

2. *Designing and enacting the detox plan*
   - The therapist builds up to a plan through a series of preliminary tasks that shape and strengthen relevant family skills.
   - Consensus is obtained from family members on actual roles and schedules for detoxifying. Procedures for therapeutic and medical backup are established, where applicable.
   - The family is made knowledgeable of the requisites for helping the addict to detoxify—the pain, ploys, and other contingencies that may occur, and how to counter them.
   - Unsuccessful attempts are interpreted as "practice," and tied into a progression of trials or tasks.

3. *Maintaining the success*
   - The family successfully completes a detoxification attempt.
   - The elements of success are reviewed in detail. Family members are made to feel important, that they have done something remarkable.
   - The therapist disengages from the family, relative to this goal. They perhaps go on to work on other issues, such as individuation, job, marriage, and the like. Or, treatment is terminated, with the possibility of reconvening in the future if necessary.

# 13

# TREATING FAMILIES OF ADOLESCENT DRUG ABUSERS

H. CHARLES FISHMAN
M. DUNCAN STANTON
BERNICE L. ROSMAN

CHAPTERS 1 AND 6 emphasize the importance in drug abuse of the family life cycle stage. Since families of adolescents are at a different point in the life cycle than families of adult addicts, different treatment strategies are indicated. In the pages to follow, the similarities and differences between these two groups are addressed and the discussion is augmented with appropriate clinical vignettes and guidelines.

Heavy drug abuse by an adolescent is, itself, a serious problem. In addition, it should be noted that, unless the process is arrested, a certain proportion of young drug abusers may further progress to more serious addiction when they reach young adulthood. In such cases, adolescent drug abuse might be viewed as an early stage in the addictive process, as noted in Chapters 1 and 6. Therapy with adolescent abusers, then, not only aims at eliminating the existing problem, but in some cases may serve to prevent the occurrence of future, possibly more severe dysfunctions.

The material in this chapter is derived from the clinical experience of the first two authors (Fishman and Stanton), plus a research project on adolescent substance use directed by the third author (Rosman).* The project compared patterns, structures, and symptom function in 53 families in which a 12- to 17-year-old adolescent was referred for treatment for one of three reasons: (1) regular or habitual use of illegal drugs, (2) use of various chemical substances in making

*The project, entitled "Adolescent Substance Use in Three Family Contexts," was funded by the National Institute on Drug Abuse (Grant No. 5R01 DA 01629) and was conducted over a 3-year period, from 1977 to 1980.

suicidal attempts, or (3) cases primarily referred for delinquency problems, with secondary substance abuse. While the project was basic research, and did not include funding for treatment, 16 of the families of habitual drug abusers were seen in family therapy by 12 different therapists under the auspices of the Philadelphia Child Guidance Clinic (PCGC) Outpatient Department. The first author (Fishman) served as clinical supervisor in the treatment of these cases. For purposes of the present chapter, clinical material will be drawn from cases and therapeutic operations pertaining only to habitual abusers.*

## COMPARISONS BETWEEN ADOLESCENT ABUSERS AND ADULT ADDICTS

As might be expected, there are many similarities between families with an adolescent habitual abuser and those with an addict over age 18. Thus much of the theoretical material in Chapter 1 and the clinical principles in Chapter 6 are applicable to both groups.

On the other hand, the differences that do exist between these two clinical populations have important implications for treatment, dictating that therapy with families of adolescent abusers differ from that with young adult addicts in a number of ways.

### CHRONICITY AND/OR SEVERITY

Fewer adolescent abusers are physiologically addicted to an illegal substance such as an opioid. Consequently, their treatment is less likely to include the therapeutic trappings that accompany addiction, such as detoxification, pharmacological substitution (e.g., methadone), and the use of narcotic blocking agents (e.g., naltrexone). Since the problem with adolescents is of briefer duration, issues of chronicity and of "craving" are of less concern—the pattern is less entrenched. In many ways this simplifies considerably the treatment of families of adolescent abusers, compared to addicts in their 20s and 30s.

*Results from the research component of the program are still undergoing analysis and will be reported in future publications.

## PEER GROUP

Adult addicts are frequently involved in a drug subculture. It pervades many aspects of their daily lives, serving as a source of drugs, "friendship," and recreation. As noted in Chapter 1, they often retreat to it at times of increased family conflict, so it can serve as an integral part of the familial–interpersonal homeostatic process. In contrast, the influence of the peer subculture of adolescent abusers is less important relative to the influence of their families. While research cited in Chapter 1[e.g., 17, 76] indicates that the adolescent's peer group is influential vis-à-vis societal trends toward substance abuse (such as the occasional use of marijuana), the compulsive use of more severe, or "hard," substances is much more dependent on family relationships and patterns. In short, the mutual impact of adolescent habitual users and their peer group is of a lesser magnitude than that between older addicts and their peers.

## CRIMINAL ACTIVITY

Obviously, adolescent abusers are less likely to be as deeply involved in criminal activity than their older counterparts—partly because their drug use is less extensive and less likely to include opiates, thus requiring less money to maintain. While they may engage in minor stealing, it is unlikely that they will become imprisoned and engage in other activities that bring them into regular contact with more hard-core criminal elements such as organized crime. For instance, it is rare for such an adolescent to initiate treatment as an escape either from danger or a court sentence. Lack of such involvement thus simplifies the treatment of families with adolescents.

## MULTIPLE EXTRAFAMILIAL SYSTEMS

In addition to the drug subculture and the criminal world, adult addicts tend much more than adolescents to be directly involved with a number of extrafamilial interpersonal systems such as drug-treatment (e.g., methadone) programs, legal systems, welfare systems, unethical practitioners, vocational programs, spouse-like relationships, and so forth (see Chapter 6). These various systems can function as homeostats, undercutting family treatment or throwing it

off-track, competing among themselves and, in their effect, perpetuating the status quo. Thus the therapist must take a broad (or "meta")
view of the addict within his context and develop methods that
encompass a wide range of systems. On the other hand, treating
families of adolescent abusers less commonly requires consideration
of systems beyond the family, or if it does, the number and impact of
such systems is usually less than with adult addicts. Once again, in
terms of breadth of focus, the task with families of adolescents is less
complex and has fewer elements functioning to resist change.

## RECRUITMENT

For the most part, parents and family members of adolescent abusers
are less resistant to entering family treatment than are those of adult
addicts. Since the identified patient (IP) usually resides with them,
and the parents, in particular, feel more direct responsibility for this
young person, their involvement in the treatment program is more
likely to make sense to them. In fact, a review of the literature[152] and
a national survey[30] on family treatment for drug problems indicate
that the application of family therapy for adolescent drug abuse is
much more widespread than it is in treating adult addicts. Consequently, the therapist normally does not have to expend the same
amount of time and effort in recruiting families of adolescents that is
often required with those of older addicts. Of course, this is not
always true, and in cases where an adolescent's family is "resistant" to
coming in, the extensive material on family recruitment provided in
Chapters 3 through 5 would apply.

## LEVERAGE

The cumulative effect of the above factors is that the family therapist
usually has more *leverage* in treating families of adolescents than
with families of adult addicts. There are fewer extrafamilial systems
to contend with, the family is more likely to accept the rationale for
their involvement (since the abuser dwells within their midst), and
parents usually have more socially sanctioned control over the IP—or
such control is at least easier to establish. With such families the
therapist may not have to contend with a perception held throughout
much of society, or at least American society, that a person, once he

has reached a certain age and has perhaps moved out of his parents' home, should be seen as an *individual*. Whereas it has been pointed out in Chapter 1 that with adult addicts this is usually a "pseudo-individuation," families of older clients often continue to cling to the myth that their addicted son or daughter is an autonomous person with an individual problem, implying that their own involvement in his treatment is irrelevant and unnecessary. However, families are less likely to play this tune if their drug-abusing offspring is still an adolescent. As a result, they are easier to join, and are also more apt to respond to therapeutic interventions requiring that they, themselves, make changes.

## LIFE CYCLE STAGE AND DEVELOPMENTAL CRISES

It has been noted in Chapters 1 and 6 that, while the family of the adult addict is often struggling with a life cycle stage that involves his leaving home, families of young drug abusers have become stuck at a different transitional point (i.e., that of the onset of adolescent individuation). Adolescence is a time when the natural tendency for the person who becomes an IP is to begin assuming adult-like responsibilities and moving toward the peer group. Further, peer relationships characteristically include heterosexual activities, such as dating, and increasingly resemble adult relationships. Some families have difficulty in traversing this point of passage, and a symptom develops in one or more members. The family is in a state of crisis, and the problem manifested by one member is an attempt by the system to resolve the crisis. In other words, the symptom is indicative of or part of a "problem in living" *involving the entire family*; that is, the family encounters difficulty in navigating the requisite developmental passage.

The term "crisis" is used here in a specific way. By crisis, we refer to a breakdown of the rules that had previously governed family interactions satisfactorily. Prior to the youngster's adolescence, the family's ways of interacting and its structural composition were adequate. With adolescence, however, the youngster incurs new developmental needs that require the family to change its habitual patterns of interaction. The crisis occurs when a rule that previously functioned adequately stops working. A period of uncertainty ensues in which the family consensus has broken down. At this point, a symptom emerges. The symptom is a way of reestablishing homeostasis. It thus provides a kind of "solution" to the family's transitional dilemma.

Of course, the immediate developmental crisis does not necessarily have to occur at the point when a younster reaches adolescence. As with adult addicts it can emerge, for example, when other children leave home, a parent reaches age 30 or 40, or subsequent to the death of some important person in the system, such as a grandparent. Whatever the transitional event, however, the family system is inevitably put under pressure to transform, to operate in a different way, and with different structures, in accordance with the demands of the new situation. Families without the requisite flexibility then become dysfunctional and, in an effort to maintain the status quo, a symptom develops.

## GOALS AND DIRECTION OF THERAPY

The therapeutic plan outlined elsewhere in this book for the treatment of young adult abusers is to initially recreate a structure that is more appropriate for an earlier stage in the IP's and family's developmental span. This is done by putting the parents in charge of the young adult, even when he is not living with them. In this way their control is exaggerated. The intent is to increase intensity, leading to an escalation or "runaway," by taking a family that is already close and moving them even closer—"compressing" them[159, 162]—so that the ensuing reequilibration of the system is one in which there is real separation between parents and addict. Therapy aims at effecting the developmentally correct separation between parents and IP that the family has not heretofore achieved.

In contrast, with families of adolescents the goal of therapy is a transformation of the family system *within the existing composition*, rather than aiming for the kind of physical separation sought with families of young adults. With adolescents' families the mechanisms of control are already in place (e.g., the youngster and parents usually live together) and it is developmentally correct for the parents to be in charge. Further, societal conventions support both an "intact" family structure and the control functions of the parents. This does not mean, of course, that the parents are *exercising* their controls. As with families of older addicts, there is usually conflict between the adolescent's parents or between two or more adult figures within the system.[65] The idea is to get the parents working together in an undivided manner, while at the same time creating *modulations* in the ways in which family members deal with each other. The desired result is to bolster the family hierarchy while increasing members' repertories so that they can respond more appropriately both to developmental needs and the vicissitudes of life.

Treating families of adolescents does not usually involve as great a level of intensity as does therapy with families of adult addicts. There is usually less hopelessness and the stakes are generally not as high with families of adolescent abusers. Movement toward differentiation between parents and the adolescent is taken only to the edge of the family's outer boundary. Given the family's developmental stage, there is normally no need for a permanent expulsion or "explosion"[162] at this time (although temporary exclusion may be used to effect parental control, as noted below). Expansion of the system to consolidate appropriate external and internal systems, such as increasing the adolescent's affiliation with his peer subsystem as well as his siblings, is also done more gently. Consequently, interventions more in line with structural than strategic methodology are appropriate.

## THERAPEUTIC TECHNIQUES

The remainder of this chapter deals with various techniques we have found useful in treating families of adolescent drug abusers. Minimum space is given to basic operations that apply in the treatment of families with all kinds of problems, since these have been presented in earlier publications,[5, 100] and most recently in Minuchin and Fishman's book *Family Therapy Techniques.**

### RESISTANCE TO FAMILY INVOLVEMENT

Occasionally an adolescent drug abuser will appear alone for treatment and show resistance to including his family. He may claim that they know nothing of his drug use, or that they are already "hassling" him too much and he wants no more of it. As noted in Chapter 5, these

*Published by Harvard University Press, Cambridge, Mass., 1981.

responses should be viewed as protective moves on his part, as a way of blocking the therapist from entering (and challenging) the family system. In such instances, many of the techniques set forth in Chapter 3 for initiating family involvement with adult addicts also apply here. In addition, there are other options available.

One such option is to get into a gentle disagreement with the IP about how much he cares about his parents. The client may state that he wants nothing to do with them, or that he hates them. If the therapist has gathered enough information about the client and family, he can counter with a noble ascription by stating, "You're not kidding me. You really care about those people. They're important to you and you don't want to see them hurt or made upset. You know they're going through tough times and you would like to make it easier for them. That's the sign of a caring son [or daughter]." This tack can help to lessen defensiveness in the client as to his part in the family problem. It also conveys to him that the therapist will be able to empathize with his parents, meaning that their engagement in therapy need not include their being attacked by the therapist. Thus the client may be able to lower the shield with which he protects the family.

Another approach is to empathize with the adolescent as to how tough things are for him. The therapist draws him out about all the pressures he gets from his family—the conflicts and demands. However, the therapist must beware of blaming the family here, remaining empathic with the effect on the adolescent and joining him only in terms of all the difficulties he faces. Eventually the therapist can shift his emphasis to one of resignation, perhaps stating, "You know, it looks like no matter what you do, your family is involved in some way. They hold all the cards. You've been saying how you'd like more reasonable curfew hours and to be left alone once in a while. But so far you haven't been able to get them to hear you properly. And you still have to go home to a situation that hasn't changed. But I'm thinking that there may be another way to handle this. One of the things we do at this Clinic is to work with family members toward negotiating reasonable arrangements with each other. Now my guess is that your parents are a lot more reasonable than you're thinking right now, because you are kind of stuck. How about if we bring them in and see what can be negotiated, so that you can get some of the things you want and they can feel better and can let up the pressure a little. They sound like pretty good people to me." If at this point the client still resists, the therapist can say, "Well, maybe you're right. But I don't see any way you can get out of it easily. They're still your family and you love them. Maybe you can figure out a way to change the situation for the better, but it's a pretty tough job. What do you plan to do?" From here the therapist can work with the client on his plans for change, especially if they involve changing his own behavior toward the family. He should also caution the patient that there will be a reaction to his new behavior, if for no other reason than that it is new and the family may not believe or trust it. Should the patient be unsuccessful during the next week, the therapist will have more leverage for including the family in subsequent meetings.

A third tack is a version of "strategic disengagement".[161] (It is greatly facilitated if the therapist's agency has a policy, as we do at the PCGC, of not allowing therapy to continue beyond two sessions with the adolescent alone; his family must be involved directly after two sessions, even if therapy later reverts to individual sessions with him.) The therapist joins considerably with the client in the first two sessions. He tries some of the above approaches, but still encounters massive resistance. If the therapist has joined the adolescent well enough he can then say, "You know, I've got a problem. My bosses won't let us continue to meet with someone beyond two sessions unless the family comes in. But you're still not ready for that. Why don't we recess until you feel strong enough to let me give them a call." With this move, the therapist plays on the young person's fear of abandonment. Given sufficient joining, the client may panic at the thought of losing the therapist, subsequently giving permission to involve his family members. Of course, proper use of this technique demands a certain amount of skill on the part of the therapist, including sensitivity to the ongoing interaction and feedback process between therapist and client, plus acumen in identifying what may be occurring within the client's family.

The above example demonstrates the use of "strategic impotence," in which the therapist joins with the client against an impersonal third party.* In this case it dovetails with an adolescent's sense of powerlessness, thus facilitating joining. Of course, another option is for the therapist to plead impotence without invoking this sort of third party, such as claiming his "hands are tied" unless the client allows his family to be engaged.

*Another example of strategic impotence is given in Vignette 11, Chapter 5.

Once the therapist gains permission, through strategies such as the above, to contact the family, he can utilize the various principles for engaging families discussed in Chapter 5. He has at least made it over the first hurdle. While this hurdle may be less difficult than with adult addicts, overcoming it is still an accomplishment.

## REFRAMING

This technique is based on the notion that reality is always partial. Whenever a person describes reality, he describes only part of the picture, which usually represents a social consensus. Reality, then, is confirmation by significant others. Since the therapist, as the leader of the therapeutic system, is a significant person, he is able to use reframing to provide alternative realities that allow change in the ways members interact. In this sense, reality is used as a therapeutic tool.

As in treating families of adult addicts, the therapist will often want to deal with the family of the adolescent by reframing the IP's drug-using behavior as misbehavior rather than as a manifestation of illness. This allows the parents to achieve the distance necessary to effectively establish a generational hierarchy.

As with treating adult drug abusers, the therapist also wants to establish a counterpoint of competence: "Your youngster is conning you. . . . You [to son] are a very good con man." For example, a 16-year-old who had been mainlining heroin for 2 years was seen with his parents. This youngster had been sickly as a child and was still seen by his mother, with whom he was extremely overinvolved, as a boy who was sick rather than bad. Even when he stole his grandmother's jewelry and fenced it, his mother saw him as unable to change his behavior because of the fact that he "lost a father when he was very young." The therapist (Fishman) reframed his behavior as voluntary and delinquent, asking the mother whether the child was crazy or bad. The mother was forced to say that she didn't think her son was crazy. That left only one alternative, an alternative that provided a frame for increased distance. At the same time, the therapist under-scored the fact that the youngster could and did act differently in other contexts—at work and even in the session. This message conveyed hope as well as the idea that the boy could operate effectively; it thus helped to attenuate the parent's overconcern for the boy.

This different framing of reality allowed the mother to join the boy's stepfather, demand different behavior, and implement consequences for his misbehavior. At the same time, the new perspective conveyed a message to the boy of greater respect, challenging him to act in a more competent, differentiated manner. The goal in this therapy is not to create an exaggerated hierarchy that leads to separation, but, instead, one that is maintained by the *mutual accommodation* of both sides. Toward this end, the therapist engaged the youngster as a "cotherapist" right in the session to help him in the implementation of the new family organization. This was done by allying with the boy, by supporting him at appropriate points, and by challenging him to do his part in implementing change so that the family could fulfill more of his needs regarding autonomy, peer relations, and competence.

## ENACTMENT

This technique involves bringing the dysfunctional family interactional pattern right into the therapy room so that more *functional* patterns and structures can then be *directly* introduced. It has been primarily developed by Minuchin[68, 100, 103] and merits heavy use in the treatment of families with an adolescent drug abuser, particularly because Minuchin's work relies on the developmental perspective consistent with the needs of this younger age group.

One example of enactment comes from the treatment of a youngster who had stolen over 20 cars in the few months prior to treatment and used marijuana and amphetamines heavily. During the session he consistently laughed as his father spoke. The therapist (Jody Cox, MSW) asked the father if he was comfortable with the way his son was behaving. The father said that he was not, but felt that his son could do no differently. The mother, who was more peripheral (while the father was overinvolved and supportive of the youngster's delinquency), was livid.The therapist then gave the parents the challenge of doing whatever was necessary, right in the session, to get their son to act respectfully toward them.

The stage was thus set for the enactment of different interactions. The previous pattern, in which the father supported the child regardless of his behavior, was changed as it occurred in the room. The handling of the youngster's smiling became the fulcrum for change. At the point in which the father and mother joined together, agreeing that the son was being insolent, the young man began taking their words more seriously. A new structure, one in which the parents were together and a functional hierarchy was in place, had been introduced.

Enactments are utilized in numerous ways throughout the course of therapy. Since, with adolescent abusers, the system is usually less rigid than with young adult addicts, the therapist does not need to use a single, high-intensity problem (i.e., addiction) as a change fulcrum. Instead he can opt to use either drug-related or non-drug-related issues to create enactments.

## BOUNDARY MAKING

Structure can be regarded in terms of boundaries. In the prototypic family discussed throughout this book, one might describe the dysfunction as that in which the boundary around the parental spouse subsystem is overly permeable—the addict and a parent are inappropriately close. Generally, in families of both older addicts and adolescent abusers the boundary between the parental subsystem and the offspring subsystem tends to be dysfunctional and overly permeable. In particular, one or both of the parents are apt to support the youngster in his drug-taking behavior.

The technique of boundary making is a way of operationalizing changes in structure. There are numerous interventions that can be used to create boundaries. An important one is getting the parents to form a united front, thereby bolstering the boundary around the parental subsystem. This implicitly strengthens the boundary around the spouse subsystem as well. Another important technique, particularly since this is a therapy that seeks to work toward the adolescent's developmental goals, is to enhance the boundary around the teenager and his peer group. This can be done through such interventions as (1) using another teenager as a cotherapist, (2) seeing the youngster and his siblings together, and (3) giving the parents tasks that create distance between them and the youngster, such as going on vacation as a couple.

### Diminishing Overcontrol

It is not uncommon in families with an adolescent drug abuser for one or both parents to expend great energy (or at least to devote considerable worry) toward gaining or maintaining complete control over all aspects of the young person's life. They fret when he is in school, out of school, alone in his room, with friends, visiting relatives, and on and on. They plague him with questions concerning his activities and whereabouts. They check his dresser drawers. They "know" his is up to no good most of the time.

In such instances the therapist needs to find a way to establish boundaries that are appropriate, that is, those that delineate a domain over which parents can realistically establish control. Otherwise the parents will continue to waste energy over areas that they have little or no ability to control.

The therapist first approaches this issue by tracking and probing. He checks the parents' response to subtle hints about how difficult their task is, how hard it must be to be precluded from information about the IP's activities, and so forth. If the therapist senses that he is well enough joined, and the parents will not resist him too energetically, he may then move to establish the correct boundary directly, with firmness. He might tell the parents that, try as they may, there is no way they are going to be able to stay on top of their child 24 hours a day. He follows this assertion with examples to reinforce his argument. He does not blame them, but his tone conveys strength; he cannot project an anxious or uneasy demeanor, as if he is unsure of his position. In this way he restructures forcefully, establishing a workable reality around boundaries that are feasible and manageable.

In situations where resistance is extremely high (i.e., intensity is great and the parents will hear no arguments for limiting their attempts to overcontrol) the therapist might take an alternative, more strategic tack. The rationale underlying this tack is to join the parents and draw them out in their position, to (paradoxically) take it to its logical extreme with the idea that eventually they will be forced to realize the limitations of their control. The therapist might ask the parents what more they could do to insure that they can keep on top of the IP's activities. He could plan the IP's daily schedule with them, and then suggest that one or both parents be with the adolescent at every point: accompanying him to school, remaining in the school, chaperoning his dates, checking his dresser twice a day, and so forth. This schedule can be constructed with the parents alone, or, if the adolescent is present, in such a way that the therapist can silence the IP's inevitable protests. Usually at some point one or both parents will state something like, "I can't do all that! I've got too much to do at work [or home]." The therapist does not relent easily here, however, stating that if the parents are to feel secure in their knowledge about their youngster, they will need to stay on top of things. The therapist takes a stance such that the parents must convince him unequivocally of their limitations before he agrees to back off. By going through this process several times, involving several content areas, the parents and therapist may eventually reach a set of boundaries that are workable. This technique shares many elements with the approach described elsewhere in this volume of bringing the parents and IP closer, that is, increasing the intensification to the point of rebound so that the subsystems naturally reequilibrate with more proper distance.[162]

### Establishing Parental Control

As a complement to the above, when treating families of adolescent drug abusers it is frequently necessary for the therapist to help the parents establish control over their domain. Usually this is the home in which they live, and it is necessary to set up "house rules" by which offspring must abide (an example is given in Chapter 7). The therapist wants to help the family negotiate appropriate rules and also the *consequences* if these rules are broken. The interaction may revolve around duties to be performed by offspring, the hours they are allowed to keep, and so forth. Generally the therapist will tend to take the side of the parents in such negotiations, especially at first. This is done to firm up the boundary around the parental subsystem and insure that the parents' authority is strengthened; if they can be assisted in working together, the chances that they will enforce the rules (rather than one of them breaking ranks and "going soft") are increased. In one case (treated by Stanton) the abusing adolescent regularly returned home at all hours of the night while one or both parents waited up for him. The therapist worked out an agreement with them that followed three steps: first, appropriate hours were negotiated between parents and son. Second, the son was required to turn in his house key and the parents also agreed to secure all other entrances to the home, including the cellar windows. Third, the parents were to lock the house tightly at the agreed upon hour each night (alternating in this responsiblity) and to go to bed, even if they could not fall asleep. In other words, the son would be locked out of the house if he returned home late. The therapist warned the parents that their son probably would not take this boundary at face value and that they should expect him to challenge it. An agreement was also reached that if the son broke into the house, he would repair all damages and lose all privileges for a week. The parents followed the task and two nights later the son came home an hour late. The parents stuck to their guns, and when the son could not get in, he went and stayed with a friend. Thereafter during the next 3 months he was only late twice, missing his time by 10 and 5 minutes, respectively.

There is a feature of this paradigm about which therapists should be forewarned. Drug abusers' families often tend to overreact in meting out punishments. They become angry when their youngster acts out or misbehaves and respond with massive punishment—such as removing a year's privileges for a 40-minute lateness. In the face of such capital punishment, the young person feels he has nothing to lose by continuing to misbehave, since he will get the full punishment no matter what he does—if one is going to get 10 years for stealing a loaf of bread, he might as well rob a bank and make the crime worthwhile. Of course, with such extreme threats the parents cannot follow through. As a result, their reaction leads to no net change and is therefore homeostatic.

To break this homeostatic sequence, the therapist has to tread the thin line of helping parents to establish reasonable consequences,* while at the same time not undercutting their authority by making their decisions look foolish. Sometimes it is prudent not to challenge an unreasonable rule at all, especially if it is the first time one or both parents have become assertive. In such a situation, the therapist might go along with the rule, but terminate the discussion with a statement to the parents like, "OK. Why don't you give it a try? Since you are sort of experimenting, you can see how it works and then decide next time which way you want to go with it." This message does not denigrate the parents or imply that they are wrong, but does connote the "experimental" nature of the exercise and that the parents are capable of being reasonable and flexible. Or, if the therapist does not want to embarrass the parents in front of their children, he can meet with them separately ("The adults should get together on this") and discuss the merits of a relative balance between crime and punishment.

*Separated Parents*

In some cases the parents are separated or divorced and the adolescent lives with one of them, or shuttles between two households. Such

---

*Of course, this is a principle that is exercised routinely by behavioral therapists who work with child and adolescent problems in the context of the family.

parents are often wary of being brought together to deal with their youngster, partly because they may think the therapist is going to attempt to put their marriage back together. If they do both attend the same session, the therapist should state very clearly that reconciliation is not his intention, and that they have been convened *only* to help the adolescent. If this issue still seems salient, and, as is often the case, the adolescent has a fantasy that he can bring his parents together, the therapist might even ask him about it. After the therapist has stated that he is not attempting to resurrect the marriage, he can ask the IP, "Do you think you can get your parents back together? How? What have you tried? What else do you think you might try?" This is done to get either a firm denial from the adolescent, or, if he wavers, to get the parents to state unequivocally that such a rapprochement is not possible, thereby making the nature and extent of the boundaries more clear. On the other hand, if the parents display ambivalence about staying apart, the therapist might consider informing them that such a topic should be postponed until after some progress is made in the presenting problem, which brought them to treatment.

One way of viewing the adolescent's role in such entanglements is that if he is without problems while living with one parent, the other parent may feel he or she has "lost" him.* His failure in one household reflects negatively on the parent with whom he lives, indicating to the other parent that the former spouse is not doing that well without him or her. This is an area where firm boundaries must be established as to which parent is to be in charge of what and when, and under what conditions should the other parent be in control (e.g., during visitations). Further, it is rarely helpful to deny the fact that the adolescent holds allegiance to both parents by discounting the absent parent, especially if the more distant parent is giving signals that he or she wants continued contact with the youngster. Such a move only triangulates the adolescent further,

---

*Sometimes it is even helpful to ascribe noble intentions to the adolescent, stating, "Your getting in trouble while living with your father is a lovely way to let your mother know she has not lost you. As long as things don't go too well between you and Dad, Mom knows you are still loyal. If everything was fine at home, she might wonder whether she would ever see you again, or whether you had disowned her and gone over to Dad completely. On the other hand, you don't cause Dad so much trouble that he would want to throw you out. So he doesn't have to lose you either. This is a very thoughtful and creative thing you are doing."

making his position even less tenable. A better alternative is to accept the triad as such and aim toward changing the rules to make them more workable.

As an example, a family of a 14-year-old drug abuser was seen in which the parents had been divorced for 10 years and were rarely in contact. The family wanted nothing to do with the therapy. The only time the adolescent saw his father was when he and his mother had a fight, whereupon he would storm out of the house and go to reside with his father for a few days. The approach taken by the therapist (Stanton) was to gently assert to the mother (individually) that her son was inescapably the son of her ex-husband also. The therapist suggested to her that perhaps it was time for him to get to know his father in a new way, a way that did not include his running to his father and telling him negative things about her. The therapist and mother agreed upon a plan with the following elements: (1) she was to tell her son that she recognized that he and his father were important to one another; (2) she was to suggest that the son make more regular, scheduled visits to the father, perhaps even spending part of the summer vacation with him; (3) she should not level any blame toward either son or father; (4) in talking to the son she was to try to avoid conveying any suppressed anger, overt nervousness, or ambivalence about these ideas, since the son would then not believe her; instead, she should talk in benevolent tones and a positive manner. (In fact, steps were taken to insure this by having the mother rehearse her message in the session, with the therapist present.) The mother carried out the task competently, and the son, after an initial reaction of disbelief, expressed relief. However, the mother had to press her position several times at home before her son would finally agree to visit his father. It should be noted that this intervention had several therapeutic effects: (1) through the mother's initiative, long-term conflict between the parents was reduced, at least as it directly affected and triangulated the son; (2) the mother relaxed her overinvolvement with her son, allowing new options to emerge—the system was derigidified; and (3) a new sequence was set in motion that did not include a crisis cycle involving escalation between mother and son. This process, along with other, concomitant interventions (e.g., establishing a support system for the mother, helping her get control of her household, etc.), eventually resulted in the son's ceasing his heavy use of drugs, attending school regularly, and coming home at appropriate hours.

## INTENSITY

Ours is a therapy of challenge to the family organization. To be effective, a challenge must have impact. Intensity is the technique by which the therapist controls the degree of impact, so that the message goes above the family's homeostatic threshold. Intensity can be varied in a number of ways, such as by increasing the affect, the duration of an enactment, or the cognitive frame (e.g., predicting dire consequences if the family doesn't change). Making the family responsible for carrying out the detoxification of a young adult, regardless of how difficult, is an intervention of tremendous intensity. With families of adolescent drug abusers, lower intensity interventions are usually sufficient. This is because the symptom is less severe, and because more moderate reorganization of existing structures is usually adequate, as compared to the older abuser group. Furthermore, since we are interested in maintaining the continuity of the present unit, the intensity can be of a more gentle sort.

In one family with divorced parents the IP was using marijuana very heavily. The therapist (Fishman) saw the IP as not receiving sufficient nurturance and attention from his parents. His father was battling leukemia, while his mother was changing careers. The parents were floundering, as they struggled with their life crises. The boy's symptom served both to bring the parents together so that they supported each other, and to provide him with an emotional involvement, since he had been isolated from his parents and peers. On the transactional level, the symptom was maintained by shifting coalitions between either parent and the youngster—first one parent, then the other, joined the boy in resisting the other parent.

The therapist worked with the adults toward engaging each of their respective social networks in order to give them more support in their struggles. Concurrently, the therapist worked individually with the youngster, as well as with the youngster and both parents, to support both sides of the hierarchy: the son was given the challenge of winning more autonomy, while the adults were helped to pull together as parents. After a brief "honeymoon" period, the boy was caught using marijuana at school. An uproar ensued in which the parents reverted to their previous pattern of initially undermining each other, followed by their losing interest in the boy's difficulties. The therapist utilized an intensity intervention—one of duration—and had three sessions a week in which he mobilized the family and gently pressured all parties involved to make the changes necessary. By following process, the therapist mounted a prolonged challenge to the family rules, while supporting and maintaining the members in proximity around the task. Signals from the system to move to another topic were ignored until the goal was achieved.

## UNBALANCING

This is the technique in which the therapist upsets the homeostasis by siding with one individual or subsystem. Breaking with the tradition of formal (if not real) neutrality, the therapist preferentially allies with one side.

The approach described with older abusers hinges on an intervention of unbalancing. The therapist sides with the parental subsystem, supporting the need for control of the addict. This support from the therapist creates a greatly strengthened parental hierarchy.

With younger adolescents, since the therapeutic goal is the continued maintenance of the present system, the therapist attempts to support the parental subsystem toward control of the youngster, while at the same time giving salience to the child's need for enhanced autonomy. In a sense, as Minuchin puts it, the therapist "works both sides of the street."*

What results is a therapy in which both sides of the hierarchy are supported and, while at points in the course of treatment there may be more support for one side, overall there is a softer, more equitable unbalancing. This type of unbalancing facilitates continued work with the entire therapeutic unit, since, in our experience, it is always necessary to join and support an adolescent. Furthermore, if this unit is going to maintain its cohesion, each side must recognize the legitimacy of the other's position.

As an example, a family came to therapy because their 17-year-old daughter used soft drugs heavily, stayed out to all hours (ignoring curfews set by the parents), and acted out sexually. The father and daughter were extremely overinvolved with one another. They shared an interest in music and spent many evenings listening to jazz. The father was extremely concerned over his daughter's outside activities. He questioned her in elaborate detail and attempted to mandate her every move—even to dictating the clothes she should wear.

*Salvador Minuchin (personal communication, April 1980).

The year that the father was laid off from his job, having still more time available to attend to his daughter as well as to disagree with his wife, all hell broke loose. The girl refused to follow the father's mandates. The parents told her that she must either follow the rules or she could move out. She chose the second option and went to live in a dangerous part of the city.

Presenting for the first session were a despondent, lonely, and pseudomature teenage girl, a depressed father, and a mother who was isolated and angry. As the family began speaking about the problem the father started to cry. Soon the girl was also welling up, while the mother became more and more taciturn.

The therapist intervened by supporting the parents' right to have control over their daughter's activities to the extent that they could be assured that she was safe. For the youngster, the therapist supported her right to have areas of autonomy. She needed emancipation from her father's intrusive and overcontrolling parenting.

By "working both sides of the street," the therapist was able to create a therapy where both the parents and daughter felt supported. Each advocated their position with increased forcefulness. The pattern of unmodulated flare-up, rapid retreat, and consequent lack of resolution was changed. Instead, compromise was attained. The parents told the daughter that she must come home—they would not allow her to continue to live on the streets. For her own part, the girl was able to negotiate more interpersonal space while in the parents' home. She was no longer obliged to fulfill her age-appropriate needs in the previously unmodulated and dangerous ways.

## SEARCH FOR STRENGTH

As demonstrated in Chapters 10 and 12, in this approach the therapist needs to search for competence, looking for areas of untapped strength and resources of the individual, as well as demonstrating to the family that each member has more skills and breadth than the family perceives. One aspect of this process is to dediagnose, that is, to destigmatize the IP while, at the same time, spreading the problem to underline the complementary familial correlates of the youngster's symptom. The therapist searches for those areas of strength in the child as well as in the other family members. This process both enhances joining and facilitates the adolescent's developmental need for individuation and differentiation.

Through the search for competence, both youngster and parents are engaged in the establishment and maintenance of new hierarchies. The drug-taking behavior can be seen as serving a function in the family, while the family operates to maintain the youngster as symptomatic and undifferentiated. Searching for competence allows family members enough distance to hold the child accountable and stop the ways in which they are supporting the youngster in the abuse. As with the example below, the youngster, by experiencing greater strength and competence both in the session and at home, separates from the family to some extent, becomes less available for defusing family conflicts, and gains the confidence to operate in other contexts in a more functional way. These changes thus challenge the dysfunctional family patterns and introduce new alternatives.

## COMPLEMENTARITY

Every member of a family is both a protagonist and an antagonist, both a responder and a creator of responses in others. For every behavior there is a reciprocal behavior in other significant people in a context that maintains the existent status quo. The question then becomes: If a person is taking drugs, what is the family doing to maintain that person as a drug taker? If one is depressed, the question becomes who is depressing him? By inquiring into the ways the person's context participates in maintaining him as he is, complementarity addresses the ultimate question of family therapy. Then the corollary question naturally arises: How can the context change so that different, more functional facets of the individual are called forth and rendered salient?

To illustrate, a family appeared for treatment in which the 14-year-old daughter had increasingly been using marijuana and sniffing glue, as well as having overdosed on her anticonvulsant medications as part of a suicide attempt. It was learned that the father, a blue collar worker, had recently been laid off. He remained at home all day, moping and drinking. Mother worked as a domestic and was the sole breadwinner, while the IP, who was mildly retarded, had become increasingly isolated from her friends over the past few months. Because of her overdose, she was obliged by the family, on the advice of mental health professionals, to stay at home. She and the father spent many hours together, while the mother grew increasingly disengaged from the family. The therapist (Fishman) challenged the family around the areas of complementarity: How could the parents act differently so the youngster would change? Conversely, how could the youngster change her behavior so that she had a different experience of herself and so that the parents, especially her father, would need to spend less time at home supervising her? In addition, the therapist utilized boundary-making techniques to help engage this quite isolated youngster with her peers. He used a teenager as a cotherapist in a few sessions, thereby creating norms for age-appropriate, peer-related behaviors. This helped to separate father and daughter. At the same time, the therapist exhorted father to seek vocational rehabilitation.

The search for strength was utilized by challenging the family's picture of the daughter as frail, mentally retarded, and socially inept. The therapist observed that when he interacted with the girl in a playful yet challenging way, she responded by being more socially appropriate, brighter, and even somewhat saucy. The therapist, using himself as an agent of change, sought to evoke more of these positive attributes in the girl. While the parents looked on, their daughter emerged as charming, warm, and loving—a person with extensive social skills, even though she was intellectually limited. Thus the therapist, by engaging the daughter in the session, provided the family with the experience of the youngster as socially poised, extroverted, and warm. The rules of the family organization tended to suppress such facets, but the therapist, challenging these rules, demonstrated to the family that the girl was more competent than they had perceived. This different experience led family members to make changes in the ways they interacted with the girl, ways that had maintained her as immature.* In this case, the immaturity and overprotection clashed with the developmental pressure of adolescence, which called for more autonomy and increased peer relationships. Drugs, then, provided a paradoxical resolution to these conflicting demands (see Chapter 1). With a change in the family pattern, the youngster no longer needed drugs for resolution, since the family allowed her more freedom to have experiences outside the family, thereby increasing her confidence. Her parents were then able to resolve some of their own difficulties. Father, since he no longer had

---

*Once the parents have recognized the positive features in their offspring, such changes can often be strengthened by giving the parents at least partial credit for the strengths. In this way the parents can bask in the praise and are less likely to counter the therapist if they see him as competing for their youngster.[160]

to stay home and take care of his daughter, was able and obliged to tend to his own developmental needs, including facing the demands of a midlife job change.

## SUMMARY

While many of the family patterns and therapeutic techniques discussed elsewhere in this book are applicable to families of both young adult addicts and adolescent drug abusers, there are also a number of clear differences between these two groups. In contrast to adult addicts, treatment of adolescent abusers is geared to a different developmental stage; rather than working for a separation between IP and parents, the family is kept intact, and shifts are effected within the given composition. This dictates the predominent use of techniques that are more typically structural in nature (e.g., enactment, unbalancing), in line with the structural emphasis on the developmental process in families with younger offspring. With both groups, great importance is attached to getting parents to work together, reinforcing the family's generational hierarchy. However, in families of young adults, emphasizing parental control is usually a transitional stage within the process of leaving home, while the goal with adolescent abusers is to achieve an intact, in-the-home hierarchy that remains in place at the end of therapy. Further, in treating this younger population the crisis aspects and level of intensity necessary for change are usually less extreme. Within this therapeutic framework, the therapist has many options for bringing about organizational and transformational change in the family—a number of which are illustrated here through clinical case examples. Our experience indicates that the approach described can be very effective in attaining desired goals and in producing beneficial change in families with an adolescent drug abuser.

# 14

## SUPERVISORS' VIEWS ON
## THE SPECIAL REQUIREMENTS OF
## FAMILY THERAPY WITH
## DRUG ABUSERS

THOMAS C. TODD
HENRY BERGER
GARY LANDE

THIS CHAPTER takes the form of a discussion between authors Todd, Berger, and Lande, all of whom served as supervisors within the Addicts and Families Program (AFP). The content will be a synthesis of separate recorded meetings held both between Berger and Todd, and between Lande and Todd.

### THE ROLE OF THE SUPERVISOR

*TODD:* Why don't we begin by talking generally about the role of the clinical supervisor in the family therapy of drug abusers?

*LANDE:* One of the crucial things I see is that the clinical supervisor is constantly talking with the therapist about sharpening goals: "What are the goals, where are you going, how far are you?" That is so important in maintaining the clinical tension. In the Addicts and Families Program, the expectation of getting this work done in ten sessions was important—it put a certain pressure on the supervisor, who in turn had to put pressure on the therapist. I don't know how many therapists could keep that kind of pressure on themselves. Anorexia was different, because with anorexia there was the built-in pressure from the weight loss of the children we were seeing.* In the AFP, the research put a certain pressure on the supervisor; "Duke" [M. Duncan] Stanton would call me periodically to see if the cases were progressing. It's a new role for the supervisor because, in general, a supervisor in the Clinic is usually the last resort when administrative pressure is needed. Here, it clearly wasn't that way—I worked for Duke.

*BERGER:* I think there are two goals, really, in supervising drug cases. I guess they are always present in supervision, but much more so in working with therapists who are working with addicts and their families. Probably they are not unlike therapists who are working with schizophrenics and their families. The first thing is to try and give the therapists something concrete that they can use therapeutically—that is, strategies for the case. That is what you always try to do in supervision.

*TODD:* There is really a mixture of general principles and strategies, which are discussed earlier in this book [Chapter 6]. They include keeping the parents together as a team, getting the addict out of the middle between his parents, focusing on concrete examples of behavior, assigning "homework" between sessions, and generally following a Haley–Minuchin modified structural–strategic approach.

*BERGER:* The second thing is to keep therapists from wearing themselves out, from feeling worn out, from burning themselves out, by both trying to advise them and give them some distance, but also in trying to make the supervision a place where ideas are generated and where they feel that there is something valuable going on.

*TODD:* It sounds like a combination of stimulation and support.

*BERGER:* Right—I really think that the combination of the two is crucial. One of the things I learned was that the best way to support them was to become more involved than I initially thought I would. It wasn't until I started supervising live in some cases that I became effective as a supervisor. I then realized how difficult these cases are, and the therapists saw that I realized. That was a big turning point in supervision. It was brought home to me what they were dealing with, so I think live supervision is particularly important with these kinds of families.

I have to use the word "countertransference." These families create enormous fantasies of rescue and enormous feelings of frustra-

---

*Editors' note.* Lande had earlier worked on the Psychosomatic Research Project (described in the Preface) and anorexia nervosa was the presenting problem in the majority of the cases in that project.

tion in the therapist. I think it has something to do with the horrible nature of what is going on, the sort of slow suicide that these men get themselves into, as well as the horrible things that the addicts end up doing to their families. It is easy to become enraged at them for being so incredibly destructive, either of themselves or of their families, and to try to save them. It can overwhelm you. My most crucial experience happened when I was talking about a case of David Heard's. We talked for a while, but I just could not understand why David was spending so much time with this guy, hours and hours, it seemed. He even went to a bar once and had some drinks with the patient, and I kept asking, "What the hell's going on?"

At David's request, I stayed late a couple of evenings for live supervision. Possibly as a coincidence, or possibly as a reaction of the family to my presence as an unknown observer, the latent violence of the family exploded to the point where the patient pulled out a knife as he argued with his father. Fortunately, no one was injured, but it was obvious that the presence of that degree of danger and rage must be felt by the therapist. It naturally tends to draw him in as a needed guardian and a safeguard against overt expression.

After that, we learned something strategically, but I also developed a lot more respect for what these therapists were up against. In addition, I stopped being so grandiose about the goals, so that my expectations were not as great any more, and we began to sit back and say, "Let's see what we can do in ten weeks with these families," since that was the setup for the research design of the project. I became much more relaxed, and the clinical work became much more productive during the final half of the year that we were working. Then we had a couple of families that seemed to go fairly well. I started enjoying the supervision a lot more because I also felt less pressure on me; that case was a crucial turning point.

## AVOIDING POWER STRUGGLES

*TODD:* You probably also became more able to keep the therapists from getting locked into power struggles, becoming grandiose, et cetera.

*BERGER:* I think that in my supervision up to that point I was still thinking that you could somehow establish the right structure to control the addict. I learned through my own experience that you could not do that, which then took the pressure off the therapist. Then we started really looking for what we could do, and it became much more productive.

*TODD:* Is there anything else that went on in the supervision that you felt helped keep the therapist from getting sucked in, particularly from getting into power struggles with the addict?

*BERGER:* Well, I certainly learned a lot from that family. The reality of what you could do was driven home by that one experience, so that I no longer demanded that the therapists do something in terms of controlling this behavior, which eased the pressure on the therapist.

I guess the third thing was the intellectual stimulation. We started thinking more about these families, and at that point, I got interested. Suddenly it was more than simply a couple of hours a week. I think you have to be more committed to this kind of work—it takes a lot of effort. We started thinking about the cases; it became interesting and some fascinating things did happen, and we could talk about them among the three of us. That is where we got our rewards— instead of having to succeed or having to accomplish something with this patient, we began to get our rewards from what we were learning about these families, and so that took the pressure off.

*TODD:* And then you started to be more successful, also.

*BERGER:* Right—there was much less pressure on the supervisor, and on the therapist. Consequently, there was less pressure from the therapist on the family and the patient. Probably then the same thing happened with the families—they became more interested, more curious, or at least less enraged, less personally involved with the addict. The effect went right down the line.

*TODD:* I think avoiding power struggles is one of the most important problems with these cases. It is not completely unique to this population; I encounter it also with anorectics, which is another situation where the patient is always looking for a fight. The problem is how to avoid a very rigid power struggle between parents and patient, or between the therapist and patient.

*BERGER:* Or between supervisor and therapist. There is a kind of mirroring. Jay Haley talks about the symmetrical behavior between the supervisor and the therapist, and the therapist and the family.

*TODD:* Did you see any other ways in which that kind of mirroring took place?

*BERGER:* In terms of the AFP itself, I experienced the same kind of shift with that particular family. Until that point, I was working on the assumption that I was to be able to help the therapist, to help the addict get off methadone and get off drugs in ten weeks.

*TODD:* In "ten easy lessons."

*BERGER:* I was supposed to be able to do this—I had the same pressure. The project attitude seemed to be, "Cure 'em in ten weeks; we've got to be able to do it." It has become clearer to me that we were actually trying to see what family therapy could accomplish in ten weeks. Realizing that took a lot of pressure off me. Then my attitude became, "Let's see what these families are really like," instead of imposing some preconceived notion about what they were like.

## COMPETITION

*TODD:* Gary, I would be interested to know if you had any feelings of competition with the other supervisors in the project.

*LANDE:* No. The cases were all at different stages and we changed supervisees several times. If there was competition, it might have been among the therapists. It seemed that in this project, the "thrill of victory and the agony of defeat" would be the therapist's. I think that another reason there was little or no competition among supervisors was because the supervisors had less day-to-day organizational contact. It's interesting that the fact that the supervisors were in some ways slightly removed from the project may have helped keep the therapy focused. I was never caught up in the administrative issues—Duke protected me. Since mine was a purely clinical involvement, it allowed a certain purism in the supervision.

There has subsequently been a change at PCGC [Philadelphia Child Guidance Clinic] in the supervisory system. There is now a "core" or administrative supervisor in addition to the clinical supervisor. I think there's a certain wisdom in that, because the therapist can keep a purely positive relationship with the clinical supervisor. I think these relationships are essential and I think they do have something to do with the success of the project.

*TODD:* I was wondering if any problems were created by the fact that the AFP utilized part-time therapists and supervisors who were only available a few hours a week. Did you ever get into situations where you felt that the therapists needed you to be more available, when they were dealing with crises and might spend a whole week on a case? Did that ever get to be a problem in terms of supervision?

*LANDE:* It didn't, because I had emphasized peer support in supervision. Paul Riley, at times, really became a supervisor; often the therapists used him that way. Paul provided a great deal of live supervision, with many concrete recommendations. He would say, "Why don't you do such and such?" The other therapists trusted him, and they knew somehow that he really knew what to do. I used him explicitly as a peer supervisor, because I wasn't here full-time. Even though there weren't really that many crises that couldn't be settled on the phone, Paul was often available when I was not. That would be another reason for not using one-to-one supervision [see Chapters 6, 9, and 16].

*TODD:* Henry [Berger], earlier Gary [Lande] made a different point about the positive aspects of the pressure—he felt that it was useful to have the clear expectation of getting people off of heroin and methadone, and getting them out of the house, within a brief period. Without the unspoken competition among therapists, he did not think half as much would have ever happened.

*BERGER:* That's probably true. I guess from my point of view, I was too caught up in the other extreme, so how do you balance that? My experience was that, when the expectation was a little bit relieved, then it sort of went down the line and we didn't push quite as hard. Of course, we still pushed.

*TODD:* We still pushed the families in some kind of way. The expectation was there, and the time frame was there.

*BERGER: Something* should happen.

*TODD:* But I think that when you are free to back off a little bit, or reinterpret what it means for the addict to slip up, that makes you a lot freer, because it means that you can continue to define what success is.

*BERGER:* And you don't get into a win or lose situation, either as supervisor with the therapist, or as therapist with the patient. You can't lose. Once you get out of that bind, then the patient can't win and can't defeat you, and it becomes a whole different thing.

*TODD:* That is extremely important, because these guys are out to beat you.

*BERGER:* It's true in all therapy, but in this therapy it's extremely important. Although these patients are so inept at so many things in life, they are terrific at maneuvering this particular system around drugs. You just have to realize that compared to them, you are absolutely naive in that area, and so of course they can defeat you; there is no way around it.

*TODD:* Again, it speaks to the problem of the supervisor getting set up as an expert. It is a general principle in crisis intervention work that if there is a really rigid hierarchy, the person at the top of the hierarchy is always going to get burned, because the stress goes up the ladder. The people below are always going to say, "This guy does not understand what we have to deal with, the complexity and difficulty of it," which is exactly what the family says to the therapist.

One of the things that Gary felt strongly about was that in these cases sharing was really important, that it was the kind of situation where one-to-one supervision was a really bad idea. I think partly because of that, and partly to dilute the relationship between the therapist and the supervisor, he also emphasized peer sharing in supervision and made it much more of a partnership.

*BERGER:* I think that also evolved in our supervision. When I was able to stop being the "expert," and we all put our heads together, then the supervision went better. I don't know what it would be like if we met in one-to-one supervision. I guess you could still try to make it a peer relationship, but it's much harder to do.

## COMPARISON TO OTHER POPULATIONS

*TODD:* I would be interested in similarities and differences between these families and the families seen in other Clinic projects, particularly the Psychosomatic[101, 104] and Schizophrenia[66] projects.

*BERGER:* In the psychosomatic families, we talk about the style being "detouring protective." It's a lot easier to get sucked into being protective of or sympathetic toward a sixteen-year-old helpless girl who weighs fifty-five pounds and who is obviously being starved for affection, et cetera. Addict families are more like the families of diabetics with behavioral problems, where we talk about "detouring attacking." It's much easier to become—also inappropriately—attacking and scapegoating and blaming. You can blame the families; you can blame the addict. You can treat somebody who is sick or asthmatic, or starving and anorectic. When it comes to somebody who breaks the law, who is out there stealing and robbing, or cheating and lying, and who does the same thing to you as a therapist, that is difficult to tolerate. It is easy to get very angry about that. That is one big difference—just what it does to the therapist. It is not right to be so protective of the anorectic, and it is not effective to be so attacking or controlling in the families of addicts.

With other kinds of families, the symptoms are less dramatic and create less heat. If you work with a behavioral problem in a school-age child, it doesn't create the same feeling—you have more distance.

I think there also are some basic differences in the families themselves. It has something to do with the type of people who make up the families of an anorectic versus the kind who make up the families of these addicts. It is harder for most therapists to identify with them. The selection of the group as veterans may also make them a narrow cross-section of the population. Most of the families in the AFP were lower income and blue collar working families; alcoholism was an issue in many of them. This is in contrast to the mostly middle-class families seen in the work with anorectics. There's another aspect for me of working with Vietnam veterans, which I think played a very real role. I don't think anybody can look at a twenty-six- or twenty-eight-year-old drug addict who started his habit in Vietnam and is now having a wasted life and not make a connection to Vietnam, not get angry at what the war did to them. It may be that a lot of these men would never have begun using drugs if they hadn't been in the war.*

*TODD:* I was thinking about the whole question of violence in these families, especially the acting out and explosiveness. I personally have a real problem with that and would really be scared with some of these guys.

*BERGER:* The violence generally seemed to come primarily from the addict or his siblings. Usually the fathers were pretty placid, ineffectual, and nonviolent types. The mothers were somewhat depressed and overinvolved. The underlying threat of violence could often be felt.

It's true that it is very scary—I'm not used to people pulling a knife. I think in terms of selecting therapists, you need to have

---

*Editors' note.* In reality, only 32.5% of the AFP cases were Vietnam veterans and almost everyone in this subgroup was addicted or used drugs very heavily before his Vietnam tour. Further, 90–95% of servicemen who were addicted to heroin in Vietnam did not become readdicted upon return to the United States.[145, 156] somebody very confident; physical strength may also help. There were times when both David Heard and David Mowatt would tell me about how absolutely terrified they were, being in a room with a patient who had threatened them. The therapists who were able to handle it were able to communicate that they would not take any of that stuff.

*TODD:* It's hard to know who will be able to do that—it certainly isn't just a matter of size. I have a friend who is about five feet tall who has done an incredible amount of crisis work in the emergency room. She handles belligerent drunks even when the police are terrified. She just comes in there and grabs them by the arm and says, "Come on, Buster."

*BERGER:* She must have a tremendous amount of confidence. I don't have that much confidence—what I did when I was working in emergency rooms was simply use a show of force. If I was dealing with someone very paranoid or a very drunk guy, I would call in a couple of the staff and they would sit in the room and everything was fine and I was comfortable, so the patient was comfortable. We never had to do anything. It was when you felt cornered or threatened that the anxiety became contagious. That woman obviously has more confidence. The important thing is for the therapist to be able to call on whatever resources he needs to maintain confidence in his safety and control of the situation.

## NECESSARY QUALITIES OF THE THERAPIST

*LANDE:* The selection of therapists was a complicated issue. There were differences in the level of clinical experience among the therapists I supervised.* Working with these different therapists raised some basic issues about what the treatment required. My feeling was that addiction cases were among the hardest anybody could ever see. In terms of family structure, it may not have been obvious that they were harder. Where the difficulty resided was in gaining leverage for change. You couldn't tell the parents that the addict who was on methadone was about to die, as you might in the anorexia cases. These cases really required more than just the knowledge of what was dysfunctional in the family structure. It required a

*Editors' note.* The major considerations in selecting therapists for the AFP are presented in the Preface.

therapist who was able to convert a person away from what had been not just a destructive symptom, but a whole way of life. I told Duke that this requirement would be hard to meet, even with excellent structural therapists. It was very important to me to bring in people like Peter Urquhart and Paul Riley, who had the talents of an active therapist. I just did not believe that a cookbook approach would work or that you could develop a simple series of steps for anyone to follow. I think that was the hardest part of the therapy, and that therapists like Paul and Peter could do it (even though they had totally different styles) because they were both flexible and creative.

I don't think that structural family therapy alone is enough because it leaves out the way different therapists work. Basically, the AFP assembled a group of clinicians who were well grounded in structural family therapy. Their experience levels differed, but those who seemed more successful knew how to get people to change. The less experienced therapists had to learn some of these techniques—that was very much part of my supervision. I used Paul as a model for Jerry Kleiman, to help Jerry develop those skills.

The other thing is that this is a crisis type of therapy. The majority of cases in the Clinic weren't really like the drug cases. In most of these cases, if you stuck to basic principles of family therapy, and you kind of "hung in" with the family, that would be sufficient. Management of the PCGC day-treatment and inpatient cases was more similar to drug cases.

People used to talk about the personality of the therapist. Recently, Minuchin has pursued this, but he talks about the limits of the therapist, the style of the therapist. A therapist can't confront an addict about the results of a urine report if he feels he is going to be intimidated by threats of violence. You have to be able to really build a critical tension. I remember a couple of sessions where Jerry Kleiman was in a position where the addict was likely to hit him. It was absolutely necessary that he let the tension build to that point. Jerry was able to use, control, and help to release tension, but I can imagine that some therapists could not do so.

Duke and I talked about the different possibilities that would have been generated if the therapists had been females who were working with these male addicts. We don't know whether similar issues of violence would have been likely to be triggered with females as therapists. Some of the street addicts could be rough, and the whole task was to gain their respect—gaining their respect without talking directly about it. Paul Riley was a verbal artist. He was respected because he moved one step faster than the addicts, and thus could catch their attention. This was the beginning step. How do you train people to gain respect? It may be simpler to select therapists who can already do this naturally, rather than to try to train them in it. I think the key to the success of the therapy was the combination of training in structural principles, together with some of these special skills that the therapists brought to their work.

*BERGER:* I had some additional thoughts about the selection of therapists. I agree with Gary that many therapists are not cut out to work with these cases.

One thing I noted was that hard work and persistence were definitely not enough. If a therapist got locked into a rigid stance with a family, increasing the effort was almost completely unproductive.

At the other extreme, I saw some built-in dangers with a very creative and flexible therapist. It seems to me that one crucial aspect of this work is accountability, from project to supervisor, to therapist, to parents, to the addict. If you get a therapist who wants to bend the rules too much, this chain breaks down. Then it is likely that there will be the same struggle between the supervisor and the therapist as between the therapist and the patient. The therapist may then feel allied with the patient against the system, and may covertly encourage the patient's antisocial behavior. I also felt the supervisor should not be concerned with enforcing the project's rules. I didn't like pressure to be looking over the therapist's shoulder to see if he was working. I had a couple of meetings with Duke to say, "I'm not going to see that he does his job, I'm there as an advisor," which had not been clear.

*TODD:* I think that experience was helpful, because by the time Gary came into the Project, the split in roles was really clear, and he felt that he was free to focus on clinical issues and sympathize with people: "Yeah, it's impossible," "It's hard."

*BERGER:* That is what you need to do.

*TODD:* And play off against Duke and the administrative hierarchy and say, "Well, Duke is saying, 'You've got to do this.' You know, I understand it's almost impossible, but Duke is saying it," and that made it more palatable to the therapist. Duke made it clear that he didn't mind being portrayed as a taskmaster as long as that made the supervisor's job easier.

*BERGER:* There's a mirroring there with the family, because the therapist can turn around in working with the addict and say,

"Look, it's really a shame that you are going to get put in jail because you held that place up. I know you need the money and the dope, but the law's the law. I wish I could help you out." It's a very reciprocal thing. We divide it the same way in supervision. I was very happy to have Duke seen that way.

The third kind of therapist who is a potential problem is one who handles his difficulties with these cases by becoming extremely private and defensive about his work and not asking for help from the supervisor. With these cases, there seems to be pressures to exclude outside advice. I experienced some of these pressures as a supervisor.

At one point, we were getting very conflicting advice from Jay Haley and Sal Minuchin and other senior clinicians. It was very confusing, and you can defend and protect yourself from confusion by not asking anybody for anything: "I'm not going to let anybody confuse me. I am going to go on ahead and do what I think is right." In the long run, that doesn't work—you have to be able to pull back and say, "I don't know, I'd better ask. They may not know much more, but we better kick around some ideas." New ideas create anxiety. You have to be a strong enough person as a therapist or supervisor to take what you hear and use that part which you can incorporate and not be upset about the part that you can't incorporate—that takes a lot of flexibility.

*TODD:* Flexibility seems so important. The therapist needs to be able to move from conceptualizing and just having an intellectual curiosity about everything and then switch to being very immediate and involved—it is a very hard combination to find.

*BERGER:* That's right, you sort of move back and forth. As a supervisor, I move back and forth from sitting back and thinking about a paper, to actually seeing the family with the therapist.

*TODD:* It's interesting, because the notion of back and forth movement, particularly for people who have worked with Sal, is not new. It seems to be much more extreme in these families—when you are in there, you are *really* in there. To get back, it seems like you almost have to move farther back.

## DEALING WITH DENIAL AND DISTORTION

*LANDE:* It's really hard to separate out the crucial ingredients of the therapy. One important factor was to break down a tremendous system of denial in the families of addicts. The family members showed an incredible ability to distort the reality of what was going on, in order to excuse or overlook distasteful situations. There was a session that Gerald Hawthorne did a few years ago that was an absolute classic. The father made some statements that were totally twisted around by the addict and the mother. The father said, "I found this little plastic bag" [a heroin container]. The discussion went on for an hour, and at the end they had the father convinced that he had never even *seen* it. It was like magic, how they first started asking him about the size, what size it was, what was it made of. And by the end, they had convinced him that he had never seen the bag. The style of the therapist and the style of the supervisor had to be sensitive to the family style, in order to unobtrusively intervene into it, because neither the addict nor the family wanted to change their familiar patterns.

In the anorexia cases, the parents wanted the child to live, wanted the child to stop losing weight. Some of the drug families we saw didn't even want to be there, which raised the whole issue of what type of training was needed to recruit these reluctant families. Once the family was there, they didn't necessarily want the son to stop taking drugs. It wasn't very clear that anybody except the therapist wanted anything changed. It was a very intricate system, compared to traditional therapy. I think it required very careful supervision. Many times, the therapist would come up against such pressure, lack of cooperation, and active fighting that the only way to keep the motivation up was in supervision.

## THE PUBLIC NATURE OF THE RESULTS OF THERAPY

*LANDE:* I had worked for three years with young schizophrenics, and I had also done a lot of work with anorectics. When I think about the supervisory process, it seems much more akin to what I went through with psychosomatic and schizophrenic families. I remember I used to tell people that these cases were dramatically different from most cases, because if something went wrong, the child would be in the hospital and everybody would know whose case it was. The results were totally up front, putting absolute pressure on the therapist in a way that was very different from most other outpatient cases. In typical outpatient cases, nobody knew whether the child hit his brother last week or didn't hit his brother. The situation could easily be defined one way or the other. With AFP cases, there was always a tension that was present—if the addict overdosed, or the addict went back on heroin, the results were clear and public.

A very clever aspect of the administrative meetings was the unspoken process of making the progress (or lack of it) of the therapist's cases public [see Chapter 16]. There was always the potential of being shamed, and this set up a tremendous level of competition that no one ever talked about. The use of two people simultaneously in supervision was another aspect of keeping the therapy in the open. These cases were so difficult that just having to face your own results with your supervisor didn't give a clear enough overview of what other people were experiencing and accomplishing. I felt that this overview was an important part of supervision. I don't think a one-to-one supervision would have been as good.

*TODD:* I remember my experience with an anorectic case, where I had a very stormy lunch session. I remember very, very acutely that Sal Minuchin had said over and over, "It's impossible for a decent family therapist to fail." When you see me on the tape, it's obvious that I'm determined that I'm not going to fail, and even if it takes all afternoon we're going to stay until it's over. The other factor was that I wasn't dealing with the family by myself—there were probably six people behind the mirror. There was a lot of discussion about cases, a sense that the results were for the whole team, so no one was really alone, even though the shame would have been excruciating.

*LANDE:* I know, in terms of the supervisors in the Addicts and Families Program, that this public sharing of results was a key part of the supervision, and that nobody planned it. Without that element, much less would have happened. It reminded me very much of my own experience when I participated in competitive wrestling. There was always that dual element of trying to win for yourself and for the team. However, if you lost, you not only had to deal with a personal loss, but with compromising the team's results.

I see another similarity here to psychosomatic families. Both psychosomatic and drug cases are very difficult and they burn out a lot of people. The people who survive often end up with excellent training and strength. If they could cure *those* cases, other issues seemed easy in comparison. I felt the same way when you mentioned how much Jerry Kleiman changed. It was a combination of many qualities. He really had a lot of potential; he was enthusiastic and bright, he had good supervision, and he had a lot of encouragement. People who survive this as part of their training end up working at a more skillful level.

## STRESSES ON THE THERAPIST

*LANDE:* How do you keep people working with cases that are really very difficult and where the rewards are not that clear-cut? How do you convince therapists that they should make as many calls as necessary just to get a family to come initially to therapy? It's a fairly unique situation, not only in terms of strategy, but in maintaining the therapist's feeling that he's even doing therapy. I think part of the answer to keeping the therapist motivated was in the supervisory process and part was in the general project design. I was struck by a parallel between (1) the stress produced by the research design on the supervisors, and (2) the supervisors' stress on the therapist. You sometimes talk about supervision in terms of the parallel between what the supervisor does with the therapist and what the therapist does with the case. This was yet another level where there was a parallel in terms of administrative level, the research design level, and it seemed to carry all the way down the chain of command.

I think the high morale that was in the Addicts and Families Program was quite dramatic. The whole issue of how to keep some sense of optimism was interesting. A great deal of enthusiasm was brought in by the therapists, along with an expectation that they could do the therapy in a straightforward manner. All of them had a good background in terms of basic structural principles, and they were good in clinical theory, but they were not necessarily used to the particular pressures of working with such life-and-death matters. They have all evolved into better therapists through the program. The process of becoming competent in handling addiction cases is interesting. My view is that the supervisor can help the therapist to keep from getting hooked or locked into a power struggle with manipulative patients—he helps them to maintain some kind of flexibility or looseness. This ability of not getting hooked in a power struggle with the addict was perhaps the single most important skill for some of the therapists to learn. The addict was continually seducing and inviting the therapist into some kind of struggle—whether over methadone doses, urine results, et cetera. To the addict, these struggles were his way of life, his religion. The therapist needed to learn that in any attempt by him to confront the addict, or to manipulate him around these issues, the addict would usually win.

*TODD:* It is clear that these cases were different, because therapists placed such an emphasis on maintaining a degree of distance from the case and on obtaining additional rewards for themselves. Both of these factors seemed to contribute to the interest shown by many of the AFP therapists in publishing papers—they probably attributed more importance to this than most therapists at PCGC.

*BERGER:* Most outpatient therapists don't need that much distance—that is a good point. I think there is such a difference between a family that comes in with a ten-year-old who is having a little bit of trouble in school or wetting his bed, and somebody who is out there, robbing, selling and shooting dope, absolutely abusing all those around him and himself.

In working with drug addicts, you can't get paid enough. You'd be crazy to put all that effort in and not get something. So here we are, working on a book and you damn well need that. You have to tell the world what you've been through and what you did.

*TODD:* It's hard to generalize about which rewards were most important. I was just thinking about the role of money in the project. For some families, it was quite important. On the other hand, we had a lot of situations where family members, parents in particular, felt insulted by the money and felt, "We're not doing this for money."*

*BERGER:* But it's there. At least the [Paid] families can say to themselves, "We're not being conned once more by this guy, this addict in our midst. At least we're getting five bucks a shot." And the therapists—who got paid fifty dollars for every case they brought in [see Chapters 5 and 16]—it was not a lot of money, but at least they could say, "I'm not being taken advantage of."

*TODD:* Money did seem important, at least symbolically. I remember before the project began to generate some excitement and prestige, it seemed like this issue of money arose frequently. If somebody was being asked to work on Clinic time—just give up a day and see a couple of addicts—they resisted. But they would do it if they got extra pay—it seemed that the money helped preserve their self-respect.

*Editors' note.* Only half the families who were seen in family therapy received reimbursement. Details are provided in Chapters 2 and 17, and Appendix C.

*BERGER:* True, the money seemed to have symbolic significance. At one point there was a delay in getting staff members' checks, and it came up in the AFP team meeting. The rage, the heat, was intense—it was like a lynch mob. That seemed to me to indicate how important the money was to prevent the therapists from feeling like they were suckers or being "ripped off."

## MEDICAL SUPERVISION

*TODD:* One of the things I was struck by is that within the AFP you and Gary were the only medical people involved directly in the family therapy and were the two main supervisors. Were there any ways in which the MD became important and seemed to make a difference in the supervision?

*BERGER:* I think in a very practical way there sometimes were questions about the drugs being used, and we were kind of a resource. One problem is that there is always the temptation for the supervisor to come on like an expert, and the medical degree added to that tendency, as well as encouraging people to put things on your shoulder. On the other hand, it was certainly useful in dealing with the VA and outside agencies, who listen more to an MD. One clinical thing is that your training as a doctor keeps you from being as frightened by people who overdose or threaten suicide or are seriously ill. It's not that overwhelming to me, and I would hope that some of that got across to the therapists I was supervising. That's simply a result of being exposed to it in your medical training.

*LANDE:* I would say that one way that medical issues came up was when the therapist also became the drug counselor. I think that my being a medical doctor became an important transitional support system in this process. Another way in which being a medical doctor seemed relevant was in helping the therapist to deal with patients who were more expert with medications and drugs than they were. Here, the supervisor's medical expertise could often help the therapist to withstand the addict's manipulations and maintain a sense of reality without getting into a power struggle with the addict. I also think, like Henry, that being a medical doctor made a difference because we are used to dealing with life-threatening crises, which probably helped my supervisees to keep a perspective and not panic at critical times.

## SUMMARY AND CONCLUSIONS

*TODD:* It is clear we all agree that the families of drug abusers are among the most difficult families that a therapist may ever see, certainly as difficult as psychosomatic or psychotic cases. Many factors account for this difficulty, including the threat of violence and the potential for major crises to erupt at any moment. The families are usually resistant, not really asking for change, and tend to feel blamed very easily. Many of them had virtually abandoned hope by the time we saw them. The therapist also must deal with the knowledge that his success or failure is likely to be completely public, and that there is always the possibility of dramatic failure, such as an overdose or criminal arrest. All of these qualities combine to create powerful effects on the therapist, ranging from fear and frustration to grandiose fantasies of rescue.

These cases demand from the therapist a unique combination of emotional involvement, flexibility, and task orientation in the face of crisis. Obviously, the experience of many therapists has not prepared them for this kind of work. It is interesting, though, that the AFP therapists were not unusually experienced or highly trained. What they seemed to have in common was solid basic training in structural and strategic family therapy, plus the (natural or acquired) abilities to maneuver quickly and to motivate people to change without confrontation. It also needs to be said that therapists usually emerge from this work functioning at a much higher level of competence than before they began.

The supervisor's job is also demanding, requiring several kinds of aid to the therapist. The supervisor must help the therapist maintain a strategic overview, keeping the goals in mind. Concrete expectations are always there, ideally coupled with a relatively fixed time frame, but at times the supervisor needs to help relieve the pressure on the therapist. This is particularly important in keeping the therapist from becoming "locked in" to a power struggle with the addict or the family. The supervisor plays a key role in increasing the flexibility of the therapist by creating a supervisory climate of peer support and "brainstorming" of new ideas. Finally, the supervisor must communicate real support to the therapist by acknowledging the difficulty of the cases and, more tangibly, by being available for crises and for live supervision.

We also are saying that factors beyond the supervision are crucial to insure success. In the long run, both therapist and supervisor can burn out and become demoralized without overall support from the program. Here [and in Chapters 6 and 16] several ways in which administration can help are mentioned; these are applicable in any program and do not depend on the structure of a special research project. They include:

1. Commitment of resources. There should be some "pay-off" to the therapist for extending himself to the degree often required with these cases. Monetary rewards are not essential, although they are certainly helpful. The most critical resources are sufficient time to do the clinical work and adequate supervision. Increased prestige is also important. We talked about publications, but similar results could also be obtained by having therapists present cases and conduct training.

2. Flexibility. The program should encourage, not penalize, therapist flexibility in scheduling, making home visits, et cetera.

3. Administrative backing for the supervisor. The supervisor's job is hard enough on a clinical level without being further complicated by administrative demands. It is important to separate responsibility for administrative duties such as time sheets, record keeping, dictation, et cetera. Otherwise, the supervisor's role becomes contaminated, and power struggles between therapist and supervisor become more likely.

4. Control of the case. The supervisor's role can become impossible unless he and the therapist fit within a hierarchy such that the therapist is in charge of the crucial aspects of the case. In the AFP, this included having the family therapist also function as the drug counselor. Potential medical conflicts were probably reduced by having supervisors who were psychiatrists. Other programs should look carefully at the issue of where the family therapist fits within the treatment hierarchy.

# 15

## COMMENT ON STRATEGIES AND TECHNIQUES

THOMAS C. TODD
M. DUNCAN STANTON

IN CHAPTER 6 a comprehensive treatment model for the family therapy of drug abuse is presented. Chapters 7 through 14 offer rich clinical and theoretical amplification of this model. We anticipate that many readers, particularly those who are not sophisticated family therapists, may not always see clearly how the specific cases follow the general model and may be curious about the basis for some of the variations among the cases. The purpose of this chapter is to compare the previous cases, to discuss the basis for the differences, and finally, to illustrate how the model can be extended to other populations.

It is obvious that there are major differences among the chapters, but these differences should not obscure the underlying unity of approach. Many of the differences are simply differences in therapist style. Each of the therapists uses himself in his own way to accomplish therapeutic goals. While the particular "moves" of the therapists may differ considerably, the underlying goals are generally quite similar. There are also differences in writing style and in the focus of the chapters—some focus more on theory or commonalities across cases, while others present a more detailed examination of particular cases. Finally, the end product is dependent to a considerable degree on whether the primary author is the therapist himself, an observer or supervisor, or a nonclinician.

The reader may also be struck by the difference in tone (and, of course, the degree of formality) between Chapter 14 (on supervision) and the chapters that precede it. That chapter, and perhaps Chapter 9 (on crisis induction), describe a much more emotional side of our work. It might seem difficult to reconcile the tension and affect depicted in these chapters with the more conceptual discourse set forth elsewhere. At least two factors contributed to this contrast.

First, once a case is completed, much of the "heat" dissipates and the therapist (and his coauthors) can perhaps look back and analyze what transpired from a more "rational" perspective—a luxury he was not afforded while in the midst of the fray. Thus his writings assume a "distant" quality that may make the work look easier than it actually was. Second, supervisors obviously are more likely to be summoned at crisis points by those they supervise. They function like lightning rods for tough situations and the kind of information they receive is often screened to include only the most intense problems. This probably influences their perception of the ongoing work, and can be expected to emerge in their thinking and writing about the therapeutic process (which we suspect is partly the case in Chapter 14). In sum, the "truth" about the clinical material in Chapters 6 through 14 probably lies somewhere between these two extremes in perspective.


## DISCUSSION OF THE CASE EXAMPLES

There is no intention on our part to deny the complexity of therapy or to imply that a simple set of principles will suffice. The chapter on supervision offers particular testimony to the difficulty presented by these cases and discusses the array of specific skills and characteristics that a therapist needs either to possess or learn in order to succeed.

As we cover important clinical issues, we hope it will become more obvious that the cases show flexible application of common principles. We believe that these principles provide a common thread, or perhaps a "lifeline," that unifies the therapy and keeps the therapist from being overwhelmed by the confusing details and chaotic crises that addicts and their families present. As demonstrated in the case material, it should be apparent that the therapist needs to move strategically and stay a step or two ahead of the addict if he is to succeed in bringing about change.


### THERAPEUTIC GOALS

In Chapter 6, the three major goals of family treatment are described, in order of priority: (1) freedom from both illegal and legal drugs, including methadone; (2) productive use of time; (3) a stable living situation, not living with parents. Initially, the implementation of these goals may have seemed straightforward, but reading the clinical material in Chapters 7 through 14 should have disabused the reader of any such illusions of simplicity.

It is important to emphasize that these may initially be goals of the *therapist*. The family can be expected to display a good deal of ambivalence about the goals, and the addict may be in outright opposition to some of them. That does *not* mean that the therapist should *directly comment* on their resistance or ambivalence, but rather that the goals of therapy must be shaped gradually. In particular, it is vital to keep the parents working with the therapist and have them clearly endorse any statement of therapeutic goals. Usually, the first step is to obtain a public statement from the parents early in therapy about the ideal goals of therapy, particularly in relation to drugs. Even though the therapist knows that the initial statement is too general to be meaningful, often having the flavor of "Mom and apple pie," he knows that it can be used as a basis for more concrete elaboration as the treatment progresses.

The approach used here is in marked contrast to many of the procedures commonly applied with drug abusers in group therapy and therapeutic communities, which emphasize directness, confrontation, and genuineness. While it would be easy for a therapist to confront the addict directly on his manipulative behavior, from a family perspective this is contraindicated, since there is a high risk that it will backfire. Instead, the therapist should take special pains to bring the parents and other family members along with him and then have the confrontation come from *them*, rather than from him. Otherwise, the parents and family are apt to desert him and unite in defending the addict against this "harsh therapist."

Our ideal therapeutic goals always include full-time employment or school and the establishment of a stable living situation outside the parental home. Often the 10-session contract prevented full realization of these goals. In addition, there are marked differences among families in their readiness to accept these goals, particularly the goal of the addict leaving home.

Clinical considerations dictated many of the differences among the cases presented in the previous chapters. In Chapter 7, Kirschner deals explicitly with the issue of leaving home in the third session. Although the parents were initially resistant, he was able to get a commitment from both that their son should ultimately move out. Much of therapy became focused on the necessary steps for the addict to live successfully on his own.

Riley (Chapter 10) was faced with a situation that differed in many important ways. Ed had a common-law wife and children, with some indications that this relationship might be stabilized. On the other hand, he was an only child, with parents who were greatly invested in parenting. In addition, Ed had been accustomed to a considerable income from drug dealing. All of these factors influenced Riley's treatment strategy: (1) to strengthen the relationship between Ed and Linda, including pressure for them to have a house of their own; (2) to allow the grandparents to continue "parenting" the granddaughter, so that Ed could move out; (3) to focus on employment and education, so that Ed would not be as tempted to return to pushing.

Chapter 11 illustrates how the therapist had to modify his approach to deal with the developmental crisis presented by the father's retirement. The parents readily accepted educational and vocational goals for their son but were totally unprepared to consider his leaving home. Urquhart initially avoided direct confrontation on this issue, waiting some time before eventually introducing the goal of the addict's leaving home and having a family of his own. He noted to himself, but did not immediately challenge, the ways in which the parents undercut this eventual goal by taking care of the addict's every need.

## FOCUS ON DRUGS

The clinical chapters illustrate a diversity of strategies for handling drug-related issues. As stated in Chapter 6, drug usage is the primary criterion of success and the unifying theme in every therapeutic plan. Considerable flexibility is needed, however, depending on the pattern of drug usage shown by the addict, the response of the family, and the relationship between the therapist and the family.

As pointed out in Chapter 8, virtually all of the successful cases exhibited at least one drug-related crisis, which was generally handled by containing the crisis within the family. (The clearest exception to this was Heard's tack in the early stages of the case in Chapter 9, in which he did not oppose inpatient treatment, since he lacked the necessary leverage with the family. Instead he temporarily accommodated to the system, waiting until he could mobilize the family to block further misuse of hospitalization.)

The cases vary the most in the degree to which drugs remained a consistent focus of treatment and in the handling of relapses in drug use. At one extreme is the home detoxification case described in Chapter 12, a case in which there was a consistent focus on drug usage and detoxification throughout therapy. Such a focus was unavoidable, since substance abuse was rampant throughout the family, with *every* family member exhibiting some form of chemical misuse.

How and when to force the issue around drugs requires delicate clinical judgement. Urquhart (Chapter 11) allowed a series of dirty urines, counting on the steady build-up of cooperation from the parents. Riley (Chapter 10) felt that it was important to force the issue early. Because he could not count on the parents to take strong action, he provided most of the confrontation himself. As stated in that chapter, this is probably the riskiest strategy to adopt, since the therapist is in danger of having the parents undercut him and side with the addict.

It is important not to lose sight of the fact that it is the handling of *interpersonal* transactions that will determine the success of therapy. The cases in Chapters 7 and 9 may appear to be very different, since Kirschner focuses so little on drugs, while Heard is constantly faced with considerations of hospitalization and drugs. Careful comparison reveals, however, that there are underlying similarities—each therapist uses the prevailing themes and issues to create changes in family interaction and structure. The primary difference is one of content—leaving home in the first case and avoiding hospitalization in the second.

Relapses must also be handled in a manner consistent with the stage of therapy and what has been accomplished to date. Because of a previous pattern of success, Riley was able to virtually ignore a (supposed) relapse in the 10th session, saying to the addict, "I don't need to solve this no more, because you can handle this." Scott, on the other hand, was faced with a different situation (Chapter 12). When the first home detoxification effort failed, there was no pattern of previous success, so it was necessary to keep pushing for a breakthrough.

## TASKS AND COMPETENCE

All the therapists used tasks with their cases. These were introduced both to extend restructuring interventions from the session to the home, and to increase family members' competencies. The material in Chapter 12 is particularly detailed in explaining the rationale and method for employing tasks. The way in which a task is arrived at, and the therapist's reaction after it has been attempted, are key to effective treatment. The task is handled so that the *family feels more competent afterward*; partial successes or even "failures" are framed as positive steps rather than as setbacks. Note how Kirschner (Chapter 7) continued to underscore the helpfulness and attendant devotion in the father's attempts to remain in charge of his son, even after a detoxification attempt had failed. Scott (Chapter 12) contrasted the difference in the mother's frequency of screaming before and after she attempted to stop. A good therapist is a task "master."

## WHO SHOULD BE INVOLVED IN THERAPY

A variety of strategic considerations dictate who should be involved in therapy at different stages in treatment. Our general approach is to vary the composition of the session in accordance with structural goals, rather than routinely including all family members. This may consist of inviting particular family members to a session or dividing a session into distinct stages with different members involved.

All of the clinical cases show a common emphasis on the importance of the addict and his parents. In the case in Chapter 7, focus was almost exclusively on this triad, with strategically timed meetings with only the parents. We have frequently been asked whether it would have been preferable to have included the two younger brothers more, if only for the preventive value of keeping a new patient from appearing. We feel that it might have been ideal, but that the therapist was faced with extreme problems in keeping the therapy sessions under control. We agree with Haley[66] that the cardinal principle is for the therapist to be in control of the case, and that he should do whatever is necessary to maintain this control.

Siblings were important elements in the therapy in the cases presented in Chapters 9 and 12. Heard was able to use the sisters to help strengthen the mother in opposing the father's overprotectiveness. Scott found that the older sister was of pivotal importance in his case; her presence in the sessions was often helpful, and she also was the family member who undermined one of the efforts at home detoxification.

Riley's case (Chapter 10) is a typical example of working with the family of origin as well as the addict's marriage. In the early stages of therapy, the major emphasis is upon the family of origin; movement to the addict's spouse or girlfriend is premature without a clear go-ahead from his parents. Often, as in this case, later sessions may place more emphasis on the younger couple. Riley's sessions illustrate the typical practice of splitting sessions between the whole family and an important subgroup, in this instance the couple. This allowed Riley to maintain contact with the parents and guarantee that he continued to have their support.

## MISSING MEMBERS

There is a similar variability across chapters in the strategies adopted for dealing with family members who resist coming to therapy or miss sessions. The only general rule is that there is no general rule— the therapist makes the rules, depending on the needs of the case.

The issue of a missing member may be repeatedly emphasized by the therapist, or the parents may be given the responsibility to get the member in, as Scott did with the absent sister in Chapter 12. The therapist may take control by giving explicit permission for absence, such as Kirschner did by supporting the mother's need to take a rest. The therapist may avoid a confrontation he is afraid of losing, as Heard did when faced with overwhelming resistance to the inclusion of the grandmother. At times, it is enough for the therapist to implicitly assume that an absent member will return, as Riley did when the father did not attend because he had "had a hard day."

Several factors enter into the therapist's decision on strategy:

1. The importance of the particular family member. It was rare for therapy to continue without major efforts to reengage either parent if one of them began to miss sessions.

2. The overall strategy for the case. Some strategies focus primarily on the triad of addict and parents, while others include other family members in important coalitions. "Parental" sisters are a notable example of family members who should not be left out.

3. The prospects for success. If the odds seem to be heavily against the therapist, it often seems best to avoid a confrontation that might result in losing the case. The absence can often be relabeled and the absent member dealt with indirectly.

4. The stage in therapy. Kirschner felt comfortable in excusing the mother late in therapy, but would certainly have opposed her absence earlier in treatment.

## SESSION SPACING AND LENGTH

It was relatively rare for project therapy cases to follow exactly the ideal model of 10 weekly sessions. Certainly it would be unwise for any therapist working with drug abusers and their families to allow himself to be locked into a rigid, once-a-week schedule. As noted in Chapter 6, we feel that it is crucial for the therapist to be able to respond flexibly to crises, while it is also useful to taper off sessions toward the end of therapy.

The case examples illustrate this need for flexibility. For Kirschner's family, the initial session lasted almost 3 hours. Without this time expenditure, it would probably have been impossible to negotiate a workable therapeutic contract. Heard found it necessary to schedule a crisis session with the family in order to deal with a possible hospitalization. Although it was not emphasized in Chapter 12, home detoxification is perhaps the most demanding regimen for the therapist; it is standard practice for the therapist to be "on call" for the family during the period of detoxification.

## GHOSTS, MOURNING, AND DEATHBED INSTRUCTIONS

It may seem surprising to see consideration given within a structural-strategic framework to topics such as "ghosts," unresolved mourning, and deathbed instructions. This becomes less surprising, however, when one considers the influence of Boszormenyi-Nagy's work on one of us (Stanton) and the clinical observations summarized in Stanton's paper "The Addict as Savior: Heroin, Death and the Family."[146]

Death is an issue that clearly cannot be ignored when working with heroin addicts and their families. Not only is the possible death of the addict an important therapeutic issue, it is also frequently necessary to deal with other significant deaths. It is difficult to ascertain (and ultimately unnecessary to decide), whether other death issues become so important because of the life-and-death nature of the addiction or whether a life-threatening symptom was chosen in part to help the family deal with other deaths. Both of these (linear) views are probably "true," and the major issue for the therapist is to be alert to important deaths that still have major effects on the present situation.

The previous clinical chapters offer a variety of illustrations of our general approach to working with death issues, that is, they bring them out in a vivid way and offer therapeutic direction that will allow these issues to be laid to rest. The approach is not to gather extensive historical information, or to seek "catharsis," but rather to change the present effects of past events, often through assigning tasks for the family members.

In Chapter 10, for example, Riley kept the focus on the mysteries and sealed-over feelings regarding the death of Linda's mother. The therapist provided the additional motivation to get these ambiguities resolved and enlisted the help of Ed (thus connecting the couple even more). Ed and Linda were then given the task of going to City Hall and the morgue in order to finally learn the facts, so that these doubts would not continue to affect their relationship and their children.

In Chapter 9, Heard used the whole issue of death to break through the family's system of denial. First, the issue was heightened by discussing the addict's funeral. Soon afterward, the issue of death-bed instructions from the grandfather emerged. It was then possible to reinterpret the message from the dying grandfather in such a way that it supported necessary changes in the father's behavior.

These contrasting examples underscore the need to look carefully at each specific case. Coleman and Stanton[32] have outlined seven possible therapeutic approaches in addressing death-related issues in families of addicts: (1) confronting the reality, (2) postmortem planning, (3) planning the funeral, (4) personifying the drug and having it "die," (5) visiting a grave, (6) dealing with "ghosts," and, finally, (7) not dealing with death issues at all. Obviously, there is no cookbook approach; instead, it is crucial to note what links there are between the addict and dead family members. Only then will it be possible to design interventions that fit the needs of the particular family and are consistent with an overall plan for treatment.


## THE QUESTION OF OUTCOME

It is difficult to come up with any single simple answer to the question of outcome. As is shown systematically in Chapter 17, the overall results with this approach are quite positive, when compared to conventional treatment. All of the cases presented in Chapters 7, 9, 10, 11, and 12 showed a favorable response to family therapy, yet none of them showed perfect outcome. Judging the degree of success in a particular case depends upon the time period examined and the relative importance assigned to different outcomes.

The case in Chapter 7 is a perfect example of a highly favorable outcome that did show temporary setbacks. When therapy ended, the addict was off drugs, employed, and out of the house. Soon after that, he moved back home, apparently in response to a parental separation. Long-term follow-up indicated that he had been able to move out once again, had a steady job, and had remained off heroin. Except for the initial separation, the parents remained together.

Riley's case (Chapter 10) was also highly successful from the standpoint of drugs. As mentioned in that chapter, detoxification from methadone was not a prominent goal in that case, which was seen early in the life of the AFP. The addict was able to detoxify from methadone several months after the end of therapy and was almost completely drug-free for 3 years following treatment. He also did not resume pushing. On the other hand, despite the therapeutic work with Ed and Linda, Linda moved out and Ed remained with his parents.

A comparison of the cases mentioned in Chapters 11 and 12 is instructive, since it highlights differences in difficulty among cases (although certainly very few of them are easy). Urquhart was able to get consistently good cooperation from the addict and his parents. This was obvious from the beginning, since the family came into therapy with almost no effort by the therapist. Therapeutic outcome was consistently positive. Scott's case seemed clearly more difficult: both parents were heavy drinkers, the two sons were long-term heroin addicts, and one daughter also was found to be an addict. The degree of cooperation Scott was able to achieve is remarkable, but it is probably not surprising that the gains were not consistently maintained. The employment history was fair, with some indications of criminal activity during the first year of follow-up. The patient also returned to methadone maintenance, with periods of opiate abuse. Only during the second and third years did his drug use show much improvement.

This last case suggests the shortcomings of a short-term, time-limited contract, particularly with such an intractable, multiproblem family. As stated in Chapter 6, we favor a model that encourages the family to reengage in treatment if problems return or new problems develop. Such flexibility might have significant impact in preventing relapses after the completion of therapy.

## OTHER POPULATIONS

We are frequently asked about the extension of our clinical approach to populations other than adult male heroin addicts. We are firmly convinced that the therapeutic model we have developed is widely applicable to other family constellations, other age groups, other substances of abuse, and—particularly some of the material in Chapters 5, 6, 9, 12, and 13—to other clinical problems.

Obviously we are aware that different substances have different psychological and physical effects. We also know that the drug scene changes constantly, in response to factors such as changes in the availability and quality of street drugs, changes in the social fabric of the society, and even to passing fads. In view of these changes, any treatment approach, including a chemical antagonist, that is specifically tied to a particular drug of abuse invites rapid obsolescence. Our experience indicates that the *function* of the drug in an interpersonal context is much more important than its specific pharmacological properties. It seems clear that a wide range of drugs (including alcohol) can serve similar functions. Even in our population of heroin abusers, there were frequent periods of polydrug abuse or substitution of a nonopiate drug.

Some differences between drugs do have significance for treatment. The addictive properties may make withdrawal more or less stressful; some drugs, such as barbiturates, are unsuitable for home detoxification because of the danger involved. Chemical properties also make some drugs more difficult to detect, which can affect treatment strategies that require monitoring drug usage. Whether drugs are legal or illegal and how socially acceptable they are can have implications for the goals of treatment—abstinence or use within socially acceptable limits.

### SINGLE-PARENT FAMILIES

Chapter 6, under "Restructuring," deals with the extension of this model to single-parent families. Some of the modifications in technique, which stem from Minuchin's[100] earlier work, are elaborated therein. However, the reader should not overlook the applicability to single-parent families of much of the AFP clinical material, despite the technical requirement that AFP families either have two parents or a parent and a parent surrogate. We feel there are many similarities among (1) two-parent families where one parent is peripheral, (2) single-parent families with an added parent surrogate, and (3) single-parent families where there is another important adult involved, such as an aunt, uncle, or grandparent.

## FEMALE ADDICTS

In the AFP, experience with female addicts has been limited to families of male addicts that also included an addicted spouse or sister. However, we have upon occasion seen female addicts in other contexts, and our impression is that many of the dynamics are similar to those for males, as are the therapeutic strategies.

One difference is that often it appears that the overinvolvement among female addicts is between father and daughter, instead of mother and son. Compared to the mother–son relationship, there is a greater tendency for the father–daughter relationship to become extremely sexualized, often to the point of overt incest. Kaufman and Kaufmann[78] and others have reported indications of high rates of incest, particularly in inner-city families where physical living conditions may be conducive to increased sexual contact. Dealing with incest becomes a critical therapeutic issue, but one that must be handled delicately because it threatens the bond between the parents and the stability of the family.

## ALCOHOL

Alcoholism, especially in young adults, presents many of the same treatment issues as heroin abuse. Again, the caution stated in the previous section applies: the therapist *must* pay close attention to the life cycle issues facing the particular family in question. Compared to heroin abusers, who are typically at the "leaving-home" stage, alcoholics often show a later onset associated with marital, parental, and vocational responsibilities. Therefore, although inclusion of the family of origin in the treatment of alcoholics has perhaps been too neglected,[158] the therapy typically involves more focus on the marital couple. [13, 74, 110, 159, 172] Whether or not a client agrees to abstinence as a treatment goal, however, the therapist usually aims toward halting an alcohol-related interactional cycle[38, 173] within the couple or family, much as he might with a heroin addict's family. On the other hand, in treating alcoholics and their families, we deviate in several ways from our "standard" treatment paradigm in that we (1) rely less on urinalysis, and (2) rely heavily on Alcoholics Anonymous and Al-Anon as collaborative support and/or treatment systems.

# OTHER DIMENSIONS OF THERAPY

# 16

# PROGRAM FLEXIBILITY AND SUPPORT

GEORGE E. WOODY
ESTHER K. CARR
M. DUNCAN STANTON
H. ELTON HARGROVE

ADMINISTRATIVE PROBLEM SOLVING and management are key aspects in treating addicts and their families. In the Addicts and Families Program (AFP), many unexpected treatment issues arose, and it was essential to develop an effective and flexible system that could respond to them. Intended not only for clinicians, but also for administrators, some of whom may be less interested in the detailed clinical applications presented elsewhere in the book, this chapter provides the reader with a summary of important programmatic issues and a description of the evolution of our attempts to deal with these issues, particularly the adjustments necessary to maximize the chance that patients would become engaged and continue in therapy.

## CONNECTING CLIENT AND THERAPIST

Psychotherapy of any kind has been notoriously difficult to carry out with drug-addicted individuals. The reason is quite simple—they have serious problems in keeping their appointments. There are probably a number of factors contributing to this, and certainly there are exceptions, but most clinicians who have worked with addicted individuals would agree that addicts all too commonly do not show up for regularly scheduled sessions. This creates an immense practical problem: how does one deliver treatment to a patient who is not there? This poor attendance, in turn, causes many therapists to become discouraged and to direct their efforts elsewhere. Thus, a family therapy program with addicts starts with two serious problems: first, how to maximize the chances that patients will keep appointments, and, second, how to help therapists maintain their enthusiasm and commitment to the program. These problems were considered in our initial planning, but their full impact was not realized for several months. Finally, when they became glaringly obvious, several changes in administrative approach took place. The evolution of these procedures is described here, after first noting certain relevant treatment and logistical features of the Drug Dependence Treatment Center (DDTC).

## THE DRUG-TREATMENT PROGRAM

A detailed description of the DDTC multimodal program is provided in Appendix B, so coverage here is limited to a few additional points applicable to the present chapter. At intake, all DDTC patients are assigned a counselor and must meet with that person. This usually occurs when the patient needs some concrete service, such as a medication change, a letter for court, or a referral to a clinic physician for evaluation of a medical or psychological problem. There is a wide variety of problems that patients discuss with their counselors, but sessions usually focus on current life problems and include the delivery of a specific service. The frequency of appointments varies widely, from once per month to three times per week, but it averages once per week. Patients attending the clinic normally sign in with the clinic secretary, receive their methadone, and then see their counselor if a session is scheduled for that day. Unscheduled, "on-the-spot" appointments are not unusual. If a medication change is to be obtained, the counselor and patient meet with a clinic physician, who evaluates the patient and prescribes medication based on information provided by both patient and counselor.

The family therapists' offices and the video rooms for family treatment were located at the Philadelphia Child Guidance Clinic (PCGC), approximately 5 minutes' walk from the DDTC.* This physical separation created an immediate problem, because a patient could receive his methadone and take advantage of other clinic services without seeing his family therapist. It was hoped that the problems

---

*While such a degree of physical separation between treatment components may be extreme, in some drug programs it is not unusual to have separate methadone and family therapy units within the same building. We did consider providing offices at the DDTC for the family therapists, but this was not feasible due to insufficient space and lack of videotaping facilities.

inherent in this separation could be overcome by stimulating the patients' interest in this new treatment, while at the same time reminding and encouraging them to keep appointments. Therapists were all hired on a part-time salaried basis; thus they were paid even if patients did not keep appointments. We hoped that this arrangement would solve some of the morale problems that might arise if patients failed to appear for therapy sessions.

## TEAM MEETINGS

We discovered fairly quickly after starting the AFP that patients would not readily keep appointments if they were merely assigned to a therapist and told to meet him at a certain time and place. Administrative steps aimed to assure that this meeting occurred became an important part of treatment. An essential activity for developing and implementing these changes was the AFP weekly team meeting. It was attended by therapists, therapy supervisors, research staff, and the principal investigators. More important, it was also attended by the DDTC Medical Director (Woody) and the Senior Drug Counselor (Hargrove). These meetings of most of the principal parties permitted (1) ongoing case management, (2) resolving differences among staff, and (3) developing new procedures aimed at plugging procedural "loopholes" and correcting administrative problems. There will always be stumbling blocks when two separate institutions collaborate, but these meetings kept communication lines open and active, serving to undercut the effects of patients' attempts to manipulate the treatment system. Whatever successes this program achieved were due in no small part to the team meetings.

## INTRODUCING CLIENT AND THERAPIST

Our first move to deal with missed appointments was to bring the drug counselor more actively into the process, so that he or she could provide the therapist with a "proper introduction" to the client. Since this made additional demands on counselors, we arranged for them to receive a $5.00 payment when the meeting between them, their client, and the therapist occurred. The client received $10.00 for making this appointment. The results of this effort were negligible, partly because of scheduling problems. Finding a convenient time for all three to meet—even if it was after work hours—was not easily done in most cases. In addition, the patients were not eager to connect with another "treater," especially if their treatment plan had been set and the new treater was requiring their family to participate. As before, they came up with innumerable excuses, such as, "I'm working and I don't have time," "I changed my mind; I want to do it on my own," "My family doesn't know I'm an addict," and so forth (see Chapters 3 through 5). Then, too, in a few instances, "turf" struggles surfaced between counselor and therapist, with the latter sometimes coming on too strong and the former being threatened by having a "smarty-pants" therapist share his or her clients.

## COMPENSATING FOR APPOINTMENT DELAYS

Another problem was the time lag between intake and the date of the appointment. The established procedure was such that the patient had received all intake processing, a medical examination, an assignment to a drug counselor, and the development of a treatment plan several days (or even a week or more) before arrangements to meet the family therapist were made. We first responded to this by making the therapists available to be called *immediately* upon intake of an eligible client (Principle 5, Chapter 5). Thus they were usually able to go to the DDTC that same day and meet the client, or soon thereafter. When they could not get to the DDTC immediately, they often called and talked to the patient by telephone. To facilitate the process, a direct telephone line was installed between PCGC and the DDTC so that phone calls did not even have to go through the main hospital switchboard (a constant source of delay). As mentioned in Chapter 5, we eventually improved the procedures further by equipping therapists with beepers so that they could be reached at all times during working hours. These latter steps (immediate response and utilization of telephone and beepers) eliminated much of the slippage, and increased the probability that therapist and client would get connected early in the process.

The third, and most important, adjustment we made was to change the role of the family therapist. This is discussed below.

## THE DUAL ROLE

As the program progressed, it became increasingly clear that the patients were not seeing their family therapists because they did not perceive them as helpers. The physical separation between the DDTC and PCGC was a strong contributing factor, but it was not the primary one. It was apparent that, above and beyond all else (at least initially), the patients perceived methadone as their major treatment. Obviously, receiving a dose of methadone was simpler and easier than facing therapy with the family. The family therapists, being in a separate building, were not identified with methadone in any way. Patients did not even have to see them to receive methadone. Since some of the key staff members did not consider it ethical to require patients to see their therapists as a condition for receiving methadone, some other way had to be found to bridge the gap.

Another factor was the potential for slippage in the coordination between drug counselors and therapists in the ongoing management of their (shared) cases. The counselor's job was to negotiate dosages and a treatment plan with the client. On the other hand, the family therapist was trying to shift responsibility for such matters to the family. Sometimes decisions were made in one of these realms without coordination with the other (e.g., the case in Chapter 7). If the family made a treatment decision without the counselor's input, he felt undercut, while counselor–client decisions made outside the family context diminished the role of both family and therapist. Although these difficulties were overcome satisfactorily in some cases, in others they resulted in intrastaff, family, and client antagonisms—as if we could not get our act together. In fact, a few cases were lost to treatment entirely due to this lack of coordination. Clearly something else had to be done.

To deal with these problems, approximately 5 months into the program a major decision was made by the Medical Director (Woody) and the DDTC Director, Charles P. O'Brien. This was to make the family therapist also the drug counselor for any cases assigned to family treatment, giving him the additional responsibilities of a drug counselor. Thus he wore *both* hats, serving in a kind of "dual role." This was a crucial change, which effectively turned the situation around. It gave the family therapist primary responsibility for his cases. All patients' petitions for medications (methadone, sleeping medications, weekend take-home doses, etc.) had to go through the family therapist, who then discussed them with a DDTC physician (usually following negotiation with the family). Thus, both the therapist and the family were brought into the medication-dispensing system. Adoption of the dual role neutralized earlier difficulties in connecting with the client and integrating the family into the treatment process. As noted in Chapter 5, it also increased significantly the number of cases in which whole families (including *both* parents or parent surrogates) became engaged in treatment—the percentage of successfully recruited families rising from 56% before the dual role to 77% after it was instituted—and doubled the cost-efficiency. Stanton and Todd have stated elsewhere[167] (see also Chapter 6) that treatment with these clients is unlikely to succeed without this provision.

## MEDICAL SUPPORT

It may be obvious from the foregoing that the support of family therapists by the medical staff was key to the success of the AFP. This was partly facilitated by restricting medical input on family therapy cases, whenever possible, to the several DDTC physicians who were most familiar with the family program—particularly the Medical Director (since he attended the weekly AFP team meetings).

Medical support extended across several dimensions. In addition to providing underpinnings to family therapists on medication and treatment decisions, it included giving them a certain amount of latitude within the treatment process. Medical staff became sensitive to issues surrounding the involvement of parents and family in the therapeutic plan. They appreciated the rationale for this and made a sincere effort not to undercut therapist–family decisions. Their back-up included supporting therapists in obtaining additional urine tests (when initial tests were questionable) and, on a few occasions, in explaining directly to the parents and family why a therapist might be taking a given position on a particular medication. All of these efforts helped treatment proceed more smoothly, and made the family crises that did occur more manageable.

## TRIANGULATION AND MANIPULATION BY PATIENTS

As implied above, much of the effort that went into monitoring and revising administrative procedures was done to counteract manipulative behaviors by patients. Many of them were trying to beat the system and to play off staff members against each other—much as they did within their families. In the early stages of the program, they were sometimes successful at this, especially if the therapist and drug counselor were not in accord. A patient might approach a therapist by saying, "My counselor said I could have a raise [in methadone dosage]," or approach a counselor with, "My family therapist said I should get a take-home this weekend." Obviously such ploys were destructive both to treatment and intrastaff relations. Team meetings and regular contact between therapists and counselors helped to counteract these attempts.

Similar actions occurred after the dual role was implemented, but this time they more commonly included therapists and physicians rather than therapists and drug counselors. In one case, the family, patient, and therapist agreed on a dosage change. The next day the patient visited the Medical Director to renegotiate the dosage to an entirely different level. This "flanking move" might have worked if the Medical Director had not refused to discuss the issue. Instead, he referred the patient back to the therapist. Actually, after several patients had failed at such attempts, the frequency of these moves decreased considerably; the patients had tested the system and it had held up.

## INCENTIVES FOR FAMILIES

We also introduced a number of procedures to facilitate families coming to the clinic. In addition to application of the clinical techniques described in Chapters 3 through 5, these included (1) providing parking for them, or covering their parking fees, and (2) reimbursing some families for travel costs, especially if they had to come some distance for sessions.* (Travel reimbursement was allowed only if the family was a particularly large one, or was financially destitute.) All of these steps helped to increase regular attendance and attenuate the dropout rate.

## THERAPIST FACTORS

### AVAILABILITY

The therapists in the AFP were allowed considerable flexibility in establishing their own schedules. We wanted them to be able to

---

*These additional reimbursements were not offered if a family was in the Paid Family Therapy group or the Movie group.

respond as quickly as possible to changing clinical situations, such as when a crisis occurred in the patient and/or the family. They also needed latitude in recruiting families for initial sessions and in holding treatment sessions during evening hours, since most families with working members could not readily keep daytime appointments (see Principle 20, Chapter 5). Sometimes they made home visits on weekends or needed to hold lengthy telephone conversations at odd hours, especially during detoxification crises. When such situations arose, the therapists were given compensatory time. As noted in Chapter 5, this sort of program dictates that the treatment agency not be overly rigid (such as requiring therapists to punch a time clock). It is our experience that therapists doing this kind of work should be given a certain amount of trust. If they are hassled by bureaucratic punctiliousness they will neither make the extra effort nor apply the sort of creativity usually required in treating these families.

## EFFICIENCY

Too much rigidity regarding clinical procedures can also be counter-productive. For instance, requiring that therapy sessions be limited to 1 hour in length, or to once a week, is usually not conducive to effective family treatment. Addicts' families tend to generate crises readily, and the therapist may have to see them several times and/or for somewhat longer sessions during such periods. An agency thus needs to set case requirements that allow a balance between more demanding and less demanding cases, rather than (1) setting a fixed quota of weekly, time-limited sessions, or (2) indiscriminantly increasing caseloads without giving consideration to the therapists' current situations.

On the other hand, there are ways of assuring that the work gets done. At our weekly team meetings we took regular stock of case progress. So that therapists did not grow lax in engaging new families, thus letting them slip away, we regularly monitored all recruitment efforts, probing with such questions as, "Have you met the father yet?" "When are they coming in?" and, "What are you going to do to make them less frightened of treatment?" Similar attention was paid to the progress of ongoing cases, especially if there had been a time lapse since the last session. These issues were raised both in supervisory sessions (Chapter 14) and in team meetings.

Since the family recruitment endeavor required so much effort on the part of therapists, we made a portion of their pay contingent upon its success (see Principle 17, Chapter 5). We provided them with monetary incentives for bringing complete families (including both parents or parent surrogates) into the clinic. This tied the reward more directly to the effort and proved to be effective in motivating therapists to accomplish these tasks.

## MORALE

A number of steps can be taken to maintain the morale of therapists (some of which have been discussed in Chapters 14 and 15). For instance, when the procedural changes described earlier for connecting therapist and client were implemented, the therapists began to be perceived as more essential by patients, who began keeping appointments two or three times as often. Ironically, we also found that as patients saw their therapists more often, they became more engaged in the process of therapy and the intensity of their initial focus on medication diminished. Therapists' morale thus began to improve because they felt more important and effective.

Obviously, introduction of the dual role raised therapists' morale considerably. This tied in with increasing support from a number of figures higher in the program structure; the therapists now knew they had firm backing in their work. This is in contrast to some programs in which family therapists are seen as a necessary evil at best, and are only marginally tolerated or supported.

The weekly AFP team meetings also helped to buttress morale. They were the setting within which a support group of fellow clinicians—with similar goals—could coalesce. They also allowed the airing of grievances and the working through of difficulties. One particularly meaningful session occurred following a patient's death by a drug overdose. The group provided the kind of support and clarification necessary to help the therapist deal with his own feelings in this very trying situation.

As emphasized in Chapters 6, 9 (Editors' note), and 14, having a support group of one or more therapists observing sessions live and making suggestions can also be helpful and boost morale, especially for therapists who are new to this kind of work. It also increases the chances for effective therapy.

There was one additional aspect to this program that, although hard to document, did indeed seem to emerge. It concerned perceptions by the staff at PCGC and DDTC of the therapists in our program. At the outset, little was known about our work, and some of us were new to our respective institutions, having come aboard specifically for this work. As might be expected, there was distrust, and perhaps a certain amount of envy within PCGC because we were granted a coveted suite of offices. Over a 2- to 3-year period, however, the curiosity of other staff became increasingly aroused, while at the same time we began to receive recognition from outside our two institutions. Toward the third and fourth years, the therapists were being accorded an increasing amount of respect by their peers. Concomitantly, a number of therapists not previously associated with the AFP approached the Principal Investigator about joining our staff. The upshot of this ironic turn of events was that being a therapist in the program eventually came to be seen as a kind of status symbol. This provided a definite boost to therapists' morale during this later period.

## CONCLUSION

This chapter presents some administrative and procedural factors that can optimize the family-treatment effort with addiction. The two primary factors are (1) program flexibility and (2) support of therapists. The former requires the ability to adjust procedures as needed and to avoid shackling therapists with rigid time and case requirements. The latter includes facilitating the therapist–client connection, providing therapists with authority over case management and medications (the dual role), providing them with a clinical support group, and concretely backing them up both medically and administratively. While we refer to "optimizing" the treatment effort, our situation was hardly optimal. Some programs will not encounter the problems that we did. Others will face different obstacles. This does not, however, preclude an effort to revise and adjust. Administrative flexibility plays a pivotal role in the success or failure of family therapy with drug abusers.

# 17

# TREATMENT OUTCOME

M. DUNCAN STANTON/THOMAS C. TODD/FREDERICK STEIER/
JOHN M. VAN DEUSEN/LINDA COOK

SO FAR OUR THRUST has been toward explicating principles and techniques for conducting effective family treatment with drug abusers. The question naturally arises as to the degree of success that can be expected when this therapy paradigm is applied. Over the years, psychotherapy with addicts has not had an enviable track record, which is one reason for the prevailing use of pharmacological substitutes such as methadone.[40] Even nonpsychotherapy methods have, at best, enjoyed a "spotty" reputation with clients of this type, especially if drug-free or nonaddicted status is embraced as the primary goal. Consequently, many who work with the addictions have adopted a (not unreasonable) posture of skepticism when "new" or "untried" psychotherapeutic methods are brought to their attention. This chapter answers at least some of the questions about treatment effectiveness that might logically arise.

The general procedure compares outcomes across our four treatment conditions: Nonfamily Treatment ($n = 53$) (methadone and individual counseling); Family Movie Treatment ($n = 19$); Unpaid Family Therapy ($n = 25$); and Paid Family Therapy ($n = 21$). These treatment conditions are briefly discussed in Chapter 2. A more detailed description of them, and the research design of which they were a part, appears in Appendix C. The data are examined from two perspectives. First, an analysis is presented of the basic outcome variable—days a patient is free of (various) drugs. Second, comparisons are made using a more inclusive outcome schema, which we have termed "Levels of Success"; it is a set of parameters that, among other things, takes into account patients who died between the date of intake and the end of the follow-up period.

Appreciation is extended to Robert Rosoff for assistance in preparation of the data and to Gene Zug and Emanual Johnson for obtaining the follow-up interviews.

## DRUG-FREE DAYS

### *METHOD*

#### *Outcome Variables*

In this analysis the generic outcome measure employed was the percentage of days that a patient did not use a particular drug (or drugs) during the posttreatment follow-up period, henceforth referred to as "days free." Separate values for days free were derived for the following five drug categories: (1) Legal Opiates (primarily methadone); (2) Illegal Opiates; (3) All Nonopiate Illegal Drugs except Marijuana; (4) Marijuana; (5) Alcohol.

Employment and/or enrollment in school were also assessed. The measure was the percentage of "working" days (excluding weekends) spent working or in full-time school during the follow-up period; part-time work and part-time school were recalculated to the equivalent number of full-time days worked, based on an 8-hour work day.

Estimates of days free were derived from the following six sources: (1) Drug Dependence Treatment Center (DDTC) records and/or charts, (2) urinalysis results from the DDTC and from client follow-up interviews, (3) DDTC drug counselor reports, (4) client self-reports, (5) family member reports (usually parents), and (6) spouse reports.

#### *Follow-Ups*

Because it was realized that some patients would drop out of the DDTC program soon after intake, and that the cumulative number of dropouts would obviously increase over time, it was important to establish a follow-up procedure that would allow accurate assessment of client drug use (and work or school activities) within the posttreatment period. Previous studies[e.g., 9, 33, 97, 174] have indicated that, for the most part, addicts will truthfully report drug use in the context of a posttreatment follow-up interview if they understand they have nothing to lose. Our method was to obtain "sets" of follow-up interviews (defined below) on clients in all four groups. These were given by two interviewers who worked in the field and had no involvement in the treatment. Some interviews were held in the clinic, while others involved home visits. The race of the interviewer and family were matched—a Black interviewer seeing Black families and a White interviewer seeing White families. Each client was paid $15.00 and each family member and spouse $10.00 for the interview.

The total follow-up period assessed was 1 year.* For the three Family groups, it extended from the end of family treatment (averaging approximately 18 weeks from intake date) to a point 1 year post-treatment. For the Nonfamily group, a parallel time span of 1 year was examined. This was done in a manner that allowed comparability of follow-up periods between it and the three Family treatments: subjects in the Nonfamily group were assessed across the period from 5 to 17 months after intake, whether or not their original treatment extended into this 12-month span. The general design was to obtain sets of follow-up interviews from all 118 cases during the 6th and 12th months of their respective 1-year periods.

A "set" of follow-up data usually included interviews with the client and one or both of his parents. To verify the information obtained, supplementary interviews were often held with spouses, siblings, important relatives, employers, parole officers, and drug counselors or therapists. All interviews with addicts included urine samples taken at the time of the interview and subsequently analyzed. At each interview, signed permission was obtained to meet for another interview in 6 months. The 40- to 90-minute interview followed a structured format covering drug and alcohol use by the client and other family members, employment or school progress of client, living arrangements, family contacts of client, medical problems, legal problems, and any other positive or negative changes that may have occurred in the family during the period under assessment. Although some of the information was qualitative, most of it could be coded and quantified.

## Determination of Outcome Data

While an attempt was made to get complete data on all subjects, in some cases this was not possible, because (1) not all sources were available for all subjects, (2) some sources did not provide information on all drug variables, and (3) the sources did not appear to be

---

*These follow-ups are continuing over a 4-year period, but subsequent data have not been collected and/or have not been analyzed.

equally reliable. These factors complicated the process of computing outcome figures in particular cases, so a procedure was developed for utilization of the "best estimate" of a client's drug use in such cases. Two general rules were followed:

1. The best available source of days-free information for each drug was established for each month in the subjects' follow-up period, and the estimate of that source was used exclusively. The best source was defined as the available source most likely to be valid. Our order of ranking, from most to least valid, was: urine report, counselor report, client self-report, DDTC record and/or chart, spouse report, family member report. If there was only one source of drug-use information available for a specific month, that source was used.

2. If the best available source had some information for a specific month, but there were gaps (no information for part of the month), a decision was made either to use that source in conjunction with a set of rules[171] to fill in the gaps, or to use another source, on the basis of the folowing rule: if a less preferred source was judged more accurate, it was used instead of a more preferred source that had gaps.

One might wonder why parent and family member reports were ranked so low as to their potential validity, especially since Stephens'[174] data with 17 cases indicated that family member reports are generally accurate. In fact, we began this research with such an idea in mind, expecting that family members would provide the best corroboration available, since they were so closely in touch with clients' lives and day-to-day activities. However, we found the opposite to be true. We examined parents' reports closely and ran analyses to compare them with urinalysis data. While some parents seemed to be accurate, most were either extremely vague, having "no idea" about their sons' drug use (e.g., "I don't know what he's doing," or, "I guess he's on something, sometimes, but I never can tell"), or their estimates were simply wrong. All of the correlations that emerged between (1) days-free figures derived from individual family member estimates, and (2) urines, were very low (none above .10), and some were even negative.* As a result, we had to revise our thinking about

---

*One might speculate that a parent who "thinks" a son is using drugs (whether he is or not), or who ignores this matter completely, may not only be reflecting an opinion but may also be giving the subtle message that he should continue to use drugs.

parents as estimators (or revealers) of their son's drug use, and depend on more (apparently) valid sources.

After a days-free value was calculated for each month of the first year follow-up period on each of the five drug categories, we calculated total numbers of days free for the full 12 months of the follow-up period. One-way analyses of variance (ANOVA) were then performed for these five variables and also for a sixth variable—days employed or in school. Of the 118 subjects involved in the study, 104 are included in the days-free analyses. At this time, sufficient drug-use information has not been obtained for the 14 remaining clients (including 3 who were deceased).

## RESULTS

The results in this section are presented as comparisons between the four treatment groups in terms of the mean percentage of days free for each of five drug categories, plus the percentage of days working or in school during the first 12 months posttreatment.

Analyses of variance revealed statistically significant group differences at the .10 level or better in 3 of the 5 drug category comparisons. One of these was significant at the .009 level, with two others at the .06 level. Differences between groups in the number of days spent at work or in school were not significant. These results are presented in Table 3.

Pursuing our original hypotheses, the "expected" direction of the group means, from greater to lesser percentage of days free, was: Paid Family Therapy, Unpaid Family Therapy, (paid) Family Movie, and Nonfamily Treatment. Results indicated that for all of the drug-use variables except Alcohol, this hypothesis of direction was strictly upheld.

### Special Problems with Alcohol Measures

The groups did not differ significantly in terms of days free of alcohol for the year. It is not clear, however, if this is due to the nature of alcohol as a socially acceptable drug, or to the difficulty of applying a days-free measure to alcohol use. For example, a client who has one beer every day after work would show no days free, while another client who drank a bottle of scotch every other day would show 15 days free each month, even though his pattern of alcohol use was more extreme.

An alternative, more sensitive, alcohol measure is the conventional frequency–quantity index,[106, 175] in which the amount of pure alcohol consumed during a given period of time is computed (e.g., the consumption of two cans of beer every day for a week would yield a total of 2 [cans] × 12 [ounces per can] × .04 [4% alcohol in beer] × 7 [days] = 6.7 ounces of alcohol per week). Consequently, we undertook an analysis using client self-reports of amounts of alcohol consumed, and applied the frequency–quantity index.* We computed the average number of ounces of alcohol consumed by patients in each of the four treatment groups during the 1-year follow-up period. The figures were as follows: Nonfamily, 816 ounces; Movie, 386 ounces; Unpaid Family therapy, 667 ounces; Paid Family Therapy, 655 ounces. An analysis of variance showed that, as with days free of alcohol, the differences between these means were not statistically significant, partly due to the considerable variability shown among the subjects.

## COVARIATES

Although random assignment of patients to treatment conditions was used, it is still possible that, even with this procedure, certain groups may have garnered more patients with characteristics related to successful (or unsuccessful) outcome than others, thus making the group differences more, or less, statistically significant than would otherwise have occurred. Fortunately, such factors (covariates) can be identified and statistically controlled through application of analysis of covariance (ANACOVA).

Drawing from (1) the relevant literature, (2) the results of our pretreatment comparisons,[171] and (3) our experience, we selected 16 variables for statistical examination as potential covariates. Our purpose here was to develop a "set" of covariates composed of variables that significantly altered the significance levels of the main effects across treatment groups. The rationale was that such a combination could most effectively partial out the contribution of important nontreatment variables and determine the extent to which differences (or lack of them) between groups were truly due to treatment conditions.

---

*Initially, we also examined counselor reports to obtain these data (urinalysis, the preferred source for other drugs, did not, of course, provide information on alcohol levels). However, we found that client self-reports were much more clear and specific on alcohol use than counselor reports, especially concerning quantity of drinking. Interestingly, clients almost invariably reported greater frequency of drinking for themselves than did their counselors.

After entering each potential covariate in an analysis of co-variance with each of the five drug variables, we chose a set of four covariates that effected the greatest changes (positively or negatively) in the significance levels of the main effects across treatment groups. These covariates were (1) age of the client at first opiate use, (2) the client's employment status at time of intake, (3) whether the client had ever been married, and (4) educational level of the client's father (highest grade completed).*

Analyses of covariance were performed for each of the five drug variables and for the Work–School variable using the above covariate set.

## Results

By introducing the four (pretreatment) variables as a covariate set, we found all of the group differences to shift toward greater signifi-cance. This is especially noteworthy, since the covariates were se-lected for inclusion in this set if they affected significance greatly in either direction. Results of the analyses of covariance are presented in Table 3.

In particular, days free of Legal Opiates, of Illegal Opiates, and of Marijuana all shifted to become significant at better than the .05 level (.03, .01, and .015, respectively), and group differences on days free of All Nonopiate Illegal Drugs except Marijuana shifted very slightly and remained highly significant (.001). Thus, by statistically con-trolling the possible group differences on a set of pretreatment variables, we find statistically significant differences emerging be-tween groups on four of the five drug measures. Only the Alcohol variable (examined both in terms of days free and frequency–quantity), in addition to Work–School, remained nonsignificant.

## LEVELS OF SUCCESS

A close examination of the distribution of the data within each group prompted a slightly different approach to the analysis of treatment

---

*These four variables clearly stood out in individual covariate analyses. A fifth variable ("currently married") also fell into this group, but was not included because of its high correlation with "ever married." In addition, all four variables met the usual requirements for use in covariate analyses.

*Table 3.* Analyses of Variance and Covariance of Mean Percentage of Days Free of Various Drugs and Work–School: 1-Year Follow-Up[a]

| DEPENDENT VARIABLE | NONFAMILY[b] (n = 43) | FAMILY MOVIE (n = 17) | UNPAID FAMILY THERAPY (n = 23) | PAID FAMILY THERAPY (n = 21) | LEVEL OF SIGNIFICANCE[c] | |
|---|---|---|---|---|---|---|
| | | | | | ANOVA | ANACOVA |
| Legal Opiates | 43 | 43 | 61 | 69 | .06 | .03 |
| Illegal Opiates | 62 | 66 | 76 | 81 | .06 | .01 |
| All Nonopiate Illegal Drugs except Marijuana[d] | 75 | 79 | 85 | 88 | .009 | .001 |
| Marijuana | 54[e] | 59 | 69 | 75 | NS | .015 |
| Alcohol | 41 | 54 | 45 | 56 | NS | NS |
| Work–School[f] | 39 | 41 | 44 | 37 | NS | NS |

[a]All means are presented in terms of the percentage of days free of a particular drug during a given period of 12 months. Deceased clients are not included in the analyses.

[b]Methadone and individual counseling.

[c]ANOVA, without covariates; ANACOVA, with covariates.

[d]Due to heterogeneity of variance, the following transformation was applied to the number of days free for these data: $x' = \log(361 - x)$.

[e]For this variable, $n$ for Nonfamily group = 40.

[f]Rather than days free, this variable depicts the percentage of "working" days patients actually worked or were in school.

410

outcome. There were two reasons for its implementation. First, one of the problems with the days-free estimates is that they do not take into account patients who have died between date of intake and the end of the follow-up period, whether from drug overdose or other reasons. This selective analysis may thus be excluding clients who had poor drug outcomes at the time of death, given that many addicts who die prematurely do so for drug-related reasons. However, if the treatment groups were divided into more gross categories according to general Level of Success (Good, Fair, Poor), the deceased cases might legitimately be combined with other cases in the "Poor" outcome classification (assuming that a dead client represents a poor treatment outcome). This procedure allows merging of these two different outcome variables—extent of drug use and whether living or not—plus days incarcerated (see below). However, the living–deceased category would only enter the analysis if a particular patient had died, and, in such a case, he would only be included in the "Poor" category. In this way, an additional and relevant variable is drawn into the analysis.*

The importance for treatment outcome research of accounting for deceased subjects, especially in a youthful client population such as this, cannot be overemphasized. For example, a recent examination of data for the addicts on our own sample shows that over an average period stretching from intake to a point 31 months posttreatment, 8 of the total 118 patients had died. We suspected that the rate was lower for the 46 family therapy cases and, looking more closely, we found that only 1 of these 8 deceased clients actually had participated in family therapy (an addict in Unpaid Family Therapy in which the family had attended a single session). Five of the 7 others were among the 53 Nonfamily cases and 2 were among the 19 Movie cases (although one of the latter died of an overdose before the first Movie session). In other words, the mortality rate for family therapy cases (Paid, Unpaid) was 2%, while for cases that were not treated in family therapy (Nonfamily, Movie) it was 10%. The differential may even be greater than this, since we know whether all the family therapy and Movie clients are living or not, but have not determined this for all of the Nonfamily cases. This finding—that the rate for premature deaths was five times greater for cases not treated by

---

*While some clients might die from non-drug-related causes, it is assumed that cases such as this would distribute randomly across treatment groups (see following).

family therapy (a difference significant at the .05 level*)—is one that may have important implications for prevention, and certainly merits further investigation.

A second benefit of analyzing results in terms of Levels of Success is that it can take into account clients who were incarcerated for all or part of the follow-up period. Although such clients may be "cleaner" in jail than if they are unconstrained, a reduction in drug use because of incarceration seems a potentially misleading measure of the effectiveness of therapy. Further, incarceration for continued criminal activity itself certainly may be regarded as an undesirable outcome of treatment. Therefore, for the purposes of the Levels of Success analysis, the time a patient spent incarcerated for criminal activity committed *after* admission to treatment was categorized as a "Poor" outcome (i.e., as though he were "dirty" for all drugs during the period of incarceration). If a patient was imprisoned during the follow-up period for crimes committed *before* he entered treatment, his level of success, in percentage of days free, was computed based only on the time during the follow-up period that he was *not* incarcerated (i.e., it was prorated). Put differently, the period of incarceration for these cases was not included in the analysis and their drug-use estimates are based on the days when they were not in prison.

The third reason for a Levels of Success analysis has to do with clarification of how many patients are helped, to what extent, by which treatments. Categorizing clients in this way permits the drawing of such conclusions as "approximately X% of the patients had good outcomes under treatment Y," as opposed to simply providing means, which do not show the distribution of outcomes within groups.

## METHOD

The first step in this analysis was to obtain frequency distributions by dividing the days-free data into class intervals of 10% (0–10%, 10.1–20%, etc.). This was done across all drug categories and treatment groups. It allowed determination of the levels at which clients

---

*This result is based upon a $z$ test for the difference between two proportions, using a one-tailed test here because of our a priori hypothesis of the direction of the results.

seemed to cluster—for instance, in bimodal form. We suspected beforehand that the greatest proportion of subjects would fall into the 0–20% and 80.1–100% days-free categories. This proved to be so. These two class intervals were thus chosen, representing, respectively, what we labeled as "Poor" and "Good" outcomes. The remaining interval range, 20.1–80% days free, was termed a "Fair" outcome range. Deceased cases were added to the "Poor" category within their respective treatment groups, under the assumption that if deaths were randomly distributed across conditions, the level of statistical significance would not be affected. If, on the other hand, deaths were nonrandomly distributed among groups, this would enter into the group differences that might emerge, and was important information to take into account.

For the analysis of alcohol use, we used the frequency–quantity of alcohol consumed rather than days free of alcohol. We considered a "Good" outcome to be the consumption of less than 130 ounces of alcohol during the 1-year follow-up period ("light" drinkers and abstainers); this was equivalent to an intake of less than four drinks per week. A "Poor" outcome entailed the consumption of 1000 ounces or more of alcohol ("heavy" drinking), or the death of the client during the follow-up period; 1000 ounces per year is approximately equivalent to an intake of one six-pack of beer a day. The consumption of intermediate amounts of alcohol was considered to be "moderate" drinking, and a "Fair" outcome. While our categorization is consistent with that of Cahalan et al.,[20] their "heavy" drinker category includes individuals who drink large amounts infrequently ("binge" drinkers). We analyzed our data for binge drinkers and found no one who had not already been categorized as a "heavy" drinker based on total ounces alone.

Within the period examined here (the approximate 5-month treatment span plus 12 months' posttreatment), three deaths occurred, one in the Movie group and two in the Nonfamily group. These were included in the Levels of Success comparisons, bringing the total $n$ for this analysis to 107. Because we were interested in the *distribution* of cases across categories, chi-square analyses were applied to the data.

Since our primary concern is in the comparison between family therapy versus nonfamily therapy, and because it is inappropriate to perform a chi-square test of independence on a table with 12 cells ($4 \times 3$) for this sample size, the Paid and Unpaid groups were combined to form one category (Family Therapy), while the Movie and Nonfamily groups were combined to form the other category (Nonfamily Therapy). Statistical comparisons were thus made between these two "combined" treatment conditions.

## RESULTS

Table 4 presents the data analyses for the Levels of Success comparisons. Inspection reveals that the chi-square results between Family Therapy and Nonfamily Therapy were significant at the .05 level for four of the five drug categories (i.e., the dependent variables). Results for Alcohol and Work–School were not significant.

## GENERAL DISCUSSION

The analyses show that the Paid Family Therapy group had a greater average percentage of days free in all five different drug categories than did the other three groups; the Nonfamily treatment group had the lowest average percentage of days free in all five categories. When analyses of covariance (using a set of four covariates) were performed on the days-free data, the differences between the four treatment groups were significant at the .05 level or better for four of the five drug variables.

In earlier reports[148, 166, 171] we compared the four groups using only the first 6 months of follow-up data. The differences observed in these earlier reports were even more striking than the results presented here. Examining the first and second 6-month periods showed that the Paid Family Therapy group remained fairly constant in terms of total days free, while the other three groups tended to increase their proportions of days free in the second 6 months. This phenomenon has been noted by Frank[49] for outcome research with other forms of psychotherapy; that is, results for more successful types of therapy tend to hold up or stabilize, while initially less successful modes show gradual improvement.*

---

*It would seem likely that a greater proportion of cases that did not do well (more of whom were, proportionally, in the Nonfamily and Movie groups) sought additional treatment at a later point during the follow-up year. This would, of course, bring them more in line with the Good outcome cases by year's end. However, at this writing, data on the extent to which subjects reentered treatment have not been analyzed.

An important issue that must be addressed here is the extent to which success in the reduction or elimination of drug use might be offset by "switching" to the heavy use of alcohol. That is, did those who reduced legal and illegal drug use merely transfer their addiction to alcohol, as has been shown in other studies?[e.g., 120] A careful examination, done separately for each group, of the relationship between (1) days free of all illegal drugs and legal opioids (e.g., methadone, LAAM*) and (2) changes in frequency–quantity of alcohol revealed this not to be the case, however, as no clear pattern of relationship (i.e., no correlation) emerged.

There was no significant difference among groups in the amount of time spent working or in school. This result can be attributed to the fact that getting the client back to work or school was not a major treatment goal for many of the clients in the three family groups. Rather, the major emphasis in these groups tended to be to try to get the client off illegal drugs; goals related to work or school tended to be of secondary importance, given the constraint of a 10-session paradigm (see Chapter 6). Because therapists had different goals for different families, it is not possible to tell how much effort was expended on getting the client back to work or school, and how successful this effort was.

We were concerned that a greater percentage of the Nonfamily treatment group might be dropping out of the study and that we were losing some of the "worst" cases from the comparison. The percentages of clients across the four groups for whom we did not obtain data† were: Nonfamily, 15%; Movie, 5%; Unpaid Family Therapy, 8%; Paid Family Therapy, 0%. A statistical analysis of these rates showed them to not differ significantly. Nonetheless, the percentage of cases on which follow-ups were obtained was lowest for the Nonfamily group, and it seems fair to assume that addicts who have not been located following treatment, or have been uncooperative, are more likely to demonstrate poor outcomes than those who are easily found and who readily cooperate in follow-up interviews. It is our opinion that differences in the proportions of clients on which data were obtained affected comparisons between the Nonfamily and

*Levo-alpha-acetylmethadol.

†Of the 11 clients not included in these analyses, only three have not actually been located. Of the others, four refused to be interviewed, and four were eliminated for various reasons, such as obvious lack of veracity.

Table 4. Levels of Success over 1-Year Posttreatment[a]

| DEPENDENT VARIABLE | OUTCOME LEVEL | BASIC TREATMENT CONDITIONS | | | | COMBINED TREATMENT CONDITIONS[b] | | (A+B) VERSUS (C+D) $\chi^2$ AND LEVEL OF SIGNIFICANCE |
|---|---|---|---|---|---|---|---|---|
| | | A NONFAMILY ($n = 45$) | B FAMILY MOVIE ($n = 18$) | C UNPAID FAMILY THERAPY ($n = 23$) | D PAID FAMILY THERAPY ($n = 21$) | NONFAMILY THERAPY (A+B) ($n = 63$) | FAMILY THERAPY (C+D) ($n = 44$) | |
| Legal Opiates | Good | 26.7 (12) | 27.8 (5) | 43.5 (10) | 61.9 (13) | 27.0 | 51.2 | $\chi^2 = 7.08$ $p = .03$ |
| | Fair | 31.1 (14) | 22.2 (4) | 30.4 (7) | 4.8 (1) | 28.6 | 18.6 | |
| | Poor | 42.2 (19) | 50.0 (9) | 26.1 (6) | 33.3 (7) | 44.4 | 30.2 | |
| Illegal Opiates | Good | 33.3 (15) | 38.9 (7) | 56.5 (13) | 66.7 (14) | 34.9 | 60.5 | $\chi^2 = 7.77$ $p = .02$ |
| | Fair | 46.7 (21) | 50.0 (9) | 39.1 (9) | 23.8 (5) | 47.6 | 32.6 | |
| | Poor | 20.0 (9) | 11.1 (2) | 4.3 (1) | 9.5 (2) | 17.5 | 7.0 | |
| All Nonopiate Illegal Drugs except Marijuana | Good | 57.8 (26) | 38.9 (7) | 78.3 (18) | 81.0 (17) | 52.4 | 79.1 | $\chi^2 = 8.31$ $p = .02$ |
| | Fair | 28.9 (13) | 50.0 (9) | 21.7 (5) | 9.5 (2) | 34.9 | 16.3 | |
| | Poor | 13.3 (6) | 11.1 (2) | .0 (0) | 9.5 (2) | 12.7 | 4.7 | |

| | | | | | | | | |
|---|---|---|---|---|---|---|---|---|
| Marijuana[c] | Good | 23.8 (10) | 33.3 (6) | 43.5 (10) | 57.1 (12) | 26.7 | 48.8 | $\chi^2$ = 7.03 |
| | Fair | 45.2 (19) | 38.9 (7) | 43.5 (10) | 28.6 (6) | 43.3 | 37.2 | $p$ = .03 |
| | Poor | 31.0 (13) | 27.8 (5) | 13.0 (3) | 14.3 (3) | 30.0 | 14.0 | |
| Work–School[d] | Good | 20.5 (9) | 16.7 (3) | 20.8 (5) | 9.5 (2) | 19.4 | 15.6 | $\chi^2$ = .44 |
| | Fair | 34.1 (15) | 50.0 (9) | 37.5 (9) | 52.4 (11) | 38.7 | 44.4 | $p$ NS |
| | Poor | 45.5 (20) | 33.3 (6) | 41.7 (10) | 38.1 (8) | 41.9 | 40.0 | |
| Alcohol[e] | | | | | | | | |
| Light to abstainer | ("Good") | 25.0 (10) | 16.7 (3) | 30.0 (6) | 36.8 (7) | 22.4 | 33.3 | $\chi^2$ = 1.43 |
| Moderate | ("Fair") | 45.0 (18) | 66.7 (12) | 45.0 (9) | 42.1 (8) | 31.7 | 43.6 | $p$ NS |
| Heavy (or deceased) | ("Poor") | 30.0 (12) | 16.7 (3) | 25.0 (5) | 21.1 (4) | 25.9 | 23.1 | |

[a]Results are presented in terms of percentages of cases in a treatment group that fall within a particular outcome ("Success") level. The number of cases included is in parentheses. All analyses were done using the $n$'s, not the percentages.

[b]$n$'s within each group and level under the combined treatment conditions can be computed by adding the $n$'s from the appropriate basic treatment conditions columns (e.g., from columns A and B).

[c]For this variable, $n$ for Nonfamily Therapy (A) = 42.

[d]For this variable, $n$ for Nonfamily Therapy (A) = 44, and $n$ for Unpaid Family Therapy (C) = 24.

[e]For this variable (frequency–quantity of alcohol), $n$ for Nonfamily Therapy (A) = 40, for Movie (B) = 18, for Unpaid Family Therapy (C) = 20, and for Paid Family Therapy (D) = 19.

Paid Family Therapy groups, in particular; thus the differences we obtained are probably underestimates of the actual differences.

The Levels of Success data give perhaps the clearest picture of the differential outcome among our four treatment conditions. They provide information as to the proportions of addicts who can be helped by various methods, versus those who remain addicted or seriously drug dependent, who die prematurely, or who are incarcerated for criminal activity.

The most striking difference to be noted is between Paid Family Therapy and Nonfamily (methadone and/or individual counseling) treatment, with the Paid Family Therapy group showing nearly double the proportion of Good outcomes than those produced by the Nonfamily group on three drug variables, and 1½ times as many on a fourth. As with the days-free analysis, then, these results present a strong case in favor of the efficacy of Paid Family Therapy, with Unpaid Family Therapy running a not-too-distant second. Of particular note is the indication that both these family therapy modes show an ability to substantially increase the proportion of patients who reduce their dependence on or become free of narcotics— whether or not the drugs are illegal (heroin) or legal (methadone). While this was a major aim of all the treatment approaches, the two family therapy modes appear to have made substantial progress toward this goal, in view of outcomes usually obtained with this population of narcotics addicts.*

## GENERAL SUMMARY AND CONCLUSIONS

At this point, we are able to state unequivocally that a short-term structural–strategic family therapy approach to adult male opiate

---

*While the Nonfamily group provides a sort of baseline, it should be remembered that this was a baseline composed of fairly motivated clients, rather than of all clients who met the same selection criteria as the family groups. As noted in Chapter 2 and Appendix C, 37% of the clients in the original Nonfamily group were excluded from the study because they did not remain at the DDTC a full 30 days. Comparisons between the three family treatments and a more inclusive Nonfamily group (which included this 37%) would probably have revealed even greater differences than those shown in Tables 3 and 4. (This issue is discussed at greater length in reference 171, including a number of statistical comparisons as to pretreatment prognosis for Nonfamily cases, family treatment "refusers," and family treatment "engagers." In general, those who engaged in family treatment appeared to have slightly worse prognoses than either Nonfamily cases or refusers.)

addicts can be quite effective in reducing drug abuse. The improvements that occurred across most measures of drug taking are noteworthy, although such results did not occur in the vocational–educational area. It hardly needs to be said that the kinds of improvements demonstrated here are rarely shown by any kind of treatment with any subset of heroin addicts, either in terms of outcome or cost-efficiency.

As expected, Paid Family Therapy, in which payment was contingent on attendance and on clean urines, was somewhat (but generally not significantly) superior to Unpaid Family Therapy. A more dramatic finding was the clear superiority of Paid Family Therapy over both Movie and Nonfamily treatments. An earlier analysis[171] revealed that payment mainly functioned as an increased incentive for attendance at sessions, allowing family therapy an opportunity to become effective. This notion is supported by the fact that the payment incentive for clean urines did not significantly improve outcomes for the Movie group over the (unpaid) Nonfamily group on any variables; if the payment variable had strongly influenced drug taking, the Movie group should have shown significantly more drug-free days than the Nonfamily group.

The Family Movie group offers another kind of evidence that the outcome results are not attributable to payment per se. Families in this group received the same contingent payment as the Paid Family Therapy group. While the Movie families attended their "sessions" relatively faithfully, they showed significantly smaller therapeutic effects than both Paid and Unpaid Family Therapy. Again, the real effect of the payment seemed to be in helping to improve session attendance and reduce the dropout rate, which was its original purpose.

The much higher rate of premature deaths among addicts who did not engage in family therapy versus those who did (i.e., 10% vs. 2%) is worth noting. If such a 10% rate were to continue, more than half of the Nonfamily and Movie subjects would be dead by age 44. These data may be pointing to a preventive aspect of family therapy that has heretofore been unexplored.

While the majority of family therapy cases would probably be deemed successful by most conventional outcome and cost-effectiveness criteria, certainly there were cases in which family therapy was less successful. We would attribute the results with these later cases as due to at least five factors:

1. The AFP was an experimental program. From the start, there was testing and probing toward the development of new techniques and ways to bring about beneficial change. We had not, at the outset, established a treatment paradigm, instead waiting to let this emerge from our unfolding experience. This probably put our staff at a disadvantage, since the techniques and overall thrust of the program were not established early on, and it may have worked against the effectiveness of family therapy. In fact, it is more typical for psychotherapy researchers to have their techniques pretty much honed down before contrasting them with other treatment modes. Since we more or less "started from scratch" and needed to be innovative, waiting for a paradigm to emerge before beginning to assess outcomes was a luxury we could not afford.

2. Related to the above, most of the family therapists were not experienced in dealing with drug addicts. Only three of the nine had seen families of drug abusers prior to joining the AFP staff. Consequently, they were learning "on the job."

3. The family treatment was extremely brief, generally being confined to only 10 sessions. As noted in Chapter 6, this is a limiting paradigm, being a very short period in which to alter such severe and longstanding problems as opiate addiction.

4. The prevailing idea in the field (and among clients) that addiction is an individual problem engendered considerable resistance both to the involvement of all family members and to interventions that were family-oriented.

5. As discussed extensively in Chapters 2, 6, 7, and 16, the treatment system itself is all-important in dealing with cases of this type. Considerable energy had to be spent in responding to and rectifying administrative and procedural flaws in the system—efforts that detracted from the family therapy. In Chapter 6, the point has been made that the overall treatment system can detract substantially from the success of the therapy. This system sets the conditions for effective treatment and when it has "bugs," even the best family therapy will founder.

In view of the payment variable and the effort sometimes expended in family treatment, issues of cost-effectiveness naturally arise. Reimbursing family members to attend sessions would seem to be an expensive practice when viewed from a conventional perspective. However, these results indicate that the costs of keeping people in treatment through such means are more than compensated for by the costs saved to society. This refers to the improvement in days free from illegal drugs, which was shown by the Paid Family Therapy group. Our data indicate that addicts in this group were, on the average, kept off various drugs several more months per year than even motivated methadone clients (the Nonfamily group), a societal saving that far outweighs the costs of payment and family treatment combined. As noted in Chapter 5, even the additional costs of recruiting families were compensated for by this differential in drug use. These findings dictate that a new look be taken at the ways in which incentives are provided (or not provided) for involving addict families in treatment.

Finally, we would again point to the success rate of Paid Family Therapy as described by the Levels of Success analysis. In round figures, probably two-thirds of these cases could be considered good outcomes. This contrasts sharply with the usual rates of success for such cases (or, again, even with motivated clients, such as in the Nonfamily Treatment group), which have been much lower. It seems safe to conclude that the effectiveness of a short-term structural–strategic family therapy approach to this acknowledgedly difficult population is significant.

# 18

# DIRECTIONS FOR THE FUTURE

M. DUNCAN STANTON
THOMAS C. TODD

THE PUBLICATION of the present volume is part of a general nationwide trend toward recognition of family therapy as an appropriate treatment modality for substance abuse. This includes recent books and reviews on clinical applications[e.g., 77, 142, 152] and a survey by Coleman and Davis,[30] which showed that family therapy is now offered in some form in a high percentage of treatment programs.

For the past several years, we have been actively involved in training drug counselors and mental health professionals in the principles embodied in this book. In addition to recommending changes in clinical practice, we have pushed for changes in administration and program design, such as those outlined in Chapter 16. One of us (Stanton) has also been active in promoting policy changes at the federal level. At present some policies, most notably in the area of confidentiality, definitely work against family treatment (see below).

In terms of the future, some specific areas where we see the field heading, or where it needs to be heading, are*:

*1. The Addictive Cycle.* It should be apparent from the material presented in this book that addiction is one set of behaviors composing part of a sequence of behaviors within an intimate, interpersonal system, primarily the family system. Therefore it is a *family* addictive cycle, not an "individual" problem—whether acknowledged as such by the addict or not. Consequently, if treatment is not constructed to *intervene directly in and change the family process surrounding detoxification and readdiction*, such treatment is much less likely to succeed.

---

*Many of these points are discussed at greater length in an earlier paper by Stanton entitled "Family Treatment Approaches to Drug Abuse Problems: A Review," published in *Family Process*, 1979, *18*, 251–280.

*2. Family Recruitment.* We have emphasized the difficulty and the steps needed in getting many of these families to engage in treatment. This is partly due to their almost inherent defensiveness, and partly because they and the addict have not been led to expect family involvement. Consequently, we see a need for at least two changes in the policy of service delivery for such clients: (a) devotion of more energy and resources to outreach and educational efforts, and (b) provision of incentives and related procedures to increase the likelihood of their involvement. This also requires a change in the philosophy of who should be helped, and how (Chapter 5).

*3. Responsibility.* Families of drug abusers have too often been able to foist their addicted members on the treatment system, thereby abdicating responsibility. Further, the treatment system itself has often abetted this practice. This situation must be turned around. There is considerable need to develop methods that help families to feel more competent to care for their own. If, as Blum and Associates[17, p. 34] have stated, "the family is a force that helps resist or exaggerate the stress of other environmental factors," the need becomes clear for finding ways to strengthen the resistances and minimize the exaggerations.

*4. Confidentiality.* If drug use, especially of the heavy or compulsive variety, is seen as a family phenomenon, or as symptomatic of a larger family problem, many of the existent regulations concerning confidentiality[119] that shield abusers from family members do not make much sense. While there may be exceptions, such as in acute emergencies or in situations in which an experimenting adolescent has an adverse reaction, some of the standing regulations may serve, in the long run, to perpetuate rather than to alleviate the difficulty. To shield a person's drug problem from his family may even be an exercise in self-delusion, since they often already know about it; at the very least it results in "buying into" and rigidifying the existent family system. Drug abusers are frequently protective of their families and often protest that the problem is theirs rather than the whole family's. Confidentiality provisions can give license to this denial by officially sanctioning the identified patient as the problem and denying the importance of the family system and the significant others within it. There is a need to delineate more clearly the boundaries between confidentiality as it applies to *family members* versus the safeguards it ensures in relation to nonfamily individuals and agencies. While it is recognized that these regulations often were wrested from legislatures and government agencies at considerable cost in time, effort, sweat, and lobbying activity, consideration of the family basis underlying drug problems dictates that many of them be called into question.

*5. Treatment Systems.* Conceptualizing drug taking within an interpersonal systems or family framework is not always consonant with some of the other ways in which treatment has been administered in the drug-abuse field. This can become particularly apparent within actual clinical settings. Schwartzman and associates[131, 132] note that many programs feed into and recreate the family system of the abuser: "Unspoken conflicts between staff members frequently are acted out through individual patients and result in requests for more medication and more frequent illicit drug use."[132, p. 147] In a sense, they can reinforce the family's idea that the identified patient is "sick," incompetent, and unable to stop taking drugs. This is a very real issue, and recognizing it prompts close attention to the ways in which drug programs may be unwittingly fostering the very behaviors they are mandated to eliminate.

There appears to be a trend already underway toward incorporating family therapy methods within drug-treatment settings which have historically been neutral, or even opposed, to family involvement, such as inpatient programs and therapeutic communities. Multifamily methods (see Chapter 6) have commonly been the preferred vehicle for this integration. Family networking has great promise, but has not been explored as extensively. It will be interesting to see how this process evolves.

*6. Administrative Procedures.* The means by which administrative matters are handled within treatment systems can facilitate or negate the effectiveness of family treatment. At present, most procedures are geared to individual-oriented therapies and are not responsive to family approaches. A problem identified by Coleman and Davis[30] in their visits to drug programs was that counselors and therapists were not always allowed census credit for seeing family members. In some cases they were directly penalized, because sessions held without the identified patient present (e.g., if the parents or spouse were seen alone) were disallowed on their time sheets; they were also not given credit for the additional time required for contacting and coordinating with family members. Obviously, there is a need for allowing therapists flexibility in time and for providing them with incentives for the extra effort that may be demanded in treating families. Finally, difficulties can arise from policies and regulations established at the national level. Kleber[81] notes that current federal funding mechanisms, by supporting individual "slot" costs (as opposed to treatment unit costs), not only do not provide incentives for attendant therapies, but may induce a disincentive for provision of family and related treatments. He notes that the end result is a tendency "to penalize programs that attempt to do effective therapy with the patient and his family" (p. 271). We feel that, in terms of cost-effectiveness, changes in these existent practices will pay off and their implementation should be a high priority within the field.

7. *Training.* Training of clinicians in family treatment of addiction is a major goal of ours. The Coleman and Davis study[30] found this to be a high priority among the programs they surveyed. We would not expect this interest to abate, but rather to increase in the coming years. However, there is one caveat that should be voiced: As family systems methods become more widespread, a "fad" could develop. This might lead to inadequate training of many personnel who then proceed to do ineffective therapy. Family therapy cannot be learned overnight. Although efficient training models have been developed,[e.g., 45] and it appears to take less time to reach competence than is required for most individual modes, the orientation, content, and length of future training curricula deserve careful consideration.

8. *Prevention.* Of the various approaches to psychotherapy, family treatment has perhaps the clearest implications for prevention. This is because (a) more people are involved when one sees a family; (b) it engages people (e.g., parents) who may not otherwise have gotten into treatment themselves but who engender problems in others; and (c) if effective, a system is changed that, prior to treatment, had the potential to produce other offspring with problems. For instance, if parents are helped to improve the ways in which they handle a son or daughter with a problem, they are becoming more competent parents. Their experience should provide them with methods for dealing with younger children as these grow older; that is, the lessons learned with one offspring can be transferred to others. In fact, the work of Klein *et al.*[82] with delinquents indicates that family therapy can result in clear-cut prevention of future problems among siblings. Our own data (Chapter 17) hint that family therapy may even be preventing premature deaths. Finally, if a family situation is changed so that an addicted member is set free of the

needs of his parents and therefore, in part, his need for drugs, he is on the road to becoming a more competent person, and, in the long run, a more competent spouse and parent himself. This, then, is primary prevention, and it is our hope that its potential as a side effect of family therapy will receive increasing recognition.

Regarding our own work, to some extent the future is already upon us. In late 1980, we began a demonstration grant to further develop our treatment methods.* We are applying the home detoxification approach described in Chapters 6 and 12 on a systematic basis. The patient population is a group of male heroin (and polydrug) addicts, but the population and drug program differ in many significant ways from those of the AFP. It is our initial impression that we are dealing with a sample of "street" addicts who are significantly less motivated for treatment than our previous population. In addition, since this is not a Veterans Administration program, there are fewer supplementary programs and entitlements available to the addicts. We hope that this new project, as well as applications at other treatment centers, will extend our treatment model to other patient groups, other types of programs, and other drugs.

We feel justified in being optimistic about the future, as more programs adopt the sort of family-treatment program we present herein. The evidence seems clear that involving the family can make a substantial difference, making this one of the most promising forms of treatment of drug abuse. We should hasten to state once again that we recognize that this is not an easy road. Treatment of these families is difficult, and success will require a good deal of training, support for therapists, and significant changes in the structure of treatment programs.

*"Narcotic Detoxification in a Family and Home Context" (HEW–NIDA Grant No. R01 DA-03097).

# APPENDIX A: REVIEW OF REPORTS ON DRUG ABUSERS' FAMILY LIVING ARRANGEMENTS AND FREQUENCY OF FAMILY CONTACT

M. DUNCAN STANTON

There is a mounting accumulation of data on the family contacts and habitation patterns of "hard" drug abusers, starting with the observations of several astute investigators active in the drug-abuse field at its early stages. The first such report was in 1958 by Mason,[98] who noted an overinvolvement between male addicts and their mothers. This phenomenon was also hinted at by Chein et al.[25] in 1964. These patterns will be discussed below in two sections, dealing respectively with living arrangements and frequency of family contact.

## LIVING WITH PARENT(S)

The proportion of heroin addicts living with their families was documented in an early study by Vaillant[182] in which he found that 72% of the addicts in his sample still lived with their mothers at age 22. When those whose mothers had died prior to the addict's 16th birthday were deducted, the percentage rose to 90%. As late as age 30, 47% were living with a female blood relative (59% when corrected for those with living mothers). Ellinwood et al.[43] also noted a tendency for male addicts to be living alone with their mothers, while Bean's[12] study of 100 British drug offenders (mean age, 20.5)—two-thirds of whom were heroin users—showed that at least 33% lived with their parents. Also in Britain, Crawley[34] examined 134 opiate addicts (mean age, 21) admitted to a treatment service and found that 62% lived at home with their parents. Zahn and Ball[196] noted that 67% of a group of 108 addicts living in Puerto Rico after discharge from the national narcotics rehabilitation hospital in Lexington, Kentucky (mean age, 30.7) were living with their parents or relatives. Kolb et al.[83] determined that 61% of the heaviest drug users among a population of 903 U.S. Navy drug abusers lived with their parents upon entering the service, although the rate was slightly higher (69–72%) for those involved with addictive and illegal drugs on a lesser scale. A study of 158 heroin addicts (mean age, 25) by Eldred and Washington[42] revealed that 73% of the males and 42% of the females lived with parents or other relatives when heroin use began, and the figures were 57% and 33%, respectively, at the time of intake; this sex differential, with more males than females living with parents, has also been reported by Alexander and Dibb.[2] Further, an investigation of intakes among a group composed of approximately equal numbers of opiate, barbiturate and/or stimulant, and polydrug abusers (mean age, 24.4) by Noone and Reddig[108] indicated that 72.5% of the 323 clients either (1) lived with their families of origin at intake (62.5%), or (2) had done so within the previous year (10%). A later study by Noone[107] of 21 heroin, barbiturate, and amphetamine addicts showed that 57% lived with parents at intake, including half of the 10 married subjects. A 1972 survey by the authors (Stanton and Todd) among 85 male heroin addicts at the Philadelphia Veterans Administration Drug Dependence Treatment Center (VA DDTC), using anonymous questionnaires, found that 66% either resided with their parents or saw their mothers daily; similarly, Mintz* is gathering data in Los Angeles that show comparable rates. Findings from our own study become more striking in view of the fact that the average age of these men was 28 and all of them had previously been separated from home and in the military for at least several months. Finally, two studies in a report by Perzel and Lamon[113] apply. In the first, living arrangements of 20 psychiatric outpatients at a community mental health center were compared with those of 33 polydrug abusers. The groups did not differ significantly on a number of demographic and family variables, such as age (27 vs. 29), income, education, number of siblings, percentage of intact families of origin, parents living, and so forth. The figures for the two groups, with psychiatric patients listed first, were (1) living with one or both parents, 21% versus 48%; (2) living with both parents, 7% versus 36%; (3) living with both parents and one or more siblings, none versus 25%. The second study compared 12 heroin addicts, 13 polydrug abusers, and a group of 40 normals randomly selected from the surrounding area. The percentages of subjects who resided with one or both parents were: heroin addicts, 45%; polydrug abusers, 42%; and normals, 7%.

Of 17 reports on the extent to which drug abusers live with their parents, only two dissent from the finding that a high percentage do so. Sullivan and Fleshman[176] interviewed 28 heroin addicts undergoing detoxification and reported that they did not maintain ties with their parents; the mean age of the group was not given. The subjects were seen in

*J. Mintz, Brentwood Veterans Administration Hospital, Los Angeles, California (personal communication, January 1979).

northern California, but came from all areas of the United States, in addition to three from South America. This finding might be considered consonant with Vaillant's[182] data indicating that addicts who became abstinent lived outside their parents' homes, if detoxification can be considered at least a slight indication of better prognosis and a greater likelihood of abstinence eventually occurring.

The second study was done in Vancouver, B.C., by Alexander and Dibb,[2] who inspected 450 case files of heroin addicts to see if, at intake, they gave the same address for themselves as for their parents. This was taken as evidence of whether or not they lived with parents. The authors reported that only 23% of the males and 14% of the females did so, concluding that most addicts are not closely tied into their families of origin. However, consonant with our own experience, Noone and Reddig[108] have questioned Alexander and Dibb's study, noting that their method for gathering data is highly unreliable in that so much depends on the focus of the intake interviewer. Also, if an addict does not want his parents contacted, or has reservations about the program, he may provide an incorrect or alternative address, such as that of a girlfriend. To this point, Ross[125] found that addicts tended to operate out of two addresses, one of which was "drug-related," and the other "family-related," and it is quite possible that many of Alexander and Dibb's subjects may have reported the former when providing intake information. Further, their results are not consistent with an earlier report by Thompson,[178] who stated that an increasing and substantial minority of the addicts in Vancouver remained with their parents. In fact, Alexander has recognized some of these problems and has concurred that, indeed, his data provide "a flimsy basis for assigning a ceiling value to the proportion of addicts who are closely involved with their parents."* While it is possible that, relative to other regions, certain West Coast cities such as San Francisco and Vancouver may have attracted a segment of the addict population that is more cut off and alienated from the family of origin, such a phenomenon is in need of better documentation than presently exists in the literature.

In sum, indications are that a high proportion of addicts reside either with their parents or with older relatives—perhaps depending on which of these raised them. Further, this pattern appears to cut across international boundaries, as evidenced by the aforementioned North American, Puerto Rican, and British studies, plus reports that 80% of the heroin addicts both in Italy[3] and Thailand† live with their parents.

*B. K. Alexander, Simon Fraser University, Burnaby, B.C. (personal communication, May 1981).

†K. Choopanya, Health Department, Bankok, Thailand (personal communication, April 1978).

## FAMILY CONTACT

Despite early studies by Vaillant[182] and others, data on the frequency with which drug addicts are in contact with their families of origin are less common than data on living arrangements. This is partly because it has not occurred to many investigators to explore this area, and also because valid information of this sort is often difficult to obtain; addicts are frequently protective of their parents and may respond truthfully only if (1) they are convinced that their parents will not be contacted as a result of the information they give, (2) they have a trusting relationship with the interviewer, or (3) they are allowed to respond anonymously. When such precautions are taken, it is our experience that the reported frequency of family contacts increases markedly.

Seven reports have been located dealing with family contacts of drug abusers. In tracking addicts for long-term follow-up, Bale et al.[8] noted that these clients usually have a long-standing contact person such as a parent or relative, and Goldstein et al.[55] reported that addicts "tend to utilize a given household (usually their parents) as a constant reference point in their lives" (p. 25). These authors give examples of how even the "street" addict either regularly or periodically gets in touch with his permanent address, renews relationships with his family, and the like. Along these lines, Coleman noted in an examination of the charts of 30 male heroin addicts that the person they requested to be contacted in case of emergency was invariably the mother, and was almost never the person with whom they lived (i.e., wife or girlfriend) for clients who did not live with their mothers.* As noted above, our own research found that 66% of a sample of male addicts either lived with their parents or saw their mothers daily; 82% saw at least one parent weekly, most of the remaining 18% being older than age 35. Subsequently, the author (Stanton, unpublished study) has examined intake data on 696 Black and White, male heroin addicts (ages 20–35) who entered the VA DDTC over a 30-month period; 86% of them reported seeing one or both of their parents at least weekly.

A deficiency in the above studies is that they asked only about face-to-face contacts, neglecting to inquire about telephone calls, letters, discussions with siblings that got conveyed to parents, and such. Addicts are often tied into the family system at many points, so that communication between them and other members is routed through siblings, relatives, and spouses. Asking only about face-to-face contact provides inadequate information about the (not uncommon) addict who talks to his mother on the phone every day or two for an hour or more.[90] Perzel and Lamon[113] have made an attempt to fill

*S. B. Coleman (personal communication, March 1979).

in such information gaps by asking their subjects about both face-to-face and telephone contacts. In their first study (described above) they found that 50% of their polydrug group made daily face-to-face contact with one or both parents, compared with 29% for psychiatric outpatients. The rates for daily phone contact were 45% and 25%, respectively, although it is not clear from the report whether these latter subjects were included within, or in addition to, the face-to-face group. Perzel and Lamon's second study, which compared three different groups of subjects, showed the following daily rates for face-to-face contact: heroin addicts, 21%; polydrug abusers, 32%; normals, 6%. The data for daily telephone contact were: heroin addicts, 64%; polydrug abusers, 51%; normals, 9%. These findings are unique, and once again attest to the regular, often intense involvement that many drug abusers maintain with their families of origin.

## DISCUSSION

The phenomenon of regular involvement—either through living arrangements or contact—between most addicts and their families is one that has generally gone unrecognized in the field of drug abuse. The prevailing view has been that such people maintain distant family relationships that are minimally attended to, if at all. However, the emergent data tend to refute this idea, indicating instead that the majority of male addicts, particularly those under age 35, are involved on a regular basis with one or more of their parents or parent surrogates.

An area that needs further investigation is the definition of the drug abuser's *functional* family structure, as opposed to simple family composition. For instance, it may be spurious to ask an addict whether he sees or lives with a biological parent when he was raised by an aunt, grandmother, or stepparent. Clinicians and researchers should begin their inquiries by first determining (1) who was instrumental in rearing the abuser, and (2) whom *at present* he considers important as a parental figure. After a given addict's family network is defined, then questions of living arrangements and contact can be directed more precisely and specifically toward determination of his interpersonal involvements.

# APPENDIX B: DESCRIPTION OF THE COLLABORATING INSTITUTIONS

M. DUNCAN STANTON
CHARLES P. O'BRIEN

Most of the clinical material presented in this book was obtained within two institutions: the Philadelphia Child Guidance Clinic (PCGC) and the Philadelphia Veterans Administration (VA) Hospital Drug Dependence Treatment Center (DDTC). These institutions are described below.

## THE PHILADELPHIA CHILD GUIDANCE CLINIC

The PCGC has been in existence since 1925 and was one of the first child guidance clinics in the United States. In 1965, Salvador Minuchin assumed directorship of the Clinic. He was soon joined by two colleagues, Braulio Montalvo (in 1965) and Jay Haley (in 1967). These three worked with other staff to transform a traditional child guidance clinic into a family-oriented treatment center. They also collaborated in the development of what came to be known as "structural family therapy"[100, 103, 104] and established a program to train paraprofessional minority therapists to treat families.[62]

The PCGC is affiliated with and adjoins both the University of Pennsylvania School of Medicine and the Children's Hospital of Philadelphia. It is a large center with a staff of 300, including clinical, administrative, and research personnel, plus trainees. In addition to a sizable outpatient department, there is a 25-bed inpatient unit for brief hospitalization, two apartments for the hospitalization of whole families, a day hospital (including classrooms), and the Family Therapy Training Center. The last has provided in-depth training to hundreds of professionals and paraprofessionals over the years, plus briefer training (e.g., workshops, symposia) to thousands more. The trainees come from throughout the United States and from around the world.

Research has been an integral part of the PCGC ethic. In addition to the earlier studies of lower-income families with a juvenile delinquent member,[103] the work has encompassed psychosomatic problems,[101, 104] schizophrenia,[66] and many other patient groups.[5, 155]

The general philsophy of PCGC has been to see "psychiatric" problems that develop in children and young people as indicative of problems in and between the interpersonal *systems* within which they are embedded. Of these systems (e.g., school, work), the one seen as having greatest import for such problems is the family system. The Clinic has pioneered work in this area.

The major portion of patients at PCGC come from the lower income strata and/or from minority groups—most notably, the Black citizenry. That so much of the PCGC work had evolved with these groups had important implications for our work with drug addicts, since lower-income and Black clients have been overrepresented within the heroin addict population.

## THE DRUG DEPENDENCE TREATMENT CENTER

The DDTC is a major treatment service within the Philadelphia VA Hospital complex.* Like PCGC, it is affiliated with the University of Pennsylvania School of Medicine, and PCGC and DDTC are separated by a 5-minute walk. The DDTC was founded in 1971 for the purpose of providing a full range of services to drug-dependent veterans. The program began with the philosophy that treatment of addictive diseases had been a poorly developed and studied endeavor that would benefit from a clinical research approach. Accordingly, this center was set up with intricate data collection facilities and the intention of measuring treatment outcome as carefully as possible. The program was originally envisioned as being a small facility for intensive treatment and clinical research. However, it began during a peak period of returning Vietnam veterans, which had created a high political interest in the drug-abuse problem. Accordingly, the initial staff of one full-time psychiatrist, a psychiatric social worker, and four counselors grew rapidly to its present size of approximately 70 staff members, including six psychiatrists, four psychologists, four social workers, a nurse practitioner, two staff nurses, and three pharmacists, the remainder being rehabilitation counselors, psychotherapists, research technicians, and administrative personnel. The number of patients in the program during the course of the family therapy study consisted of 300–350 active outpatients. There were 10 inpatient beds.

The overall treatment approach is strongly multimodal. At the time of intake the patients are informed of the various treatment possibilities and priority is given to "drug-free" approaches. The program was initially

*The name of this facility has subsequently been changed to the "Drug Dependence Treatment and Research Service," but for purposes of this book the original title (DDTC) has been retained.

founded with the intention of minimizing the importance of methadone maintenance, and in fact, initially, methadone maintenance was only available via a contract with another facility. Eventually it became apparent, however, that even in a multimodal program where drug-free approaches are emphasized, methadone remains the central form of treatment. Methadone is the treatment that is attractive to the vast majority of patients and, unless it is made available, most will not even apply for treatment. The available modalities include inpatient detoxification, outpatient detoxification, methadone or LAAM* maintenance, naltrexone treatment, and drug-free therapeutic community. The therapeutic community is integrated with the outpatient program, but it is located approximately 35 miles outside of Philadelphia. Follow-up treatment for graduates of the therapeutic community is conducted at the DDTC in Philadelphia. There is an active interchange between patients receiving outpatient, inpatient, and therapeutic community treatment.

In addition to the basic treatment modalities, other treatments are given to patients independent of the basic program to which a patient belongs. It would be incorrect to call these ancillary treatments, because in fact they are considered integral parts of the treatment program. However, they function within the structure of the particular program—methadone treatment, LAAM treatment, and so forth. In a true sense, methadone is considered to be a means of getting a patient engaged in some of these additional treatments. Such treatments include individual psychotherapy (usually cognitive–behavioral or supportive–expressive), group therapy, family therapy, vocational counseling, relaxation therapy, electrosleep therapy, and psychotropic medication (depending on the patient's psychiatric diagnosis). Job counseling is considered to be an essential part of this program and virtually all patients receive some form of vocational counseling. In addition, a job bank is maintained and many patients receive vocational or even college training through the program.

The patient population consists of 95–98% veterans. The only non-veterans are involved in research treatments funded through the University of Pennsylvania. The population is 99% male, 60% Black, and averages 26–27 years of age. Ninety percent are narcotics addicts. Typically, the VA patients are somewhat better educated than patients in nonveteran drug-treatment programs. Most are high school graduates. This reflects the selection process that occurred when the patients entered the armed forces.

Family therapy was already being practiced at the DDTC prior to the inception of the Addicts and Families Program in 1974. (The founder and director of the program [O'Brien] was trained in family therapy at PCGC in 1968 and has subsequently continued in the active practice of family therapy.)

*Levo-alpha-acetylmethadol (a long-acting derivative of methadone).

The DDTC patients have always been encouraged to bring in their families for both family evaluations and continuing family therapy; however, there has generally been a great deal of resistance to this. In those cases where this resistance could be overcome, family therapy was actively practiced. It therefore seemed logical that an outcome study of family therapy using a specific family therapy approach, namely structural–strategic family therapy, should be conducted in this program. The presence of a large supply of relatively homogeneous patients was also an important asset for an outcome study. Strict selection criteria could be employed, including age of patient, duration of addiction, detoxification history, and geographical relationship to parents.

Treatment in the DDTC program is organized along the lines of a psychiatric residency training program, in the sense that it makes use of a primary therapist under close supervision, with periodic case conferences. Each patient is assigned to a rehabilitation counselor. A counselor may have from 15 to 30 clients. Approximately 60% of these are on methadone or LAAM maintenance; however, a few are on naltrexone (a narcotic antagonist) or are drug-free. Each week the counselor presents his problem cases to his supervisor, who may be a psychiatrist, psychologist, or psychiatric social worker. In addition to presentation of problem cases, all patients are reviewed periodically and a treatment plan is established. This review is conducted in team meetings where counselors, psychiatrists, social workers, and nurses are represented. Physical examinations are conducted by nurse practitioners supervised by physicians. Psychiatrists are constantly available for consultation regarding psychiatric diagnosis and possible prescription of psychoactive medication. The clinic is open 7 days per week. Emergencies after hours are handled through the VA Medical Center duty physician, with a DDTC physician always available by telephone.

Approximately 60% of the DDTC methadone patients attend the clinic daily, the remainder coming in five or six times per week and receiving methadone "take-home" doses for the other days. Patients give a urine specimen that is tested for illegal drugs at least once a week. The testing days are selected at random, in accordance with Food and Drug Administration regulations, and patients do not know until their arrival if they are scheduled to give a urine sample on a given day.

In addition to providing treatment for approximately 1000 patients per year, the DDTC also provides the setting for a wide variety of research activities. These range from basic biochemical studies of addiction and endorphins in animals, to conditioning studies in addicted humans and animals, to controlled clinical outcome studies of different types of psychotherapy or psychoactive medication. In 1980, there were 22 active research projects within the program, producing 20 to 25 publications per year. The program receives funding as a research center through the VA as well as additional funding through the National Institute on Drug Abuse and other sources. The treatment staff is well trained and sophisticated. Thus, the background treatment to which the Addicts and Families Program was added was already highly regarded and effective. The possibility that structural–strategic family therapy could have an impact in this setting by demonstrating further patient improvement was viewed enthusiastically.

It is important to note that patients and staff of this program are accustomed to research activities. Particularly since Jim Mintz, PhD, became Research Director in 1972, questionnaires, rating forms, follow-up interviews, and random urine tests have been routine. In addition, patients have been accustomed to being reimbursed for participating in many of these research activities. Thus the patients and clinical staff showed minimal resistance to the demands of the research protocol, with its attendant measurements and cross-checks.

# APPENDIX C: RESEARCH DESIGN OF THE ADDICTS AND FAMILIES PROGRAM

M. DUNCAN STANTON
THOMAS C. TODD
CHARLES P. O'BRIEN

The case material in this book dealing with adult opiate addicts derived primarily from a clinical research project involving 118 patients, conducted within the Philadelphia Child Guidance Clinic (PCGC) Addicts and Families Program (AFP). It was a collaborative effort with the Drug Dependence Treatment Center (DDTC) of the Philadelphia Veterans Administration (VA) Hospital.

This appendix presents a general outline of the research design, giving particular highlights relevant to the clinical context. The overall design (including information on the Family Evaluation Session, comparisons with "normal" subjects, etc.) has been presented in greater detail in an earlier publication.[171]

Four different treatment conditions (described below) were involved. All subjects in these conditions were patients at the DDTC. If assigned to family therapy, this therapy became adjunct to (but an integral part of) their overall treatment regimen.

To be eligible for the study, the patients had to meet the following criteria: (1) be under age 36; (2) be male; (3) have been addicted to heroin at least 2 years (all but one subject had been addicted for 2 years or more: range, 1–16 years); (4) have made two or more previous attempts to detoxify; (5) be on methadone, at least initially; (6) have family living within 1 hour's drive of the DDTC; (7) have no history of psychosis (although it was later learned that two family-treatment subjects actually had such a history); (8) have no siblings enrolled in the same drug program; (9) be in regular, face-to-face contact with two parents or parent surrogates (e.g., stepmother, stepfather, mother's boyfriend), at least weekly contact with one and monthly with the other; and (10) have not been treated previously in family therapy. Approximately one-third of the way through the study, two additional criteria were added: (11) have parents or parent surrogates living in the same household, and (12) could not have a VA medical disability of 30% or more.

We were interested in determining whether patients who met these criteria had a different prognosis from the DDTC patient population as a whole. We suspected, a priori, that patients in the AFP would have better prognoses, since a high percentage of them had intact families. However, this did not turn out to be the case. When we followed a group of 20 patients who qualified but did not go into family treatment because no therapist was available, we were surprised to find that they did worse than the overall DDTC population. In general, they tended to drop out of treatment earlier—70% leaving by the end of 4 months—and were more likely than the total population to maintain "dirty" urines during their tenure within the program. Thus the family treatment seemed to be involving a group of "poor prognosis" patients.

## ADDICT INTAKE AND ASSIGNMENT PROCEDURE

All patients who appeared for treatment at the DDTC over a 30-month period were administered an intake interview to determine their eligibility for this study. They were seen by an intake counselor and a psychiatrist. They were also asked to sign a form agreeing to follow-up interviews, for which they would receive payment. Twenty-seven percent were eligible, the major reasons for exclusion being age, deceased parent(s), infrequent parent contact, or nonaddiction to heroin. If judged eligible, they were asked for additional information about their drug use, job history, family demographics, and so forth. The AFP was then contacted by direct telephone line to see if any openings existed. If not, nothing was said to these patients about family treatment and they became part of a "Nonfamily Treatment" group. If an opening or openings did exist, they were assigned randomly to the available therapist(s), also attempting to hold race of therapist and family constant—Black therapist with Black family and White therapist with White family—a goal that we were able to accomplish in 86% of the cases. (While this is not a totally random assignment procedure, we had no a priori evidence or reason to believe that patients would be assigned to either family or nonfamily treatment, or, for that matter, to any therapist, in any systematic or biased way. This procedure was employed because we were concerned from the outset with getting enough cases on a regular basis to fill our family-treatment groups.)

The patient assigned to family treatment was given the name of his therapist.* At approximately the same time the therapist was contacted and given the name of and information about the patient. An appointment was made for them to meet. Whenever possible, the therapist saw the patient or talked to him over the telephone that same day. It was the therapist's job to explain to the patient that family treatment would be part of his program, with the patient, of course, having the option of refusing after the therapist had tried to enlist him. The therapist had two responsibilities in the initial stage of treatment: one was to oversee the patient's drug-treatment plan, such as adjusting methadone dosage and the like, and the other was to bring in the family for treatment (Chapters 3, 4, and 5). He might have had the patient call his family right from the office and introduce them to him. His goal was to have both parents or parent surrogates, as well as any siblings age 12 or older living nearby, come in with the patient for the Family Evaluation Session—a nontherapy research exercise. The therapist did not know to which of the three family-treatment conditions the family would be assigned. He did not find this out until they were actually in the Family Evaluation Session. At that time he was given a sealed envelope containing a note that designated the treatment group. Families were randomly assigned to the three family-treatment conditions—Paid Family Therapy, Unpaid Family Therapy, or Family Movie Treatment.

The Family Evaluation Session is described in more detail in another publication.[171] It had two phases. In the first phase, the family wore microphones and performed four (videotaped) interactional tasks together. The second phase consisted of two family perceptual measures administered to the family as a group, but not videotaped. Each family member age 12 or older was paid $10.00 for participating in the exercise. Treatment proceeded following this session. After either 10 sessions or 10 weeks had elapsed, whichever occurred later, the family engaged in a second, posttreatment Family Evaluation Session (with payment), in order to determine whether changes had occurred consequent to therapy.

## THERAPISTS

Nine male therapists were involved in recruiting families for the three family-treatment groups and in treating the two family therapy (Paid, Unpaid) groups described below. Usually four of them—two Black and two White therapists—were working for the AFP at any given time. Their academic credentials ranged widely. Three had no academic degrees, one had a BA, one an MSW, one an EdD, and three were recent PhD psychologists. Five were under age 30, while the mean age was 34. Their clinical credentials were modest: when they joined the project, their experience as family

---

*In the final 71% of the cases, the family therapist served as the client's drug counselor, a "dual role" discussed extensively in Chapters 5, 6, and 16.

therapists averaged 3.3 years (three had only had 1 year of experience). Three had previous clinical experience in working with drug abusers and their families prior to entering the project. Three were Black and six were White. During their tenure they had weekly supervision and met weekly with the entire AFP staff to discuss a mixture of administrative and clinical issues.


## TREATMENT CONDITIONS

Four treatment groups were employed, three of which included the families of the addicts during treatment. The fourth included family members only for follow-up interviews. The treatment period (intake to termination) for family groups averaged 4½ to 5 months in length. The therapists (or, in the case of the Movie group, the drug counselors) wrote weekly progress notes and an overall evaluation at termination of treatment. The treatment groups or conditions were:

1. *Paid Family Therapy* ($n = 21$). At the end of the Family Evaluation Session a contract was made with the family to attend 10 family therapy sessions (brief family therapy).* The usual rationale given was that the family is important for helping the addict get off and stay off of drugs. Sessions usually included most or all of the family—especially in the beginning phases—and all sessions were videotaped. All families attended at least four sessions, while 17 (81%) completed 10 or more sessions; three (14%) participated beyond 10 sessions, usually because a crisis occurred near the normal termination point. The major components of the therapeutic approach are presented in Chapter 6.

This therapy mode also included a reimbursement aspect, primarily instituted to counteract the low motivation for treatment that these families have historically shown. In brief, every family member age 12 or older received $5.00 at each session he attended. He also got a chance to increase his payment if the addict member had been "clean" that week, that is, if the addict's urine tests showed no use or abuse of illegal drugs. This was done by means of a random drawing by all family members, supervised by a research assistant, following each session. The therapist was not involved in this exercise, in order to remove him from a paymaster role. For every family member present, $5.00 was added to the sum to be drawn for, so that the

---

*There were several cases in this group and in the Unpaid group in which a full 10-session program was not necessary, and treatment terminated earlier. In these cases the family was doing well, and insisting that they continue to come would have been counter productive, as it would have conveyed the message that they were not as competent as they were actually demonstrating.

total was as high as $30.00, for example, if six members attended. If it was a "dirty" week, the sum was held over until the next week, at which time a drawing was held for the combined total for both weeks. A "dirty" urine during the second week resulted in the elimination of the first week's sum and a carrying over to the third week of the second week's sum. The drawing and payment were discontinued after 10 sessions, even if a family continued therapy beyond that point. This method of drawing for money had a number of advantages. It raised the incentive for each member to come to the sessions. It also mobilized all family members to put pressure on each other to attend and specific pressure on the addict to attend and to abstain from drug use. The more members present, the larger the sum, and if the addict got consecutive "dirty" urines, all members stood to lose in the drawing. Further, the use of clean urines as a contingency for reimbursement served as a check against the misuse of payment sums by the addict for the purchase and abuse of illegal drugs.

2. *Unpaid Family Therapy* ($n = 25$). Procedures for this group were identical to those for the Paid Family Therapy group except that no money was provided to the family (aside from that given for the two Family Evaluation Sessions). This group allows determination of whether reimbursement is important in (1) getting people into treatment, (2) keeping them in, and (3) producing improvement. Two of these families (8%) did not attend any family therapy sessions following the Family Evaluation Session, 10 (40%) attended between one and three sessions, and 13 (52%) completed at least four sessions. Of this last group of 13, three completed fewer than 10 sessions, seven completed exactly 10 sessions, and three went beyond 10 family sessions.*

3. *Family Movie Treatment* ($n = 19$). This program required the family to come in once a week for 10 weeks to view 10 different, noncontroversial, anthropology movies about people in various foreign cultures. The rationale given to the families was, "We find the families that at times have difficulties can be helped by seeing how people in other cultures and societies live and work together, because it gives them a perspective." Movies were selected according to their plausibility, interest, and generally innocuous content. We used movies for the control group because, in contrast to family therapy, they did not permit much interaction among family members while the family was at the research site. A research assistant administered the movies. Instead of being assigned to a family therapist, the addicts in this group became patients of the VA DDTC Senior Drug Counselor, who worked intimately with our program and received

*It should be obvious that reimbursing members for coming to sessions significantly improved attendance and reduced the number of dropouts, as shown by a comparison between the Paid and Unpaid groups on this variable.[165, 171]

partial salary support. These families were paid and got urinalysis reports in the same manner as the Paid Family Therapy group. Seventeen (94%) of the families attended six or more sessions, 14 (78%) came eight or more times, and 10 (56%) attended the requisite 10 sessions.*

The movie group thus served as a comparison or control for the effects of reimbursement per se and also for the effect on the family of attending weekly sessions together at the clinic. The importance of this latter aspect should not be overlooked, since most of these families rarely got together for family activities. In this respect the movie program was definitely a family intervention.

4. *Nonfamily (Methadone and/or Individual Counseling) Treatment* (*n* = 53). These were addicts at the DDTC who met all of our criteria for inclusion in the study but were not selected for one of the family-treatment groups. Nothing was said to them about family treatment. Instead they underwent the usual DDTC treatment procedures and received methadone maintenance, individual counseling, and other services; they were assigned a drug counselor. However, to be included in our study they had to remain in the methadone program for at least 30 days (see below). Their progress in the DDTC program was followed to the same extent that addicts in the family groups were followed. In comparison with family-treatment patients, this group provides us with a baseline estimate of the treatment outcomes that can be expected with similar, fairly motivated subjects in an ongoing "standard" multimodal methadone program.†

It should be noted that this was a standard, or "treatment as usual," condition. Consequently, family members were intentionally not recruited for a Family Evaluation Session or engaged in "pretherapy" contact. To do so would have been a clear family intervention (as the recruitment process usually demanded a good deal of effort to organize the family), and would have ruled them out as either "nonfamily" or as "standard treatment" cases. Conversely, the engagement process for the family cases should be viewed as an integral part of their treatment (see Chapters 4 and 5), rather than a "pretherapy" exercise.

---

*These percentages are based on a sample size (*n*) of 18 (rather than 19) because one patient died of an overdose before treatment could begin.

†These 53 patients are not all the patients eligible for the Nonfamily group, but are a sample of the total set of eligibles. Funding did not permit us to follow up the whole group. Consequently, the group was divided into 6-month cohorts and the 53 cases were randomly selected from each cohort in the same proportions as there were subjects assigned to the three family groups from those cohorts. This procedure permitted comparability across all four groups in terms of the time periods when their subjects entered treatment.

## EARLY DROPOUTS AND REFUSERS

There were, in addition, three groups of patients who were eligible at intake for the study but were later excluded. These were (1) 39 "family-treatment" patients (30% of those assigned to family treatment) who terminated from the DDTC prematurely, that is, within a few days from intake, and usually left before having been seen by a therapist (however, if these patients reentered the program they were still eligible, which happened in five cases); (2) 27 "family" cases, discussed in Chapter 5 and elsewhere,[168, 169] who refused to become involved in family treatment—in 19 cases because the patient would not let us contact his family, plus 8 cases in which the family refused to participate; (3) 31 nonfamily cases (i.e., 37% of those so assigned) who dropped out of the DDTC before they had been in treatment 30 days. This last group was excluded because it was judged by DDTC personnel that it would be unfair to use for comparison a nonfamily metha-done group of patients who had not been on methadone at least 30 days.

# REFERENCES

1. Africano, A., Fortunato, M., & Padow, E. The impact of program treatment on marital unions in a methadone-maintained patient population. In *Proceedings of the Fifth National Conference on Methadone Treatment* (Vol. 1). New York: National Association for the Prevention of Addiction to Narcotics, 1973.

2. Alexander, B. K., & Dibb, G. S. Opiate addicts and their parents. *Family Process*, 1975, *14*, 499–514.

3. Andreoli, V. *Current drug abuse treatment approaches in Italy.* Paper presented at the National Drug Abuse Conference, Seattle, Wash., April 1978.

4. Annis, H. M. Patterns of intra-familial drug use. *British Journal of the Addictions*, 1974, *69*, 361–369.

5. Aponte, H. J., & Van Deusen, J. M. Structural family therapy. In A. S. Gurman & D. P. Kniskern (Eds.), *Handbook of family therapy.* New York: Brunner/Mazel, 1981.

6. Attardo, N. Psychodynamic factors in the mother–child relationship in adolescent drug addiction: A comparison of mothers of schizophrenics and mothers of normal adolescent sons. *Psychotherapeutic Psychosomatics*, 1965, *13*, 249–255.

7. Balaban, B. J., & Melchionda, R. Outreach redefined: The impact on staff attitudes of a family education project. *International Journal of the Addictions*, 1979, *14*, 833–846.

8. Bale, R., Cabrera, S., & Brown, J. Follow-up evaluation of drug abuse treatment. *American Journal of Drug and Alcohol Abuse*, 1977, *4*, 233–249.

9. Ball, J. C. The reliability and validity of interview data obtained from 59 narcotic drug addicts. *American Journal of Sociology*, 1967, *72*, 650–654.

10. Barr, H. L., & Cohen, A. *The problem-drinking drug addict* (National Institute on Drug Abuse, Services Research Report; DHEW Pub. No. [ADM] 79-893). Washington, D.C.: U.S. Government Printing Office, 1979.

11. Bateson, G. *Mind and nature: A necessary unity.* New York: Dutton, 1979.

12. Bean, P. Social aspects of drug abuse: A criminological study of a group of London drug offenders. *Journal of Criminal Law, Criminology and Police Science*, 1971, *62*, 80–86.

13. Berenson, D. The therapist's relationship with couples with an alcoholic member. In E. Kaufman & P. Kaufmann (Eds.), *Family therapy of drug and alcohol abuse.* New York: Gardner Press, 1979.

14. Berg, B., & Rosenblum, N. Fathers in family therapy: A survey of family therapists. *Journal of Marriage and Family Counseling*, 1977, *3*, 85–91.

15. Berliner, A. K. Narcotic addiction, the institution and the community. *International Journal of the Addictions*, 1966–67, *1–2*, 74–85.

16. Blum, R., & Associates. *Students and drugs*. San Francisco: Jossey-Bass, 1970.

17. Blum, R., & Associates. *Horatio Alger's children*. San Francisco: Jossey-Bass, 1972.

18. Bonnheim, M. L., & Korman, M. *Family interaction and acculturation in Mexican-American inhalant users*. Unpublished research, University of Texas Health Science Center at Dallas, 1980.

19. Boszormenyi-Nagy, I., & Spark, G. M. *Invisible loyalties*. New York: Harper & Row, 1973.

20. Cahalan, D., Cisin, I., & Crossley, H. *American drinking practices* (Publications Division, Rutgers Center of Alcohol Studies, New Brunswick, N.J.). New Haven, Conn.: College & University Press, 1969.

21. Callan, D., Garrison, J., & Zerger, F. Working with the families and social networks of drug abusers. *Journal of Psychedelic Drugs*, 1975, 7, 19–25.

22. Cannon, S. R. *Social functioning patterns in families of offspring receiving treatment for drug abuse*. Roslyn Heights, N.Y.: Libra, 1976.

23. Carter, E. A., & McGoldrick, M. *The family life cycle: A framework for family therapy*. New York: Gardner Press, 1980.

24. Chein, I. Narcotics use among juveniles. *Social Work*, 1956, 1, 50–60.

25. Chein, I., Gerard, D., Lee, R., & Rosenfeld, E. *The road to H*. New York: Basic Books, 1964.

26. Chessick, R. D. The "pharmacogenic orgasm" in the drug addict. *Archives of General Psychiatry*, 1960, 3, 545–556.

27. Clark, J. S., Capel, W. C., Goldsmith, B. M., & Stewart, G. T. Marriage and methadone: Spouse behavior patterns in heroin addicts maintained on methadone. *Journal of Marriage and the Family*, 1972, 34, 496–501.

28. Coleman, A. F. How to enlist the family as an ally. *American Journal of Drug and Alcohol Abuse*, 1976, 3, 167–173.

29. Coleman, S. B. *Death—The facilitator of family integration*. Paper presented at the meetings of the American Psychological Association, Chicago, September 1975.

30. Coleman, S. B., & Davis, D. I. Family therapy and drug abuse: A national survey. *Family Process*, 1978, 17, 21–29.

31. Coleman, S. B., & Stanton, M. D. An index for measuring agency involvement in family therapy. *Family Process*, 1978, 17, 479–483.

32. Coleman, S. B., & Stanton, M. D. The role of death in the addict family. *Journal of Marriage and Family Counseling*, 1978, 4, 79–91.

33. Cox, T. J., & Longwell, B. Reliability of interview data concerning current heroin use from heroin addicts on methadone. *International Journal of the Addictions*, 1974, 9, 161–165.

34. Crawley, J. A. A case-note study of 134 outpatient drug addicts over a 17-month period. *British Journal of Addiction*, 1971, 66, 209–218.

35. Cummings, N. A. Turning bread into stones: Our modern antimiracle. *American Psychologist*, 1979, 34, 1119–1129.

36. Cuskey, W. R., Richardson, A. H., & Berger, L. H. *Specialized therapeutic community program for female addicts* (National Institute on Drug Abuse, Services Research Report; DHEW Pub. No. [ADM] 79-880). Washington, D.C.: U.S. Government Printing Office, 1979.

37. Davis, D. I. Forum: Family therapy for the drug user: Conceptual and practical considerations. *Drug Forum*, 1977-78, *6*, 197-199.

38. Davis, D. I., Berenson, D., Steinglass, P., & Davis, S. The adaptive consequences of drinking. *Psychiatry*, 1974, *37*, 209-215.

39. Dennehy, C. M. Childhood bereavement and psychiatric illness. *British Journal of Psychiatry*, 1966, *112*, 1049-1069.

40. Dole, V. Addictive behavior. *Scientific American*, 1980, *243*(6), 138-154.

41. Eldred, C. A., Brown, B. S., & Mahabir, C. Heroin addict clients' description of their families of origin. *International Journal of the Addictions*, 1974, *9*, 315-320.

42. Eldred, C. A., & Washington, M. N. Interpersonal relationships in heroin use by men and women and their role in treatment outcome. *International Journal of the Addictions*, 1976, *11*, 117-130.

43. Ellinwood, E. G., Smith, W. G., & Vaillant, G. E. Narcotic addiction in males and females: A comparison. *International Journal of the Addictions*, 1966, *1*, 33-45.

44. Entin, A. D., & Schumann, M. D. An exploratory study of the families of drug-using adolescents. In J. O. Bradt & C. J. Moynihan (Eds.), *Systems therapy*. Washington, D.C.: Groome Child Guidance Center, 1971.

45. Flomenhaft, K., & Carter, R. Family therapy training: Program and outcome. *Family Process*, 1977, *16*, 211-218.

46. Forrest, T. Treatment of the father in family therapy. *Family Process*, 1969, *8*, 106-108.

47. Fort, J. Heroin addiction among young men. *Psychiatry*, 1954, *17*, 251-259.

48. Fram, D. H., & Hoffman, H. A. Family therapy in the treatment of the heroin addict. In *Proceedings of the Fifth National Conference on Methadone Treatment* (Vol. 1). New York: National Association for the Prevention of Addiction to Narcotics, 1973.

49. Frank, J. D. The present status of outcome studies. *Journal of Consulting and Clinical Psychology*, 1979, *47*, 310-316.

50. Frazier, T. L. Treating young drug users: A casework approach. *Social Work*, 1962, *7*, 94-101.

51. Ganger, R., & Shugart, G. The heroin addict's pseudoassertive behavior and family dynamics. *Social Casework*, 1966, *47*, 643-649.

52. Gerard, D. L., & Kornetsky, C. A social and psychiatric study of adolescent opiate addicts. *Psychiatric Quarterly*, 1954, *28*, 113-125.

53. Glick, I. D., & Haley, J. *Family therapy and research: An annotated bibliography*. New York: Grune & Stratton, 1971.

54. Glover, E. On the etiology of drug addiction. In E. Glover (Ed.), *On the early development of mind*. New York: International Universities Press, 1956.

55. Goldstein, P. J., Abbott, W., Paige, W., Sobel, I., & Soto, F. Tracking procedures in follow-up studies of drug abusers. *American Journal of Drug and Alcohol Abuse*, 1977, *4*, 21-30.

56. Gurman, A. S., & Kniskern, D. P. Deterioration in marital and family therapy: Empirical, clinical and conceptual issues. *Family Process*, 1978, *17*, 3-20.

57. Gurman, A. S., & Kniskern, D. P. Research on marital and family therapy: Progress, perspective and prospect. In S. L. Garfield & A. E. Bergin (Eds.), *Handbook of psychotherapy and behavior change: An empirical analysis* (2nd ed.). New York: Wiley, 1978.

58. Haastrup, S., & Thomsen, K. The social backgrounds of young addicts as elicited in interviews with their parents. *Acta Psychiatrica Scandinavica*, 1972, *48*, 146–173.

59. Haley, J. *Strategies of psychotherapy*. New York: Grune & Stratton, 1963.

60. Haley, J. Toward a theory of pathological systems. In G. H. Zuk & I. Boszormenyi-Nagy (Eds.), *Family therapy and disturbed families*. Palo Alto, Calif.: Science & Behavior Books, 1967.

61. Haley, J. A review of the family therapy field. In J. Haley (Ed.), *Changing families*. New York: Grune & Stratton, 1971.

62. Haley, J. We became family therapists. In A. Ferber, M. Mendelsohn, & A. Napier (Eds.), *The book of family therapy*. New York: Science House, 1972.

63. Haley, J. Strategic therapy when a child is presented as the problem. *Journal of the American Academy of Child Psychiatry*, 1973, *12*, 641–659.

64. Haley, J. *Uncommon therapy*. New York: Norton, 1973.

65. Haley, J. *Problem-solving therapy*. San Francisco: Jossey-Bass, 1976.

66. Haley, J. *Leaving home: Therapy with disturbed young people*. New York: McGraw-Hill, 1980.

67. Harbin, H. T., & Maziar, H. M. The families of drug abusers: A literature review. *Family Process*, 1975, *14*, 411–431.

68. Hoffman, L. Breaking the homeostatic cycle. In P. Guerin (Ed.), *Family therapy: Theory and practice*. New York: Gardner Press, 1976.

69. Hollingshead, A. B., & Redlich, F. C. *Social class and mental illness*. New York: Wiley, 1958.

70. Huberty, D. J. Treating the adolescent drug abuser: A family affair. *Contemporary Drug Problems*, 1975, *4*, 179–194.

71. Jackson, D. D. The question of family homeostasis. *Psychiatric Quarterly Supplement* (Part 1), 1957, *31*, 79–90.

72. Jackson, D. D. The study of the family. *Family Process*, 1965, *4*, 1–20.

73. Jaffe, J. H. Drug addiction and drug abuse. In L. S. Goodman & A. Gilman (Eds.), *The pharmacological basis of therapeutics* (5th ed.). New York: Macmillan, 1975.

74. Janzen, C. Families in the treatment of alcoholism. *Journal of Studies on Alcohol*, 1977, *38*, 114–130.

75. Johnson, T. F. Hooking the involuntary family into treatment: Family therapy in a juvenile court setting. *Family Therapy*, 1974, *1*, 79–82.

76. Kandel, D. B., Treiman, D., Faust, R., & Single, E. Adolescent involvement in legal and illegal drug use: A multiple classification analysis. *Social Forces*, 1976, *55*, 438–458.

77. Kaufman, E., & Kaufmann, P. (Eds.). *Family therapy of drug and alcohol abuse*. New York: Gardner Press, 1979.

78. Kaufman, E., & Kaufmann, P. From a psychodynamic orientation to a structural family therapy approach in the treatment of drug dependency. In E. Kaufman & P. Kaufmann (Eds.), *Family therapy of drug and alcohol abuse*. New York: Gardner Press, 1979.

79. Kaufman, E., & Kaufmann, P. Multiple family therapy with drug abusers. In E. Kaufman & P. Kaufmann (Eds.), *Family therapy of drug and alcohol abuse*. New York: Gardner Press, 1979.

80. Klagsbrun, M., & Davis, D. I. Substance abuse and family interaction. *Family Process*, 1977, *16*, 149–173.

81. Kleber, H. D. Methadone maintenance treatment—A reply. *American Journal of Drug and Alcohol Abuse*, 1977, *4*, 267–272.

82. Klein, N. C., Alexander, J. F., & Parsons, B. V. Impact of family systems intervention on recidivism and sibling delinquency: A model of primary prevention and program evaluation. *Journal of Consulting and Clinical Psychology*, 1977, *45*, 469–474.

83. Kolb, D., Gunderson, E.K.E., & Nail, R. L. Preservice drug abuse: Family and social history characteristics. *Journal of Community Psychology*, 1974, *2*, 278–282.

84. Kolb, D., Nail, R. L., & Gunderson, E.K.E. Differences in family characteristics of heroin injectors and inhalers. *Journal of Nervous and Mental Disease*, 1974, *158*, 446–449.

85. Krystal, H., & Raskin, H. A. *Drug dependence: Aspects of ego functions.* Detroit, Mich.: Wayne State University Press, 1970.

86. L'Abate, L. Pathogenic role rigidity in fathers: Some observations. *Journal of Marriage and Family Counseling*, 1975, *1*, 69–79.

87. L'Abate, L. A positive approach to marital and family intervention. In L. R. Wolberg & M. L. Aronson (Eds.), *Group therapy: 1975.* New York: Stratton Intercontinental, 1975.

88. Langsley, D. G., & Kaplan, D. M. *The treatment of families in conflict.* New York: Grune & Stratton, 1968.

89. Langsley, D. G., Machotka, P., & Flomenhaft, K. Avoiding mental hospital admission: A follow-up study. *American Journal of Psychiatry*, 1971, *127*, 1391–1394.

90. Leichter, H. J., & Mitchell, W. E. Jewish extended familism. In R. F. Winch & L. W. Goodman (Eds.), *Selected studies in marriage and family.* New York: Holt, Rinehart & Winston, 1968.

91. Levitt, E. E. Research on psychotherapy with children. In A. E. Bergin & S. L. Garfield (Eds.), *Handbook of psychotherapy and behavior change.* New York: Wiley, 1971.

92. Levy, B. Five years after: A follow-up of 50 narcotic addicts. *American Journal of Psychiatry*, 1972, *7*, 102–106.

93. Lieberman, J. J. The drug addict and the "cop-out" father. *Adolescence*, 1974, *9*, 7–14.

94. MACRO Systems, Inc. *Three-year follow-up study of clients enrolled in treatment programs in New York City: Phase III—Final report.* Report submitted to the National Institute on Drug Abuse, June 1975.

95. Madanes, C., Dukes, J., & Harbin, H. Family ties of heroin addicts. *Archives of General Psychiatry*, 1980, *37*, 889–894.

96. Madanes, C., & Haley, J. Dimensions of family therapy. *Journal of Nervous and Mental Disease*, 1977, *165*, 88–98.

97. Maddux, J. F., & Desmond, D. P. Reliability and validity of information from chronic heroin users. *Journal of Psychiatric Research*, 1975, *12*, 87–95.

98. Mason, P. The mother of the addict. *Psychiatric Quarterly Supplement*, 1958, *32*(Part 2), 189–199.

99. McClelland, D. C., Davis, W. N., Kalin, R., & Wanner, E. *The drinking man: Alcohol and human motivation.* New York: Free Press, 1972.

100. Minuchin, S. *Families and family therapy.* Cambridge, Mass.: Harvard University Press, 1974.

101. Minuchin, S., Baker, L., Rosman, B. L., Liebman, R., Milman, L., & Todd, T. C. A conceptual model of psychosomatic illness in children. *Archives of General Psychiatry,* 1975, *32,* 1031–1038.

102. Minuchin, S., & Barcai, A. Therapeutically induced family crisis. In J. Masserman (Ed.), *Science and psychoanalysis: Childhood and adolescence* (Vol. 14). New York: Grune & Stratton, 1969.

103. Minuchin, S., Montalvo, B., Guerney, B. G., Rosman, B. L., & Schumer, F. *Families of the slums.* New York: Basic Books, 1967.

104. Minuchin, S., Rosman, B. L., & Baker, L. *Psychosomatic families.* Cambridge, Mass.: Harvard University Press, 1978.

105. Modlin, H. C., & Montes, A. Narcotics addiction in physicians. *American Journal of Psychiatry,* 1964, *121,* 358–365.

106. Mulford, H. A., & Miller, D. E. Drinking in Iowa: II. The extent of drinking and selected sociocultural categories. *Quarterly Journal of Studies on Alcohol,* 1960, *21,* 26–39.

107. Noone, R. J. *Drug abuse behavior in relation to change in the family structure.* Paper presented at the Third Pittsburgh Family Systems Symposium, Western Psychiatric Institute and Clinic, University of Pittsburgh, April 1979.

108. Noone, R. J., & Reddig, R. L. Case studies in the family treatment of drug abuse. *Family Process,* 1976, *15,* 325–332.

109. O'Donnell, J. A. *Narcotic addicts in Kentucky.* Washington, D.C.: U.S. Government Printing Office, 1969.

110. Olson, D. H., Russell, C. S., & Sprenkle, D. H. Marital and family therapy: A decade review. *Journal of Marriage and the Family,* 1980, *42,* 973–993.

111. Oltman, J. E., & Friedman, S. Parental deprivation in psychiatric conditions: III. In personality disorders and other conditions. *Diseases of the Nervous System,* 1967, *28,* 298–303.

112. Papp, P. The Greek chorus and other techniques of paradoxical therapy. *Family Process,* 1980, *19,* 45–57.

113. Perzel, J. F., & Lamon, S. *Enmeshment within families of polydrug abusers.* Paper presented at the National Drug Abuse Conference, New Orleans, August 1979.

114. Pittman, F. S., Langsley, D. G., Flomenhaft, K., DeYoung, C., Machotka, P., & Kaplan, D. M. Therapy techniques of the family treatment unit. In J. Haley (Ed.), *Changing families.* New York: Grune & Stratton, 1971.

115. Rado, S. The psychoanalysis of pharmacothymia (drug addiction). *Psychoanalytic Quarterly,* 1933, *2,* 1–23.

116. Rado, S. Narcotic bondage: A general theory of the dependence on narcotic drugs. *American Journal of Psychiatry,* 1957, *114,* 165–170.

117. Rado, S. Fighting narcotic bondage and other forms of narcotic disorders. *Comprehensive Psychiatry,* 1963, *4,* 160–167.

118. Reilly, D. M. Family factors in the etiology and treatment of youthful drug abuse. *Family Therapy,* 1975, *2,* 149–171.

119. Rinella, V. J., & Goldstein, M. R. Family therapy with substance abusers: Legal considerations regarding confidentiality. *Journal of Marital and Family Therapy,* 1980, *6,* 319–326.

120. Riordan, C. E., Mezritz, M., Slobetz, F., & Kleber, H. D. Successful detoxification from methadone maintenance: A follow-up study of 38 patients. *Journal of the American Medical Association*, 1976, *235*, 2604–2607.

121. Rohrbaugh, M., Tennen, H., Press, S., & White, L. Compliance, defiance and therapeutic paradox: Guidelines for strategic use of paradoxical interventions. *American Journal of Orthopsychiatry*, 1981, *51*, 454–467.

122. Rosenberg, C. M. Young drug addicts: Background and personality. *Journal of Nervous and Mental Disease*, 1969, *148*, 65–73.

123. Rosenberg, C. M. The young addict and his family. *British Journal of Psychiatry*, 1971, *118*, 469–470.

124. Rosenfeld, H. A. On drug addiction. *International Journal of Psychoanalysis*, 1960, *41*, 467–475.

125. Ross, S. A study of living and residence patterns of former heroin addicts as a result of their participation in a methadone treatment program. In *Proceedings of the Fifth National Conference on Methadone Treatment* (Vol. 1). New York: National Association for the Prevention of Addiction to Narcotics, 1973.

126. Sager, C. J., Masters, Y. J., Ronall, R. E., & Normand, W. C. Selection and engagement of patients in family therapy. *American Journal of Orthopsychiatry*, 1968, *38*, 715–723.

127. Salmon, R., & Salmon, S. The causes of heroin addiction—A review of the literature. Part II. *International Journal of the Addictions*, 1977, *12*, 937–951.

128. Savitt, R. A. Psychoanalytic studies on addiction: Ego structure in narcotic addiction. *Psychoanalytic Quarterly*, 1963, *32*, 43–57.

129. Scher, J. Patterns and profiles of addiction and drug abuse. *Archives of General Psychiatry*, 1966, *15*, 539–551.

130. Schwartzman, J. The addict, abstinence and the family. *American Journal of Psychiatry*, 1975, *132*, 154–157.

131. Schwartzman, J., & Bokos, P. Methadone maintenance: The addict's family recreated. *International Journal of Family Therapy*, 1979, *4*, 338–355.

132. Schwartzman, J., & Kroll, L. Methadone maintenance and addict abstinence. *International Journal of the Addictions*, 1977, *12*, 497–507.

133. Scopetta, M. A., King, O. E., & Szapocznik, J. *Relationship of acculturation, incidence of drug abuse and effective treatment of Cuban-Americans: Final report* (National Institute on Drug Abuse Contract No. 271-75-4136), 1977.

134. Seldin, N. E. The family of the addict: A review of the literature. *International Journal of the Addictions*, 1972, *7*, 97–107.

135. Selvini-Palazzoli, M., Boscolo, L., Cecchin, G., & Prata, G. *Paradox and counterparadox*. New York: Jason Aronson, 1978.

136. Selvini-Palazzoli, M., Boscolo, L., Cecchin, G., & Prata, G. A ritualized prescription in family therapy: Odd days and even days. *Journal of Marriage and Family Counseling*, 1978, *4*, 3–9.

137. Shapiro, R. J., & Budman, S. H. Defection, termination, and continuation in family and individual therapy. *Family Process*, 1973, *12*, 55–67.

138. Slipp, S., Ellis, S., & Kressel, K. Factors associated with engagement in family therapy. *Family Process*, 1974, *13*, 413–427.

139. Smart, R. G., Fejer, D., & White, J. *Drug use trends among metropolitan Toronto students: A study of changes from 1968 to 1972*. Unpublished manuscript, Addiction Research Foundation, Toronto, 1972.

140. Sonne, J. C., Speck, R. V., & Jungreis, J. E. The absent-member maneuver as a resistance in family therapy of schizophrenia. *Family Process*, 1962, *1*, 44–62.

141. Soper, P. H., & L'Abate, L. Paradox as a therapeutic technique: A review. *International Journal of Family Counseling*, 1977, *5*, 10–21.

142. Sowder, B., Dickey, S., & Glynn, T. J. *Family therapy: A summary of selected literature* (National Institute on Drug Abuse; DHEW Pub. No. [ADM] 80-944). Washington, D.C.: U.S. Government Printing Office, 1980.

143. Speck, R. V., & Attneave, C. L. *Family networks*. New York: Pantheon, 1973.

144. Stanton, M. D. Drug use in Vietnam: A survey among Army personnel in the two northern corps. *Archives of General Psychiatry*, 1972, *26*, 270–286.

145. Stanton, M. D. Drugs, Vietnam and the Vietnam veteran: An overview. *American Journal of Drug and Alcohol Abuse*, 1976, *3*, 557–570.

146. Stanton, M. D. The addict as savior: Heroin, death and the family. *Family process*, 1977, *16*, 191–197.

147. Stanton, M. D. The family and drug misuse: A bibliography. *American Journal of Drug and Alcohol Abuse*, 1978, *5*, 151–170.

148. Stanton, M. D. Some outcome results and aspects of structural family therapy with drug addicts. In D. Smith, S. Anderson, M. Buxton, T. Chung, N. Gottlieb, & W. Harvey (Eds.), *A multicultural view of drug abuse: The proceedings of the National Drug Abuse Conference—1977*. Cambridge, Mass.: Hall/Schenkman, 1978.

149. Stanton, M. D. The client as family member: Aspects of continuing treatment. In B. S. Brown (Ed.), *Addicts and aftercare: Community integration of the former drug user*. Beverly Hills, Calif.: Sage, 1979.

150. Stanton, M. D. Drugs and the family: A review of the recent literature. *Marriage and Family Review*, 1979, *2*, 1–10.

151. Stanton, M. D. *Family structure and drug abuse: A review*. Report prepared for the Office of Program Development and Analysis, National Institute on Drug Abuse, December 1979.

152. Stanton, M. D. Family treatment approaches to drug abuse problems: A review. *Family Process*, 1979, *18*, 251–280.

153. Stanton, M. D. A critique of Kaufman's "Myth and Reality in the Family Patterns and Treatment of Substance Abusers." *American Journal of Drug and Alcohol Abuse*, 1980, *7*(3, 4), 281–289.

154. Stanton, M. D. A family theory of drug abuse. In D. Lettieri, M. Sayers, & H. Pearson (Eds.), *Theories on drug abuse: Selected contemporary perspectives* (National Institute on Drug Abuse Research Monograph Series No. 30). Washington, D.C.: U.S. Government Printing Office, 1980.

155. Stanton, M. D. Family therapy: Systems approaches. In G. P. Sholevar, R. M. Benson, & B. J. Blinder (Eds.), *Emotional disorders in children and adolescents: Medical and psychological approaches to treatment*. Jamaica, N.Y.: S. P. Medical & Scientific Books, 1980.

156. Stanton, M. D. The hooked serviceman: Drug use in and after Vietnam. In C. R. Figley & S. Leventman (Eds.), *Strangers at home: Vietnam veterans since the war*. New York: Praeger, 1980.

157. Stanton, M. D. Some overlooked aspects of the family and drug abuse. In B. G. Ellis (Ed.), *Drug abuse from the family perspective* (National Institute on

Drug Abuse; DHHS Pub. No. [ADM] 80-910). Washington, D.C.: U.S. Government Printing Office, 1980.

158. Stanton, M. D. Marital therapy from a structural/strategic viewpoint. In G. P. Sholevar (Ed.), *Handbook of marriage and marital therapy*. Jamaica, N.Y.: S. P. Medical & Scientific Books, 1981.

159. Stanton, M. D. Strategic approaches to family therapy. In A. S. Gurman & D. P. Kniskern (Eds.), *Handbook of family therapy*. New York: Brunner/Mazel, 1981.

160. Stanton, M. D. Who should get credit for change which occurs in therapy? In A. S. Gurman (Ed.), *Questions and answers in the practice of family therapy*. New York: Brunner/Mazel, 1981.

161. Stanton, M. D. An integrated structural/strategic approach to family therapy. *Journal of Marital and Family Therapy*, 1981, *7*, 427–439.

162. Stanton, M. D. *Fusion, compression, expansion, and the workings of paradox: A theory of therapeutic/systemic change*. Paper submitted for publication, 1982.

163. Stanton, M. D., & Coleman, S. B. The participatory aspects of indirect self-destructive behavior: The addict family as a model. In N. L. Faberow (Ed.), *The many faces of suicide*. New York: McGraw-Hill, 1980.

164. Stanton, M. D., & Rosoff, R. J. *Drinking problems in parents of drug addicts: A new look*. Paper in preparation, 1982.

165. Stanton, M. D., Steier, F., & Todd, T. C. *Reduction of family therapy dropout rates through reimbursement: A study with addict families*. Paper presented at the National Council on Family Relations, Philadelphia, October 1978.

166. Stanton, M. D., & Todd, T. C. *Structural family therapy with heroin addicts: Some outcome data*. Paper presented at the Society for Psychotherapy Research, San Diego, June 1976.

167. Stanton, M. D., & Todd, T. C. Structural family therapy with drug addicts. In E. Kaufman & P. Kaufmann (Eds.), *Family therapy of drug and alcohol abuse*. New York: Gardner Press, 1979.

168. Stanton, M. D., & Todd, T. C. Engaging "resistant" families in treatment: II. Principles and techniques in recruitment. *Family Process*, 1981, *20*, 261–280.

169. Stanton, M. D., & Todd, T. C. Engaging "resistant" families in treatment: III. Factors in success and cost-effectiveness. *Family Process*, 1981, *20*, 280–293.

170. Stanton, M. D., Todd, T. C., Heard, D. B., Kirschner, S., Kleiman, J. I., Mowatt, D. T., Riley, P., Scott, S. M., & Van Deusen, J. M. Heroin addiction as a family phenomenon: A new conceptual model. *American Journal of Drug and Alcohol Abuse*, 1978, *5*, 125–150.

171. Stanton, M. D., Todd, T. C., Steier, F., Van Deusen, J. M., Marder, L. R., Rosoff, R. J., Seaman, S. F., & Skibinski, E. *Family characteristics and family therapy of heroin addicts: Final report, 1974–1978*. Report to the National Institute on Drug Abuse (Grant No. R01 DA 01119) by the Philadelphia Child Guidance Clinic, 1979.

172. Steinglass, P. Family therapy for alcoholism. In B. Kissin & H. Begleiter (Eds.), *The biology of alcoholism* (Vol. 5). New York: Plenum, 1976.

173. Steinglass, P., Davis, D. I., & Berenson, D. Observations of conjointly hospitalized "alcoholic couples" during sobriety and intoxication: Implications for theory and therapy. *Family Process*, 1977, *16*, 1–16.

174. Stephens, R. The truthfulness of addict respondents in research projects. *International Journal of the Addictions*, 1972, *7*, 549–558.

175. Straus, R., & Bacon, S. D. *Drinking in college.* New Haven: Yale University Press, 1953.

176. Sullivan, N. D., & Fleshman, R. P. Paternal deprivation in male heroin addicts. *Drug Forum,* 1975–76, *5,* 75–79.

177. Taylor, S. D., Wilbur, M., & Osnos, R. The wives of drug addicts. *American Journal of Psychiatry,* 1966, *123,* 585–591.

178. Thompson, P. Family of the addict explored. *The Journal* (Addiction Research Foundation, Toronto), 1973, *2,* 8.

179. Torda, C. Comments on the character structure and psychodynamic processes of heroin addicts. *Perceptual Motor Skills,* 1968, *27,* 143–146.

180. Vaglum, P. The patient-centered family working group—A medium for collaboration with "unmotivated" family members: A model and an example. *Scandinavian Journal of Social Medicine,* 1973, *1,* 69–75.

181. Vaillant, G. E. Parent–child cultural disparity and drug addiction. *Journal of Nervous and Mental Disease,* 1966, *142,* 534–539.

182. Vaillant, G. E. A 12-year follow-up of New York narcotic addicts: III. Some social and psychiatric characteristics. *Archives of General Psychiatry,* 1966, *15,* 599–609.

183. Van Deusen, J. M., Stanton, M. D., Scott, S. M., & Todd, T. C. Engaging "resistant" families in treatment: I. Getting the drug addict to recruit his family members. *International Journal of the Addictions,* 1980, *15,* 1069–1089.

184. Van Kaam, A. Addiction and existence. *Review of Existential Psychology and Psychiatry,* 1968, *8,* 54–64.

185. Watzlawick, P., Beavin, J. H., & Jackson, D. D. *Pragmatics of human communication.* New York: Norton, 1967.

186. Watzlawick, P., Weakland, J., & Fisch, R. *Change: Principles of problem formation and problem resolution.* New York: Norton, 1974.

187. Weakland, J. H. Communication theory and clinical change. In P. J. Guerin (Ed.), *Family therapy: Theory and practice.* New York: Gardner Press, 1976.

188. Weakland, J. H., Fisch, R., Watzlawick, P., & Bodin, A. M. Brief therapy: Focused problem resolution. *Family Process,* 1974, *13,* 141–168.

189. Weeks, G. R., & L'Abate, L. A compilation of paradoxical methods. *American Journal of Family Therapy,* 1979, *7,* 61–76.

190. Wellisch, D. K., Gay, G. R., & McEntee, R. The easy rider syndrome: A pattern of hetero- and homosexual relationships in a heroin addict population. *Family Process,* 1970, *9,* 425–430.

191. Wikler, A. Dynamics of drug dependence. *Archives of General Psychiatry,* 1973, *28,* 611–616.

192. Winick, C. Narcotics addiction and its treatment. *Law and Contemporary Problems,* 1957, *22,* 9–33.

193. Winick, C. Maturing out of narcotic addiction. *Bulletin on Narcotics,* 1964, *16,* 1–11.

194. Wolk, R. L., & Diskind, M. H. Personality dynamics of mothers and wives of drug addicts. *Crime and Delinquency,* 1961, *7,* 148–152.

195. Wurmser, L. Psychoanalytic considerations of the etiology of compulsive drug use. *Journal of the American Psychoanalytic Association,* 1974, *22,* 820–843.

196. Zahn, M., & Ball, J. Factors related to the cure of opiate addiction among Puerto Rican addicts. *International Journal of the Addictions,* 1972, *7,* 237–245.

197. Ziegler-Driscoll, G. Family research study at Eagleville Hospital and Rehabilitation Center. *Family Process*, 1977, *16*, 175–189.

198. Ziegler-Driscoll, G. The similarities in families of drug dependents and alcoholics. In E. Kaufman & P. Kaufmann (Eds.), *Family therapy of drug and alcohol abuse.* New York: Gardner Press, 1979.

199. Zimmering, P., Toolan, J., Safrin, R., & Wortis, S. B. Heroin addiction in adolescent boys. *Journal of Nervous and Mental Disease*, 1951, *114*, 19–34.

200. Zimmering, P., Toolan, J., Safrin, R., & Wortis, S. B. Drug addiction in relation to problems in adolescence. *American Journal of Psychiatry*, 1952, *109*, 272–278.

# AUTHOR INDEX

# SUBJECT INDEX

Mourning, 15, 21, 24, 25, 67, 279–291
(*see also* Death)
unresolved, 21, 67, 228, 384, 385
Multiple family therapy (MFT), 74, 149,
150, 424
Multiple systems in drug abuse, 122, 135,
147–150, 337, 338, 381

### N

Naltrexone, 173*n.*, 174, 336, 387, 434,
435
National Institute on Alcohol Abuse and
Alcoholism, 1
National Institute on Drug Abuse, xii,
xiii*n.*, xv*n.*, 1
Negotiation, 58, 61, 62, 67, 83, 129, 143,
244, 344
for detoxification, 137, 344
of house rules, 130, 184*n.*, 208, 209, 348
of medication dosages, 142
renegotiation, 399
by parents, 129, 130
renegotiation, 23, 399
of therapeutic goals, 112, 127–129
Networking, 148, 149, 424
Noble ascriptions, 3, 95, 120, 124–127,
146, 166, 231*n.*, 350*n.* (*see also*
Joining in therapy)
Nonfamily treatment as treatment condition, 33, 34, 410, 411, 413–421,
442

### O

Observational skill, 151
Oedipal triangle, 14, 175
Opiates/opioids, 15, 18, 29, 35, 40, 123,
142, 200, 201, 336, 337, 404, 409,
410, 415–419, 427, 428
Overdoses, 7, 23, 24, 198, 199, 355, 374,
411

### P

Paid Family Therapy, 33, 34, 152*n.*, 373,
399*n.*, 403, 407, 410, 411,

413–421, 439–442 (*see also*
Money)
Panic reaction and anxiety, 209
Paradox
of addiction and individuation, 16, 19,
24, 30, 301, 356
in criticism, 304
and fathers, 304, 308
and mothers, 304, 308
and responsibility/autonomy, 16, 18,
19, 24, 30, 301, 304, 305, 306*n.*,
308, 356
therapeutic techniques using, 116, 117,
127, 127*n.*, 137, 257, 259, 347, 350
Paranoia, 366
Parents, 132
and adolescent drug abuse, 335–357
age of, 300
and alcohol use, 9, 14, 65, 85, 109, 126,
140, 141, 195, 196, 209, 319, 388,
389, 410
authoritarianism of, 9
and blame, 70, 92–95, 118, 119,
124–127, 146, 147, 166, 231*n.*, 342
(*see also* Noble ascriptions)
death of, 9, 21, 67, 279–291, 340
depression of, 132, 195, 354, 355, 365
and enactment, 132–134, 345, 346 (*see
also* Enactment in therapy)
enlistment of as allies, 39, 125
estimate of sons' drug use, 47, 406
freeing up by, 19, 26, 121, 139, 140,
257, 382, 383
and goals, 129, 133, 138, 139, 146, 147,
379
and home detoxification, 136–138,
311–334
and living arrangements, 9, 10, 40,
427–431
marital relationships of (*see* Marital
relationships, of parents)
and marital relations of addicts, 11,
17–20, 25, 26, 47, 62, 63, 93*n.*,
250, 257, 258, 382, 383
negotiation by, 129–132, 138–141, 143
and overcontrol, 8, 9, 62, 109, 110,
209–235, 346–348, 351, 388, 427

Regression, 17
Rehearsal of recruitment, 49–52, 57
Reinforcement
  of family dependence, 24
  of handicap, perception of, 110, 129,
    142, 313*n*., 424
Relabeling, 112 (*see also* Blaming
    parents, avoidance of; Joining in
    therapy; Noble ascriptions;
    Reframing in therapy)
Relapse, 30, 119, 135, 143, 171, 192, 193,
    195, 380, 381, 386, 387, 422*n*.
Relaxation therapy, 434
Repression, 118, 147
Research
  designs for, 32, 33, 40, 52, 75, 134,
    437–443
  ethic for, 37, 38
  future directions on, 28, 29, 422, 426
  and model of treatment, 8–11
  setting of, 31–38
  conclusion on, 38
Resistance to treatment (*see also*
    Engagement of families in
    treatment)
  of families, 3, 40–41, 116, 117, 123–125,
    129, 131, 137, 145, 146
  in engagement, 71–106, 144, 342
  of patients, 40, 41, 44, 48, 67, 68, 76–
    78, 131, 145, 146, 341–344,
    379
  of spouse, 266
Responsibility
  and children, 134, 245–247, 258, 266,
    270, 293
  and family, 13, 17–19, 39, 48, 49, 60, 64,
    66, 68, 72, 73, 82, 83, 96, 104,
    109–111, 133, 134, 136–138, 143,
    145, 312, 352, 369, 370, 397, 423
    (*see also* Protectiveness in drug
    abusers' families)
  and paradox, 304, 305, 306*n*., 308
  shifting of, 133, 134, 136, 143, 230, 231,
    296–298
  of therapists, 104, 112, 115, 118, 136,
    143, 291, 423
Restraining in therapy, 116, 120

Restructuring of family system, 114, 118,
    119, 130, 133, 134, 136, 138–140,
    333, 334, 340, 346–351, 352–357
Retirement, 26, 50, 66, 110, 134,
    303–309, 380
  semiretirement, 67, 68
Robitussin, 278*n*.
Roles
  dual (*see* Dual role)
  and retirement, 309
  martyr/savior (*see* Death)
  role models, 126, 149, 172
  sick role, 28, 63, 110, 117–119, 123,
    126, 129, 132, 142, 150
Rules for family in therapy, 240–243 (*see
    also* House rules)

S

Schizophrenia, 14, 15, 109, 117, 129, 370,
    375, 432
Schizophrenia Project, xiii–xv, xv*n*., 192,
    364
Self-assertion, 8, 18, 44
Self-esteem, 62
Self-help groups, 1
Separation–individuation, 8–20, 24–26,
    30, 60, 62, 67, 130, 157, 179, 184,
    190, 343, 349–351, 356
  anxiety in, 12, 13, 16, 17, 30
  avoidance of, 64
  and crises, 81, 110
  and death, 21, 24
  developmental needs for, 354
  and family life cycle, 8–20, 22, 23, 130,
    300, 301
  scale of, 15
Sequences, family behavioral, 21–23,
    28–30, 112, 116, 117, 132, 133,
    151, 157, 159, 171, 207, 348, 349,
    442 (*see also* Homeostatic model
    of addiction)
Servocontrol, 26
Sessions, frequency/length/spacing of,
    42, 50, 54, 80, 100, 101, 143, 144,
    230, 384, 386, 387, 400, 415, 420,
    440